Catatonia

Catatonia is a syndrome of motor dysregulation (mutism, characteristic postures, repetitive speech, negativism, and imitative movements), and is found in as many as 10% of acutely ill psychiatric inpatients. Although its classification has been controversial, the identification of catatonia is not difficult, but it is often missed, leading to the false notion that the syndrome is rare. Catatonia has various presentations, and may be caused by many neurologic and general medical conditions, most commonly mood disorder. Treatments are well defined, and when used, catatonia has an excellent prognosis.

This book, by two leading neuropsychiatrists, describes the features of catatonia, teaches the reader how to identify and treat the syndrome successfully, and describes its neurobiology. Patient vignettes from the authors' practices, and many from the classical literature, illustrate the principles of diagnosing and treating patients with catatonia. It is an essential clinical reference for psychiatrists and neurologists.

Max Fink, M.D. is Emeritus Professor of Psychiatry and Neurology at the State University of New York at Stony Brook, and Professor of Psychiatry at Albert Einstein College of Medicine, New York.

Michael Alan Taylor, M.D. is Professor of Psychiatry at Finch University of Health Sciences, North Chicago, and Adjunct Clinical Professor at the University of Michigan, Ann Arbor.

Catatonia

A Clinician's Guide to Diagnosis and Treatment

Max Fink, M.D.
Professor of Psychiatry and Neurology Emeritus,
SUNY at Stony Brook, New York; and Professor of Psychiatry,
Albert Einstein College of Medicine, New York

Michael Alan Taylor, M.D.
Professor of Psychiatry, Finch University of
Health Sciences, North Chicago; and
Adjunct Clinical Professor at the University of Michigan, Ann Arbor

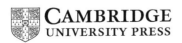
CAMBRIDGE
UNIVERSITY PRESS

CAMBRIDGE UNIVERSITY PRESS
Cambridge, New York, Melbourne, Madrid, Cape Town, Singapore, São Paulo

Cambridge University Press
The Edinburgh Building, Cambridge CB2 2RU, UK

Published in the United States of America by Cambridge University Press, New York

www.cambridge.org
Information on this title: www.cambridge.org/9780521822268

First published 2003
This digitally printed first paperback version 2006

A catalogue record for this publication is available from the British Library

Library of Congress Cataloguing in Publication data
Fink, Max, 1923–
Catatonia : a clinician's guide to diagnosis and treatment / Max Fink and Michael A. Taylor.
    p. ; cm.
Includes bibliographical references and index.
ISBN 0-521-82226-2 (HB : alk. paper)
1. Catatonia.   I. Taylor, Michael Alan, 1940–   II. Title.
[DNLM: 1. Catatonia – physiopathology.   2. Catatonia – therapy.   3. Diagnosis,
Differential. WM 197 F499c 2002]
RC376.5 .F54 2002
616.8′3 – dc21   2002067692

ISBN-13 978-0-521-82226-8 hardback
ISBN-10 0-521-82226-2 hardback

ISBN-13 978-0-521-03236-0 paperback
ISBN-10 0-521-03236-9 paperback

Contents

Patient vignettes

Preface

Few phenomena in psychiatry or neurology are as enigmatic as catatonia. This is a fact in large part due to the many contradictions surrounding the concept. Catatonia has been described as a disease, but also as a syndrome. It has been considered to be a subtype of schizophrenia, and yet has been claimed to be more common in affective disorders. It has been reported to be both caused and ameliorated by neuroleptic drugs. It has been reported to represent a state of stupor so profound that its sufferers die from medical complications, and has also been reported to represent a state of excitement so marked that physical restraints are necessary.   (Lohr and Wisniewski, 1987: 201)

Catatonia is a cluster of motor features that appears in many recognized psychiatric illnesses. The classic signs are mutism, a rigid posture, fixed staring, stereotypic movements, and stupor. Catatonia was initially described in the first half of the 19th Century, but its name and our ideas about it are credited to the German psychopathologist Karl Ludwig Kahlbaum.[1] In psychiatric disease classifications (such as the American Psychiatric Association's Diagnostic Statistical Manual and the World Health Organization's International Classification of Diseases), catatonia is traditionally linked to schizophrenia (American Psychiatric Association, 1952, 1980, 1987, 1994; World Health Organization, 1992). Today, however, we recognize that catatonia consists of identifiable and quantifiable motor signs that are part of a broad psychopathology that includes most of the major diagnostic classes. It is a syndrome that warrants consideration and recognition in its own right. Its many forms have been given numerous labels, but they likely reflect a common pathophysiology.

The limited association of catatonia to a subtype of schizophrenia, with the negative prognosis and treatment implications that schizophrenia evokes, serves catatonic patients poorly. Catatonia is often benign and transient, but we find instances of such severity that the outcome is fatal. Such results are tragic because catatonia is eminently treatable when it is recognized. We describe the different forms of catatonia, offer guides to its recognition and to its treatment, and seek to explain its origins within our present-day concepts of brain organization, physiology, and chemistry. We seek to enhance its appreciation as a separate category in our psychiatric classification systems.

One of us (MAT) described catatonia as a feature of mania and brought this forgotten association to professional attention in the mid-1970s.[2] His interest was stimulated by a 63-year-old woman in manic delirium who intermittently postured and showed several other catatonic features. She recovered with lithium carbonate treatment. MAT subsequently delineated the signs, neuroanatomy, and pathology of catatonia, and developed a neurologic model of the syndrome. He described the neuropsychiatric examination for students and has written several textbooks of neuropsychiatry.[3]

The interest of the other author (MF) was aroused in 1987 by a patient with lupus erythematosus who had been mute, rigid, and negativistic within a manic illness. After much travail, she recovered with electroconvulsive therapy.[4] This experience stimulated studies of many aspects of catatonia.[5]

When the American Psychiatric Association announced a Task Force for DSM-IV in 1990, we joined together in a plea to recognize catatonia as a unique entity, akin to the classification of delirium and dementia. We presented our image of catatonia in a challenging article *Catatonia: A separate category for DSM-IV*.[6] The Task Force members maintained catatonia as a variant of schizophrenia but added new options: *Catatonic Disorder Due to ... [Indicate the General Medical Condition]* with the code 293.89, and catatonia as a modifier of mania.[7]

As founding editors of specialty psychiatric journals, *Neuropsychiatry, Neuropsychology, and Behavioral Neurology,* and *Convulsive Therapy,* we read reports of catatonic patients that had been poorly diagnosed and inadequately treated. In 1998, we joined together to describe our experience and to present the evidence to justify greater consideration of catatonia in clinical practice.

We make the following points in this book. Catatonia and catatonic features are easily recognizable. Catatonic features are not rare phenomena but occur, several or more together, in about 10% of acutely hospitalized psychiatric patients. The features of catatonia reflect diverse brain disorders, most commonly mood disorder. Catatonia, even in its full form, is highly responsive to treatment despite the chronicity of an underlying condition.

"Responsive to treatment but often unrecognized" is a formula for clinical tragedy. We write to help physicians identify the syndrome and to treat it effectively. We write for neurologists and psychiatrists working in emergency rooms, hospital in-patient units, and consultation services. Because it expands the usual teaching texts emphasizing a readily recognizable and treatable syndrome, it should interest resident physicians and medical students. For researchers seeking homogeneous groups of patients, catatonia has a distinct psychopathology that makes it an effective and heuristic model for study.

Over the two centuries during which catatonia has been described, psychiatric terminology has changed many times. With each official Diagnostic Statistical Manual, terms are dropped (e.g., neuroses) and new ones added (e.g., body dysmorphic disorder). Well-established syndromes are given new labels the way fashion changes. Manic-depressive illness became bipolar disorder. Bipolar disorder became affective disorder, and then mood disorder. Because the old term *manic-depressive illness* is more consistent with the pre-1980 literature, and because we honor the descriptive psychiatrists who still have much to teach us, we use the older terms. We use *manic-depressive illness* for the syndrome and *mood disorder* as its descriptor, *antipsychotic* rather than neuroleptic, and *unipolar depression* rather than major depressive disorder, recurrent type. Because the mind–body dichotomy is artificial and the concept "organic" has been dropped from the DSM because all behavioral syndromes reflect brain events and are, *ipso facto*, "organic", we do not use that term or terms that reflect that notion, i.e., mental. Instead we use the terms *psychiatric* and *behavioral*.

Another convention is the term for the lethal form of catatonia. Authors define a virulent form of the illness as *lethal, malignant,* or *pernicious*. Because we can now treat the syndrome successfully and the mortality rate is much lower, we use the term *malignant catatonia* (MC). Many toxic syndromes, characterized by the main signs of MC, have been given individual names; we suggest that these be lumped together as examples of MC. We approach the neuroleptic malignant syndrome as one such toxic syndrome that is indistinguishable from MC and refer to it as *NMS* (*neuroleptic malignant syndrome*) when citing the work of other authors and as *MC/NMS* in our work.

In addition to patient vignettes that come from our clinical experience, we abstract examples from other authors. In writing each summary, we sought to present the essential relevant findings from the original report. The language is our own except where the original author's work is in quotations or italics.

References, in most instances, and additional comments are cited as end-notes in numerical order. The lists appear at the end of each relevant chapter. An overall alphabetized reference list appears at the end of the volume.

Undoubtedly there are idiosyncrasies in this book, and certainly there are strong opinions in it. But not to have strong opinions after two lifetimes of clinical experience would suggest time wasted. Readers may not agree with all that we have written, but we hope to invigorate their interest and appreciation of catatonia. If we accomplish that, patients will surely benefit.

Max Fink, M.D.
Michael Alan Taylor, M.D.

ENDNOTES

1 Kahlbaum, 1874; English translation 1973.
2 Taylor, 1990; Taylor and Abrams, 1973, 1977, 1978; Abrams and Taylor, 1976, 1979; Abrams, Taylor and Stolurow, 1979.
3 Taylor 1981, 1992, 1993, 1999, 2001.
4 Fricchione et al., 1990.
5 Systematic studies of catatonia at SUNY at Stony Brook began in 1987 with the publication of a case report describing the relief of a patient with lupus erythematosus who exhibited catatonia and mania (Fricchione et al., 1990) (*Patient 3.5*). In short order, a retrospective 5-year survey of patients diagnosed as suffering with schizophrenia, catatonic type, found 20 patients with most having concurrent diagnoses of mood disorders (Pataki et al., 1992). The studies, summarized in Petrides and Fink (2000), are published as Fink and Taylor, 1991; Fink, 1992a, 1994, 1996a,b,c, 1997a,b, 1999a; Fink and Francis, 1992; Pataki et al., 1992; Fink et al., 1993; Bush et al., 1996a, b; Francis et al., 1996, 1997; Bush et al., 1997; Fricchione et al., 1997; Petrides et al., 1997; Koch et al., 2000; Petrides and Fink, 2000.
6 Fink and Taylor, 1991.
7 American Psychiatric Association, 1994: 278–279, 382–383.

Acknowledgments

Early drafts of this book were read by Drs. Chittaranjan Andrade, Dirk Dhossche, Alfred M. Freedman, Hugh Freeman, Gregory Fricchione, Jan-Otto Ottosson, Pierre Pichot, Gabor Ungvari, and Jan Volavka. They raised useful questions and clarified our thinking. We thank them for their comments and questions, the answers to which surely improved the final product.

This book is dedicated to our patients and their families, whose faith in our efforts to help them allowed us to learn much about catatonia.

Chronology of catatonia concepts

Catatonia in psychopathology

1583	*Barrough*	"*Of Congelation*": depressive stupor and frenzy
1663	*Bayfield*	Catalepsy
1815	*Bakewell*	Negativism in manic patients
1850	*Monro*	"Cataleptoid insanity"
1863	*Kahlbaum*	*Die Gruppierung der psychischen Krankheiten und die Einteilung der Seelenstörungen.* Catatonia as a syndrome
1874	*Kahlbaum*	*Die Katatonie oder das Spannungsirresein.* The classic formulation
1877	*Kiernan*	Confirms Kahlbaum's syndrome in USA
1896	*Kraepelin*	Catatonia as a subtype of dementia praecox; psychodynamic explanation
1898	*von Schüle*	Catatonia subtypes; Kraepelin's formulation rejected
1898	*Aschaffenburg*	Dementia paralytica and catatonia separated
1912	*Urstein*	Kraepelin's restrictive formulation rejected
1913	*Kirby*	Catatonia frequent in manic-depression
1922	*Lange*	Catatonia more frequent in manic-depressive patients
1924	*Bleuler*	Dementia praecox relabeled schizophrenia; catatonia as subtype. A psychodynamic formulation of catatonia
1928	*Kleist*	Cycloid psychosis
1942	*Leonhard*	Comprehensive classification
1969	*Pauleikhoff*	Centennial anniversary of Kahlbaum's book; defines five forms of Kahlbaum's syndrome
1973	*Taylor, Abrams*	Catatonia prevalent in mania
1975	*Morrison*	Catatonia in 10% of psychotic population (Iowa 500 study)
1976	*Abrams & Taylor*	Mania and depression prevalent in manic patients
1981	*Mahendra*	Where have all the catatonics gone?

Diagnostic classification of catatonia

1874	*Kahlbaum*	*Die Katatonie oder das Spannungsirresein.* Syndrome with good prognosis, many etiologies
1896	*Kraepelin*	Catatonia as a subtype of dementia praecox; psychodynamic explanation of catatonia
1924	*Bleuler*	"Dementia praecox" becomes "schizophrenia," with catatonia as subtype. Accepts psychodynamic formulation of catatonia
1952	*APA DSM-II*	Catatonia as reaction type in schizophrenia
1980	*APA DSM-III*	Catatonia as subtype of schizophrenia
1987	*Lohr & Wisniewski*	Catatonia rating scale
1991	*Rogers*	Neurologic formulation of catatonia; new rating scale
1991	*Fink & Taylor*	Catatonia as a syndrome, not schizophrenia subtype
1994	*APA DSM IV*	Catatonia as schizophrenia subtype; secondary to medical conditions (293.89); and modifier of affective disorders
2001	*Fink & Taylor*	Many faces of catatonia

Malignant catatonia, neuroleptic malignant syndrome, delirious mania

1849	*Bell*	Delirious mania with catatonia
1934	*Stauder*	*Die tödliche Katatonie.* Malignant catatonia (MC).
1950	*Bond*	Describes delirious mania; lithium treatment
1950	*Meduna*	*Oneirophrenia*
1952	*Arnold & Stepan*	Electroconvulsive therapy (ECT) for MC
1960	*Delay*	*Syndrom malin* – neuroleptic toxic syndrome
1973	*Meltzer*	Neurotoxic syndrome secondary to depot fluphenazine
1976	*Gelenberg*	Catatonia as neurotoxic syndrome
1980	*Caroff*	"neuroleptic malignant syndrome"
1989	*Rosebush*	Neuroleptic malignant syndrome (NMS) a subtype of malignant catatonia
1991	*White*	NMS is malignant catatonia
1999	*Fink*	Delirious mania; efficacy of ECT

Catatonia treatment

1930	*Bleckwenn*	Amobarbital treatment of catatonia
1934	*Meduna*	Convulsive therapy for catatonia
1938	*Cerletti & Bini*	Electroconvulsive therapy of mania, psychosis
1950	*Bond*	Lithium treatment for delirious mania

1952	*Arnold & Stepan*	ECT for malignant catatonia
1983	*Fricchione*	Lorazepam treatment of toxic and psychogenic catatonia
1983	*McEvoy & Lohr*	Diazepam treatment of catatonia
1989	*Rosebush*	NMS as subtype of MC
1999	*Fink*	ECT for delirious mania

Other aspects of catatonia

1901	*Regis*	Oneiroid state (*Le delire onirique*)
1921	*Hoch*	*Benign Stupors.* Clinical review of retarded catatonia
1930	*de Jong & Baruk*	Experimental catatonia, bulbocapnine in cats
1932	*Gjessing*	Periodic catatonia; endocrine studies
1941	*Cairns*	Akinetic mutism
1962	*Sours*	Akinetic mutism and catatonia
1982	*Insel*	Toxic serotonin syndrome
1995	*Stöber*	Genetic basis for periodic catatonia
2001	*MacKeith*	London Conference on catatonia in childhood disorders

Catatonia: A history

The nineteenth century concept of 'disorder of motility' is one of the most difficult to grasp from the perspective of today. This tells much about the role of ideology and metaphor in descriptive psychopathology. For what might have in common clinical states as diverse as stupor, akinesia, catalepsy, psychomotor retardation, agitation, impulsions, bradyphrenia, parkinsonism, dyskinesias, akathisia, grimacing, mannerisms, posturing, stereotypes, soft neurological signs, tremors and tics except, perhaps, the fact that they all refer in a general way to human movement? Confronted with such a list, the neurologist of today might respond as he would to a medieval bestiary, i.e. with amused disbelief.

Berrios, 1996a: 378.

While we have no doubt that catatonia has long been a feature of human behavior, the first description in our literature is that of a patient in stupor by the English physician Philip Barrough in 1583, under the title *Of Congelation or Taking*.[1]

Catoche or Catalepsis in Greeke . . . The newe wryters in phisick do call it Congelatio, in English it maie be called Congelation or taking. It is a sodaine detention & taking both of mind and body, both sense and moving being lost, the sicke remaining in the same figure of bodie wherin he was taken, whither he sit or lye, or stand, or whither his eyes be open or shut. This disease is a meane betwene the lethargic and the frenesy, for it cometh of a melancholy humour for the most parte, as shalbe declared afterward . . . This evill differeth from Carus (as Galen saith) for that in it the eye liddes are ever shut, but in this disease they sometime remaine open. (Hunter and Macalpine, 1982: 26.)

A century later, in 1663, under the caption "catalepsy," Robert Bayfield wrote:

A congelation, is a sudden surprizal of all the senses, the motion, and the minde, with the which those that are seized upon, and invaded, remain and abide stiff, in the very same state and posture in which they were taken and surprized, with their eyes open and immovable . . . Galen mentioneth a story of a school-fellow of his, who when he had wearied himself with long studie, fell into a Catalepsis or Congelation; he lay (saith he) like a log all along, not to be bent, stiffe, and stretched out, and seemed to behold us with his eyes, but spake not a word: And he said, that he heard us what we said at the time, although not evidently and plainly, and told us some things that he remembered, and said, all that stood by him were seen of him, and could remember, and declare some of their gestures at that time, but could not then speak, or move one part of his body ...

Another I saw like a dead man, lying along, with neither seeing, hearing, nor feeling when he was pinched; but he breathed freely, and whatsoever was put into his mouth he presently swallowed; if he was taken out of his bed, he did stand alone, but being thrust would fall down; and which way soever his arm, hand, or leg was set, there it stood fixed, and firm; you would have taken him for a Ghost, or some rare Statue. (Hunter and Macalpine, 1982: 170.)

Individuals, once "taken", remained ill for months or years, occasionally recovering spontaneously as after a febrile illness or an epileptic seizure, but more often persisting in their condition until infection or starvation ended their lives.

A patient with negativism is eloquently described in an inquiry into the state of "madhouses" for the British House of Commons in 1815 by Thomas Bakewell.

Female, single, Age, 25. Had been six months under the care of another Keeper, when brought to me. I often said, that if ever the devil was in woman, he was surely in this one. Good heavens! When I look back upon the trouble and anxiety I underwent with this creature, I wonder how ever I got through it; her filth, her fury, disgusting language, and her almost constant nakedness for nearly two months, it being totally impossible to keep any clothes upon her, and it was scarcely possible to keep her from tearing her own flesh to pieces, as well as others; these altogether left almost without the appearance of a human being; till I had her, I thought I could manage any with the straight waistcoat; but her teeth bid defiance to every attempt to keep even that upon her. But all our extraordinary trouble arose from our not making the discovery sooner, that her particular hallucination was, had only to express the opposite of our wishes, and it was immediately done; as, Miss, you must not eat that food, it is for another person; and it was immediately taken and eaten up. Miss, you must not take that medicine, it is for such a lady, this is your's; and it was gone in an instant. Miss, you must lie still today; you must not get up, and wash you, and dress you very neatly; and up she got, and did all we bid her not to do. We therefore took care to bid her to be sure to tear her clothes all to pieces, and she remained dressed. This was certainly a departure from my usual plan of treating my patients as rational beings; but it was a case of necessity. Purgatives, tonics ... the warm bath, cold effusion, and embrocations to the head, were put in requisition: industry and perseverance may do wonders; she got quite well, and became the well-dressed, well-bred lady...After this case, I shall never think any too bad for recovery; she was under my care six months. (Hunter and Macalpine, 1982: 706.)

The image of "cataleptoid insanity" by the British physician Henry Monro in 1850 captures a catatonic patient's travail.

Cataleptoid insanity. I have been induced to apply the word cataleptoid to a certain class of insane patients who have evinced symptoms bearing a striking resemblance in some points of view to catalepsy. I will now describe this class as briefly as I can. In a large collection of insane patients we cannot help marking a few who stand in apparently profound sopor; their eyes are glued down or else staring open in a fixed manner, so immovable that you do not observe the least twinkle of the eyelid; the skin is cold and clammy; you speak to them, they will not answer; you offer them food, they will not eat. They indeed are most unwilling to move from the spot which they have taken up. You would say of them at first sight that they are in a perfectly apathetic and probably unconscious state until you try to cross their will, and then you often find a most resolute resistance. The state of the intellect in these cases is often hard to arrive at; for the mind is a prisoner; all the ordinary avenues of expression by which the caged spirit may take flight are sealed up by an influence of a numbing character, which in many points of view seems to resemble simple drowsiness. Sometimes when you lay hold suddenly of such a patient, you may shake him out of the stupor, and you find that his mind is by no means lost; that he has a clear perception of all that has been going on even during the trance; and he will argue about it as about an incubus which he could fully appreciate but could not control. I have heard the term acute dementia applied to this class of cases, but I repudiate the word on many accounts. First, it is a contradiction in terms to speak of acute dementia; the word dementia should indicate a state of fatuity which is generally the result of acute disease (the second stage as it were of madness), but is always to be applied to a passive rather than an active state; and to add the word acute to it is about equivalent to speaking of vigorous imbecility. But letting this pass, the state of mind of many of these cases is anything but demented. (Hunter and Macalpine, 1982: 988–9.)

Karl Ludwig Kahlbaum (1828–1899)

The concept of catatonia was formulated and the illness named by the German clinician Karl Ludwig Kahlbaum.

Catatonia is a brain disease with a cyclic, alternating course, in which the mental symptoms are, consecutively, melancholy, mania, stupor, confusion, and eventually dementia. One or more of these symptoms may be absent from the complete series of psychic 'symptom-complexes'. In addition to the mental symptoms, locomotor neural processes with the general character of convulsions occur as typical symptoms.[2]

Kahlbaum's clustering of the signs of catatonia into a single disease entity is his major contribution to psychiatry.[3] Early in his career, Kahlbaum developed a psychiatric nosology based on the course of illness rather than the cross-sectional picture alone. When his work received little interest from the German academic establishment, he took a position in a private sanitarium at Görlitz in 1866, became its director in 1867, and remained until his death in 1899. Numerous authors have described his life, acknowledging his contributions to the role of education in child and adolescent psychiatry and his delineation of catatonia. The most detailed biography is that of Katzenstein (1963), and his childhood and adolescence is described by Steinberg (1999). Shorter biographies by Neisser (1924), Morrison (1974a), Lanczik (1992), Bräunig and Krüger (1999, 2000), and Ahuja (2000c) praise his work. Kraepelin's assessment is described in his *History of Psychiatry:*

He [Kahlbaum] was the first to stress the necessity of juxtaposing the condition of the patient, his transitory symptoms and the basic pattern underlying his disease. The condition of one and the same patient may change often and in diverse ways, with the result that in the absence of other clues any attempt to rescue him from his plight is doomed to failure. Moreover, identical or remarkably similar symptoms can accompany wholly dissimilar diseases while their inner nature can be revealed only through their progress and termination and, in some instances, through an autopsy.

On the basis of such considerations Kahlbaum sought to delineate a second pattern of illness similar to that of paralysis and, like it, embracing both mental disorders and physical concomitants: catatonia in which muscular tension provided a basis for comparison with paralysis. Although his interpretation is faulty, Kahlbaum deserves credit for having suggested the right approach: careful attention to the progress and termination of mental disorders, information gleaned in some instances from autopsies and insight into underlying causes have made possible the juxtaposition of a vast array of evidence and often diagnosis on the basis of symptom pattern. (Kraepelin, 1919: 116–17).

Another evaluation described Kahlbaum as *"the first German psychiatrist to systematically elaborate forms of mental diseases from the pure clinical viewpoint."*[4]

Karl Jaspers (1963, quoted in Magrinat et al., 1983) praised his work:

Kahlbaum formulated two fundamental requirements: firstly, the entire course of the mental illness must be taken as basically the most important thing for any formulation of disease-entities and, secondly, one must base oneself on the total picture of the psychosis as obtained by comprehensive clinical observation. In emphasizing the course of the illness, he added a new viewpoint.

Kahlbaum presented a systematic psychopathology in *Die Gruppirung der psychischen Krankheiten und die Einteilung der Seelenstörungen* ("The divisions and classification of mental disorders") in 1863.[5] He created the terms *vesania*, *vecordia*, *dysphrenia*, and *neophrenia*, which have since been ignored, and the terms *paraphrenia*, *cyclothymia*, *hebephrenia*, and *catatonia* that are now in our nomenclature.[6] (Credit for the description of hebephrenia, another syndrome delineated by the course of illness, went to his co-worker Ewald Hecker.[7])

In a small book of 104 pages titled *Die Katatonie oder das Spannungsirresein*, Kahlbaum (1874) described his experience with 26 patients in both the stuporous and excited forms of the illness. He defined 17 signs of the syndrome following the diagnostic rules set down by Sydenham more than a hundred years earlier.[8] Rigid posture, mutism, negativism, and catalepsy initiated an illness that was soon followed by the hyperkinetic phenomena of stereotypes, verbigeration, and excitement. The illness had a progressive course:

The typical signs of the condition termed atonic melancholia may be described as a state in which the patient remains entirely motionless, without speaking, and with a rigid, masklike facies; the eyes focused at a distance; he seems devoid of any will to move or react to any stimuli; there may be fully developed "waxen" flexibility, as in cataleptic states, or only indications, distinct, nevertheless, of this striking phenomenon. The general impression conveyed by such patients is one of profound mental anguish, or an immobility induced by severe mental shock; it has been classified either among the states of depression (which explains the term atonic melancholia) or among the conditions of feeble-mindedness (stupor or dementia stupida); others have regarded it as a combination of the two.[9]

Catatonia was "a temporary stage or a part of a complex picture of various disease forms."[10] He compared catatonia to dementia paralytica, a disorder that dominated the psychiatric practice at the time:

In this newly defined group of disorders, similar to general paralysis of the insane (GPI) – with or without delusions of grandeur – clinical changes in the locomotor apparatus form the main and typical features of the disease; in addition, each disease (GPI and this disease) exhibits manifold patterns of symptoms. In GPI the paralytic components are of many varying grades of severity and type; one or other may be absent in any particular case.... In the same way as in GPI, the spastic signs in the newly described clinical form of the disease are also manifold and varied ... These muscular symptoms ... display alterations in muscular tone ... and I would like to name this disease entity the tonic-mental disorder (Spannungs-Irresein) or vesania katatonica (catatonia)...[11]

He criticized the philosophy that held abnormal behaviors to result from brain lesions.

"This anatomicopathological work produced much valuable material but contributed nothing to the basic views on the origin of mental illness or on the anatomical locus of their diverse and significant manifestations; the view is now spreading that only comprehensive clinical observation of cases can bring order and clarity into the material by using the method of clinical pathology.... It is futile to search for an anatomy of melancholy or mania, etc. because each of these forms occurs under the most varied relationships and combinations with other states, and they are just as little the expressions of an inner pathological process as the complex of symptoms called fever... How wrong it inevitably was to expect pathological anatomy alone to reform the obsolete psychiatric framework."[12]

His patients meet DSM-IV criteria for bipolar disorder, depressive mood disorder, schizophrenia, and delirium. At least seven patients were systematically ill with deliria associated with peritonitis, tuberculosis, and general paralysis of the insane.[13] The range of his patients' illnesses serves well our present image of catatonia as a syndrome in diverse psychiatric and general medical conditions.

The novelty of his presentation was quickly acknowledged. Within three years, Kiernan (1877) recognized catatonia in four patients with mania and depression. A decade later Spitzka (1883), writing from New York City's Ward's Island, described two forms of catatonia and the cyclic course of illness beginning with an initial stage of melancholia. In the same year, Neisser in Germany recognized the syndrome as a feature of mania (Neisser, 1887: 84–5).

Acknowledging catatonia as a new entity, von Schüle (1898) described six subtypes and criticized Kraepelin's adoption of catatonia as a feature of dementia praecox. In the same journal, Aschaffenberg (1898) reported an experience with 227 psychiatric patients, finding different distribution ratios among men and women for those with catatonia (men to women, 2:3) from those with dementia paralytica (3:1). An active academic industry commenting on Kahlbaum's concept quickly followed among German, French and other European as well as American authors.[14] Each effort, in samples of one to twelve patients each, confirmed Kahlbaum's descriptions and discussed the "somatic" and "psychologic" explanations for the disorder.

Catatonia purloined: Emil Kraepelin[15]

The most profound commentary on Kahlbaum's work was that of Emil Kraepelin. This leader of the German academic establishment folded Kahlbaum's descriptions of catatonia and hebephrenia into his concept of dementia praecox.[16] In successive editions of his textbook, dementia praecox became a progressive disorder that began in adolescence, deteriorating in affect and thought, ending in a state of malignant dementia. Catatonia was a phase of this unfolding pattern. Kraepelin's voice has dominated psychopathologic thought to the present day and is the basis for the classification of catatonia in DSM and ICD systems.[17]

In a distinct departure for an author writing in an age that looked to brain pathology for explanations of psychopathology, Kraepelin endorsed a psychological explanation for catatonia. He interpreted catatonic signs as *mental blocking* without a structural basis. Bleuler, using the same concepts, described mutism, negativism, and rigidity as "generalised and persistent blocking – an exaggeration of the phenomenon seen in healthy individuals when they are overwhelmed by emotional disturbance."[18] He envisioned the catatonic patient as suppressing unpleasant memories by silence (mutism), tenseness and rigidity (holds back acts that are compelled by memories), refusal to obey commands, and displacing rising emotions and tension into motor acts that shut out reality (posturing, grimacing, staring, stereotypes). Lethal catatonia was an expression of the death wish.[19]

As a corollary to these interpretations, Bleuler considered sodium amobarbital to "release" blocking, an effective therapeutic use described by Bleckwenn in 1930. Such psychodynamic thoughts are no longer fashionable today, but a recent paean to Frieda Fromm-Reichmann describes her prolonged and fruitless interactions with mute patients by "waiting them out" in months of silence.[20]

Other commentators

In a monograph on catatonia, Urstein (1912) related an experience with 30 patients. He faulted Kraepelin's adoption of catatonia as a subtype of dementia praecox, finding catatonia in patients with syphilis and other infectious diseases, toxic states, depression, mania, and delirium. The prognoses varied, being good when episodes were few, and worsening as the episodes increased in number. Thirty-eight years after Kahlbaum's book, Urstein again regretted the lack of an effective treatment.

In follow-up studies covering more than 10 years of illness, Lange (1922) reported an experience with 200 patients meeting Kraepelin's constructs for manic-depressive illness and for dementia praecox. He found catatonia to be more prominent among the manic-depressive patients than among those with dementia praecox.

In 1940, Kleist, Leonhard and Schwab re-examined a cohort of patients identified separately in two samples examined between 1921 and 1926, one initially diagnosed by Kleist and the second by Leonhard. They classified their patients into seven groups, each subdivided into typical and atypical varieties. Stupor, rigidity, akinesia, negativism, and stereotypy were identified as forms of catatonia. At the time of the follow-up, 61 patients were living and 43 had died. A progressive course was seen in 63% and a recurrent course in 37%. They claimed the diagnoses to have been stable, concluding that the course of the illness confirmed their initial diagnoses. Again, treatment was not discussed. These many forms of catatonic schizophrenia have recently been the focus of study by Beckmann and his co-workers at the University of Würzburg in their search for a genetic basis for schizophrenia.[21]

Kahlbaum described catatonia before an audience at the University of Königsberg in 1868. On the centenary of this lecture, Pauleikhoff (1969) described his 35-year-experience with 552 hospitalized psychiatric patients. He identified 353 patients as suffering from one of five forms of catatonia: Kahlbaum's catatonia (159), stupor (100), excitement (51), malignant catatonia (26), and exogenous (systemic) catatonia (17). Twelve patient histories illustrate the catatonia variants and these descriptions are consistent with the patients that we recognize today. Pauleikhoff presented his data in five-year increments, and reported a drop in the frequency of the diagnoses after 1953. He ascribed the reduced numbers of identifiable catatonic patients as the result of a change in clinic administration and in diagnostic styles, and not as a change in the incidence of the syndrome. He called attention to the deliria that were present in his patients and concluded that catatonia was a syndrome of many forms, most with favorable outcome, and not a phase of a progressive disorder with a dementia outcome.

A neurologic image of catatonia was widely discussed by French and other European authors.[22] Catatonia was one among many motor syndromes, similar to dystonia, parkinsonism, and dyskinesia. The neurologic connection was also central to the studies of epidemic encephalitis by Von Economo who described catatonia in many patients in the acute and chronic phases of the illness (Von Economo, 1931). A comment on this era stated:

The fact that an undoubted neurological disease, encephalitis lethargica, could produce a wide spectrum of psychiatric illness challenged the central idea of the so-called functional psychoses in an era that had come to be dominated by the teachings of psychoanalysis.[23]

The lesson that catatonia is a syndrome in post-encephalitic states is still ignored. In the successful book and film *Awakenings*, the patients experienced prolonged and severe motor inhibition, posturing, rigidity, and mutism. They were diagnosed as suffering from parkinsonism and their treatment with *l*-dopa was given prominence.[24] In 1996, the author Oliver Sacks was asked whether he considered the patients to have exhibited catatonic features. He averred that they did not have catatonia and that he had not considered using the treatments for catatonia for these patients.[25]

Conflicts in interpretation of catatonia between the somatic and psychologic views also marked the American experience. George Kirby (1913) pictured catatonia as typically occurring among patients with manic-depressive illness, and argued that Kraepelin had drawn the boundaries of schizophrenia much too broadly. In a monograph titled *Benign Stupors*, August Hoch (1921) described 25 psychiatric patients in stupor. Thirteen with manic-depressive illness had a favorable prognosis and 12 with general medical illnesses or schizophrenia had a poor prognosis.[26] Kirby and Hoch wrote at the time when a psychodynamic image of schizophrenia and catatonia dominated American psychiatry. Adolf Meyer, Smith Eli Jellife, and William Alanson White, who led American psychiatry, viewed schizophrenia and especially its catatonic form as evidence of the psychological basis for the psychoses.[27] Such views became the basis for the 1952 DSM classification that described abnormal behaviors as reactions to psychological and physical stressors, and not as defined syndromes.

A periodic form of catatonia with hormonal connections was described by Gjessing.[28] In the absence of effective treatment, he observed his patients for long periods, describing their spontaneous relapses and remissions.[29] Carefully examining thyroid metabolism, he reported direct associations with shifts in behavior, and an occasional treatment success with thyroid extracts. He concluded that periodic catatonia was a metabolic disorder. Similar reports of a periodic form of catatonia with a relationship to thyroid metabolism dot the literature.[30]

Another form of catatonia, with an acute onset and a malignant outcome, was described by Stauder in 27 patients. He labeled the disorder *Die tödliche Katatonie*, a term that is best translated as *lethal catatonia* (Stauder, 1934). Young adults between 18 and 26 years of age suddenly became mute, rigid, and either stuporous or severely excited. Fever and autonomic dysfunction were severe and the outcome was quickly fatal. The syndrome has been described by many authors, and is best known today as *malignant catatonia* (MC).[31] A subtype of the syndrome, associated with the use of antipsychotic drugs is widely recognized today as the neuroleptic malignant syndrome (see Chapter 3).

Catatonia disappears

The widespread acceptance, after 1930, of sodium amobarbital to relieve catatonia was the first sign of the coming era of psychopharmacology.[32] With the introduction of modern psychoactive drugs, clinical interest shifted from the detailed descriptions of behavior that had been the staple of psychiatric practice to the simpler goal of labeling the most prominent signs in order to select a medicine for its relief. Illnesses were described as depression or psychosis, and the treatments labeled antidepressant or antipsychotic. In the absence of a newly identified treatment for catatonia among the introduced patented medicines, interest in its descriptive psychopathology waned. Failing to undertake detailed examinations that identified the motor signs of catatonia led clinicians to conclude that the syndrome had disappeared. Mahendra's question in *Psychological Medicine* in 1981 "Where have all the catatonics gone?" argued that the syndrome no longer existed, and ascribed its disappearance to the efficacy of antipsychotic drugs.[33]

The new drugs were classified as *antipsychotic, antidepressant, antimanic, anxiolytic,* and *anticonvulsant.* If a patient was psychotic, one pill was prescribed; if depressed, another; if anxious, a third. Polypharmacy became widespread. Mania virtually disappeared from consideration until lithium became available, assuring a reason to identify patients with the syndrome.[34] As no medicine was labeled "anti-catatonic," catatonia was ignored. To accommodate assumed and sought differences among the medicines, and in the search for uses that could be described as "specific" for any one compound, the number of classified diagnoses increased with the publication of each new DSM classification scheme.

Another factor in the poor recognition of catatonia is the troubling awareness that the new drugs were often accompanied by disabling motor effects. The motor side-effects masked endogenous catatonic features. But an appreciation of motor side-effects for the new medicines was out of line with the enthusiasm expressed by researchers and industry leaders for their benefits. Awareness and acknowledgement of adverse motor signs was repressed.[35] Clinicians observed rigidities, tremors, dystonias, akathisias, and occasionally even the fatal *syndrom malin* in their use of the antipsychotic drugs, yet these observations were pushed out of awareness and denied. It took more than two decades for these effects to be publicly acknowledged.[36] The processes that suppressed recognition of tardive dyskinesia, tardive dystonia, and drug-induced parkinsonism served also to suppress the recognition of catatonia.

The segregation of severe psychiatrically ill patients to long-stay facilities, out of the experience of academic and research psychiatrists, also contributed to the failure to recognize catatonia. Among chronically ill patients, persistent signs of catatonia are commonplace.[37]

Interest revives

Interest in catatonia was aroused in the 1970s by studies by Morrison, Abrams and Taylor, and Gelenberg. Morrison reported that 10% of the Iowa (USA) 500 patient series had met criteria for the retarded or the excited forms of catatonia. He described catatonia as occurring more often among patients with mood disorders than among those with schizophrenia.[38]

Among patients otherwise diagnosed as suffering from mania, depression, and toxic brain states, Abrams and Taylor reported a high prevalence of catatonia.[39] They surveyed hospital admissions, reporting a prevalence of catatonia as twice as likely among patients with manic-depressive disorders as in those with schizophrenia.

Gelenberg identified catatonia in patients with neurotoxic syndromes secondary to the use of antipsychotic drugs.[40] His observations anticipated descriptions of the neuroleptic malignant syndrome and drug-induced parkinsonism.

A *syndrom malin* secondary to the use of antipsychotic drugs was described by Delay and associates (1960) and individual clinical reports followed slowly.[41] Meltzer (1973) identified a severe neurotoxic reaction to depot fluphenazine, and Weinberger and Kelly (1977) reported a syndrome of malignant catatonia secondary to neuroleptic administration. Caroff's summary of published reports captured clinical interest and his name of a *neuroleptic malignant syndrome* (NMS) was accepted (Caroff, 1980). He hypothesized that NMS resulted from excessive dopamine blockade, recommending dopamine agonists for its relief. Some patients exhibited fever and muscle weakness, suggesting a similarity to malignant hyperthermia (MH), the toxic genetic response to inhalational anesthetic agents.[42] MH was treated with the muscle relaxant dantrolene, and dantrolene and dopamine agonists were discussed as treatment for NMS (see Chapter 7).

Catatonic mutism had been relieved with barbiturates since 1930. When benzodiazepines were introduced as safer and as effective alternatives, Fricchione et al. (1983) reported lorazepam to be as effective as amobarbital in relieving catatonia. Diazepam, zolpidem and the anesthetic etomidate, for example, were soon shown to be effective.[43] The similarity of the syndrome of NMS with that of malignant catatonia was quickly recognized.[44]

That the lethal form of catatonia recognized by Bell (1849) and Stauder (1934) could be effectively treated by electroconvulsive therapy (ECT) pointed to another therapeutic direction. The report by Arnold and Stepan (1952) was confirmed by Häfner and Kasper (1982), Mann et al. (1990), and Philbrick and Rummans (1994), establishing ECT as a life-saving option for this condition. As NMS was recognized with increasing frequency, comparisons were made with malignant catatonia. Most authors could not distinguish patients with malignant catatonia from those with the neuroleptic malignant syndrome (see Chapters 3 and 7). The view of NMS as a unique dopaminergic fault on the one hand, and as a syndrome indistinguishable from malignant catatonia on the other, spurred debates as to the proper classification of NMS and malignant catatonia.[45] The reports at the end of the 20th Century find the two syndromes indistinguishable.[46]

Soon after the introduction of monamine oxidase inhibitors, a toxic serotonin syndrome (TSS) was described. The name appeared in the psychiatric literature in 1982.[47] By 1991, the syndrome was reported to have clinical hallmarks very similar to those found in NMS, except that gastrointestinal symptoms are more prominent.[48] TSS responded to the same treatments as NMS, and some investigators conclude that it is a variant of catatonia.[49]

A formal catatonia rating scale was presented by Lohr and Wisniewski in 1987, and other scales quickly followed.[50] Although none have been widely accepted or used clinically, rating scales help researchers define the incidence of the syndrome and quantify treatment progress.

The classifications of psychiatric disorders of the 20th Century took the writings of Kraepelin and Bleuler as their guides.[51] In each diagnostic system, catatonia was defined only as a subtype of schizophrenia. When DSM-IV was proposed, the writings of the German and American authors that reported catatonia in conditions other than schizophrenia and that disagreed with Kraepelin's formulation were brought to the attention of the drafters.[52] They considered the experience of limited merit, however, and continued to recognize catatonia as a subtype of schizophrenia. But they did offer a separate class for catatonia when secondary to general medical conditions, giving it a call number (293.89). They also offered catatonia as a modifier for mania and depression.[53]

An animal model for catatonia, based on the administration of bulbocapnine, was developed by de Jong and Baruk.[54] Loss of motor initiative, catalepsy, and resistance to change in position was described in mice, cats, monkeys, pigeons, and frogs. Similar effects were observed with hallucinogens. At a time when catatonia was viewed as a psychologic reaction to stress, these experiments spurred images of brain mechanisms as the basis for a common final pathway in behavior.

The neurologic aspects of catatonia were again discussed in the 1990s by Rogers in his *Motor Disorders in Psychiatry*.[55] The postures of patients suffering from encephalitis lethargica overlapped those of patients with schizophrenia. He criticized the psychodynamic paradigm and argued for a neurologic one. To identify the specific abnormalities in his populations he developed a rating scale for catatonia.

Some authors, seeing the variety of forms that catatonia took in their patients, reverted to the term *Kahlbaum syndrome* for the patients with the retarded form of catatonia.[56]

A strong interest in catatonia re-appeared among German investigators.[57] Finding Kraepelin's descriptions unhelpful in describing patients in clinical drug trials, Beckmann, Stöber, Pfuhlmann, and Franzek turned to the earlier descriptions by Wernicke, Kleist, and Leonhard for guidance. They identified family pedigrees in which catatonia was prominent, and cited an identifiable gene associated with a subtype of the syndrome.[58] They formed a society that encouraged recognition of catatonia as a syndrome among severe psychiatric illnesses.[59] Their view of catatonia as a specific form of schizophrenia sparked a debate with American authors seeing catatonia as a syndrome of diverse manifestations. Reports from the ongoing debate were recently published.[60]

Catatonia is increasingly recognized among adolescents and children, including those with mental retardation and autism. It has not always been so. Whether catatonia is to be seen in patients with mental retardation and other developmental disorders is an ongoing debate.[61] Yet, when catatonia is recognized among patients with mental retardation, it is as responsive to catatonia treatments as it is among adults.[62]

Autism, a disorder that interferes with socialization, has an onset in early childhood. Mutism, echolalia, echopraxia, odd hand postures, freezing of ongoing movements, rigidities, forced vocalizations, stereotypy, and insensitivity to pain are its hallmarks. These signs have generally been interpreted as evidence of schizophrenia, leading to the confusion between autism and schizophrenia.[63] Clinical reports now find the treatments for catatonia to be useful for the cardinal signs of autism.[64]

Adolescents exhibiting catatonia signs are described as suffering from pervasive refusal syndrome, idiopathic recurring stupor, myalgic encephalopathy, and chronic fatigue syndrome.[65] The relation of these syndromes to catatonia is a subject of recent inquiry.[66]

Present status

Kahlbaum extracted a syndrome of catatonia from his clinical experience. His syndrome was quickly incorporated into the concept of dementia praecox, a disorder formulated by Kraepelin and Bleuler. Many authors endorsed Kahlbaum's position and criticized Kraepelin's limited view of the syndrome. Despite the evidence to support the concept of catatonia as a syndrome not tied to schizophrenia, most 20th Century classifiers of psychiatric disorders follow Kraepelin and Bleuler. The recognition of catatonia among patients with diverse disorders challenges the present classifications and it is timely to develop a separate class for catatonia. Clarification is ongoing, however, in the debate on the similarities between NMS and MC, the role of catatonia in autism and other childhood disorders, and the relationship of catatonia to stupor, delirium, and diverse neurologic disorders. The search for the genetic basis for one form of catatonic schizophrenia is another example.

In the first half of the 20th Century, catatonia was interpreted in psychologic terms. Once the syndrome could be relieved by amobarbital, however, and an animal model described, a biological model took precedence and treatment algorithms were quickly developed that are remarkably effective. The efficacy of the benzodiazepines and electroconvulsive therapy (ECT) is now well defined, and this experience would be the envy of the clinicians who described the syndrome but whose knowledge provided no effective relief for their patients. The effective interventions are anti-epileptic in their action, raising seizure thresholds and stimulating the brain's GABA-ergic systems. These commonalities offer a special focus in the search for an understanding of the pathophysiology of catatonia.

But while we have made much progress in identifying the patients who have the disorder and in our ability to help them, the position of catatonic patients in our society is fraught with unnecessary peril. Despite our social commitment that the state should protect the interests of minors and the psychiatrically ill, special regulations inhibit the use of effective treatments in patients with catatonia. Patients who are mute, negativistic, in stupor, or excited are unable to give verbal or written consent for their care. In many venues the application of intravenous sedatives, and more so, the application of ECT is severely restricted, even proscribed, by demands that the patients must personally give written, signed consent to the treatments. A 22-year-old woman, without any prior psychiatric illness, developed malignant catatonia following a Cæsarean delivery.[67] The legal hurdles in place in California severely impeded her treatment for 33 days, risking her life and causing her and society great expense. Within 36 hours of treatment she no longer required special nursing care. The legislated obstacles in place in our states for the proper treatment of patients with catatonia serve our patients poorly.

ENDNOTES

1 Diethelm 1971; Hunter and Macalpine, 1982.
2 Kahlbaum, 1874; translated edition, 1973: 85. In the original: "*Die Katatonie ist eine Gehirnkrankheit mit cyklisch wechselndem Verlaufe, bei der die psychischen Symptome der Reihe nach das Bild der Melancholie, der Manie, der Stupescenz, der Verwirrtheit und schliesslich des Blödsinns darbieten, von welchen psychischen Gesammtbildern aber eins, oder mehrere fehlen können, und bei der neben den psychischen Symptomen Vorgänge in dem motorischen Nervensystem mit dem allgemeinen Charakter des Krampfes als wesentliche Symptome erscheinen.*" Kahlbaum, 1874: 87.
3 Mora, 1973: xiii. Also, Kraepelin, 1919; 1962.
4 Katzenstein, 1963.
5 Berrios, 1996b.
6 Kahlbaum, 1874.
7 Sedler, 1985.
8 Robins and Guze, 1970.
9 Kahlbaum, 1874, translated edition 1973: 8–9.
10 Kahlbaum, 1874, translated edition 1973: 26.
11 Kahlbaum, 1874, translated edition 1973: 27.
12 Kahlbaum, 1874, translated edition 1973: 2.
13 Berrios, 1996a: 382–3.
14 German authors: Neisser, 1887; von Schüle, 1898; Aschaffenburg, 1898; Urstein, 1912; Lange, 1922; Arnold and Stepan, 1952; and Pauleikhoff, 1969; and doctoral theses by Behr, 1891; Rauch, 1906; Hansen, 1908; Siroth, 1914; Winkel, 1925 (published 1929); and Maisel, 1936.
   French authors: Dide, Guiraud and LaFage, 1921 and Guiraud, 1924; Czech author: Haskovec, 1925; Danish author: Reiter, 1926; and Swiss author: Steck, 1926, 1927, 1931; are discussed by Rogers, 1990.
   American authors: Spitzka, 1883, Kiernan, 1877, Kirby, 1913, and Hoch, 1921.
15 Johnson (1993) described Kraepelin as "hijacking" these concepts.
16 Kraepelin, 1896, 1903, 1913, 1919.

17 DSM: American Psychiatric Association, 1952, 1980, 1994; ICD: World Health Organization, 1992.

18 Bleuler 1924; 1950: 211.

19 Rogers, 1991; Blacker, 1966.

20 Hornstein, 2000.

21 Beckmann et al., 1996; Stöber 2001; Stöber et al. 1995, 2000a,b,c, 2001. The genetic studies are discussed in Chapter 3.

22 Dide, Guiraud and LaFage, 1921; Guiraud, 1924; Haskovec, 1925; Reiter, 1926; Steck, 1926, 1927, 1931.

23 Johnson, 1993: 737.

24 Sacks, 1974.

25 Comment to MF, May 1996.

26 *Patient 3.15* in Chapter 3 is abstracted from his report.

27 Jelliffe and White, 1917; Jelliffe, 1940.

28 Gjessing, 1932, 1936, 1938, 1939, 1976. Also Chapter 3.

29 *Patient 3.12*, Chapter 3 is one of his patients.

30 Lindsay, 1948; Minde, 1966; Komori et al., 1997; Kinrys and Logan, 2001.

31 Chapter 3. Bell, 1849; Scheidegger, 1929; Scheid, 1937; Billig and Freeman, 1943; Arnold, 1949; Arnold and Stepan, 1952; Geller and Mappes, 1952; Huber, 1954; Pauleikhoff, 1969; Gabris and Muller, 1983.

32 Bleckwenn, 1930.

33 Also Silva et al., 1989.

34 Baldessarini, 1970.

35 Repression is the active psychologic process, an ego defense mechanism, that keeps unpleasant thoughts or observations out of awareness. (Hinsie and Campbell, 1970: 660.)

36 Gelman, 1999; Healy, 2002.

37 Turner, 1989; Bush et al., 1997.

38 Morrison 1973, 1975.

39 Abrams and Taylor, 1976; Abrams et al., 1979; Taylor and Abrams, 1973, 1977; Taylor, 1992.

40 Gelenberg 1976, 1977; Gelenberg and Mandel, 1977.

41 Lazarus et al., 1989; Gelman, 1999.

42 Lazarus, et al., 1989.

43 McEvoy and Lohr, 1983; White and Robins, 1991; White, 1992; Takeuchi, 1996; Zaw and Bates, 1997; Thomas et al., 1997.

44 Fricchione, 1985; Rosebush et al., 1990; White and Robins, 1991; White, 1992.

45 Fink, 1996a,b,c; Caroff et al., 1998a,b; Fricchione et al., 2000.

46 Davis et al., 2000; Fricchione et al., 2000; Mann et al., 2001; Fink and Taylor, 2001.

47 Insel et al., 1982.

48 Sternbach, 1991.

49 Fink, 1996b; Keck and Arnold, 2000.

50 Lohr and Wisniewski, 1987; Taylor, 1990, 1999; Rosebush et al., 1990; Rogers, 1992; Bush et al., 1996a,b; Fink, 1997a; Northoff et al., 1999b; Bräunig et al., 2000. Chapter 5.

51 Freedman, 1991.

52 Fink and Taylor, 1991.

53 American Psychiatric Association, 1994.

54 de Jong and Baruk, 1930; de Jong, 1945.

55 Rogers 1991, 1992; Rogers et al., 1991; Lund et al., 1991.
   At the MacKeith Conference in 2001, Rogers showed the same overlaps in videotapes of patients.

56 Pauleikhoff, 1969; Magrinat et al. 1983; Barnes et al., 1986; Goldar and Starkstein, 1995; Peralta et al., 1997.

57 Kindt, 1980; Hippius et al., 1987; Northoff et al., 1997; Bräunig et al., 1995a, 1998, 1999, 2000; Stöber and Ungvari, 2001; and Stöber, 2001.

58 Stöber et al. 1995, 2000a,b; Beckmann et al., 1996; Stöber et al., 2000c.

59 The WKL (Wernicke–Kleist–Leonhard) Society has met every other year for a decade.

60 Stöber and Ungvari, 2001; Riederer, 2001.

61 Earl, 1934; Turner, 1989.

62 Bates and Smeltzer, 1982; Cutajar and Wilson, 1999; Thuppal and Fink, 1999; Fink, 1999a; van Waarde et al., 2001; Friedlander and Solomons, 2002.

63 Kanner, 1943; Wing and Atwood, 1987; Mullen, 1986; Realmuto and August, 1991; Dhossche and Bouman, 1997a,b; Dhossche, 1998; Zaw et al., 1999; Wing and Shah, 2000a,b; Chaplin, 2000.

64 O'Gorman, 1970; Dhossche and Bouman, 1997a; Dhossche, 1998; Zaw et al., 1999.

65 Lask et al., 1991; Tinuper et al., 1992, 1994; Palmieri 1999.

66 A Mac Keith Conference on *Catatonia in Childhood* was held in London, September 26–27, 2001 organized by Drs. M. Prendergast and G. O'Brien of Northumberland, UK.

67 Bach-Y-Rita and De Ranieri, 1992.

2

Signs of catatonia are identifiable

Only a comprehensive and intensive application of the clinical method can enable psychiatry to progress and to increase the understanding of psychopathological processes.

Kahlbaum, 1874[1]

Catatonia is a syndrome of specific motor abnormalities closely associated with disorders in mood, affect, thought, and cognition. The principal signs of the disorder are mutism, immobility, negativism, posturing, stereotypy, and echophenomena. Dysfunctions in other motor actions have also been suggested as within the syndrome of catatonia, but the principal signs are defined in Table 2.1.[2]

Mutism and stupor are principal catatonic signs but neither alone is pathognomonic. Other motor behaviors should be present, and most patients with one sign exhibit four or more catatonic features. Because the number of features required for the diagnosis is not experimentally established, we consider two of the classic catatonia signs as sufficient to meet criteria for the syndrome. (In Table 5.1, we offer our diagnostic criteria for catatonia.)

There is also a lack of consensus about the duration of the behaviors necessary to make the diagnosis. In some patients, the signs are unstable or transient, while in others, they are present for days, weeks, or months. Writers in the 19th and early 20th centuries described patients in whom catatonia persisted for years.[3] Some clinicians accept the presence of signs for one hour as adequate for its identification, while others hold persistence for a day as necessary. We identify catatonia when features are present for an hour or longer or are reproducible on two or more occasions.

Mutism, posturing (catalepsy), automatic obedience, and stereotypy are the classic signs of catatonia. Generalized analgesia is frequent, sometimes

Table 2.1 Principal features of catatonia

Feature	Description
Mutism	Verbal unresponsiveness, not always associated with immobility
Stupor	Unresponsiveness, hypoactivity, and reduced or altered arousal during which the patient fails to respond to queries; when severe, the patient is mute, immobile, and does not withdraw from painful stimuli
Negativism (Gegenhalten)	Patient resists examiner's manipulations, whether light or vigorous, with strength equal to that applied, as if bound to the stimulus of the examiner's actions
Posturing (catalepsy)	Maintains postures for long periods. Includes facial postures, such as grimacing or *Schnauzkrampf* (lips in an exaggerated pucker). Body postures, such as *psychological pillow* (patient lying in bed with his head elevated as if on a pillow), lying in a jackknifed position, sitting with upper and lower portions of body twisted at right angles, holding arms above the head or raised in prayer-like manner, and holding fingers and hands in odd positions
Waxy flexibility	Offers initial resistance to an induced movement before gradually allowing himself to be postured, similar to bending a candle.
Stereotypy	Non-goal-directed, repetitive motor behavior. The repetition of phrases and sentences in an automatic fashion, similar to a scratched record, termed *verbigeration*, is a verbal stereotypy. The neurologic term for similar behavior is *palilalia*, during which the patient repeats the sentence just uttered, usually with increasing speed.
Automatic obedience	Despite instructions to the contrary, the patient permits the examiner's light pressure to move his limbs into a new position (posture), which may then be maintained by the patient despite instructions to the contrary.
Ambitendency	The patient appears "stuck" in an indecisive, hesitant movement, resulting from the examiner verbally contradicting his own strong non-verbal signal, such as offering his hand as if to shake hands while stating, "Don't shake my hand, I don't want you to shake it."
Echophenomena	Includes *echolalia*, in which the patient repeats the examiner's utterances, and *echopraxia*, in which the patient spontaneously copies the examiner's movements or is unable to refrain from copying the examiner's test movements, despite instruction to the contrary
Mannerisms	Odd, purposeful movements, such as holding hands as if they were handguns, saluting passersby, or exaggerations or stilted caricatures of mundane movements

even to very painful stimuli. Patients who remain in this state for long periods become malnourished, dehydrated, lose weight, and develop muscle wasting, contractures, and bed-sores. They may die as a result of venous thrombosis and pulmonary emboli.[4]

Mutism

The patient is awake and may move about, but is silent and unresponsive in speech. Stupor may be present. (Although stuporous patients have reduced motor output or are mute, many mute patients are not stuporous.) *Patient 2.1* was mute, postured for many weeks, and developed systemic complications, but eventually recovered with effective treatment.

Patient 2.1   A 40-year-old man had been treated for psychosis with antipsychotic and antimanic medications since age 16. He was attending a community clinic, and was stabilized with lithium and chlorpromazine therapy. Encouraged by the stability of his condition, his therapist prescribed olanzapine, then a new atypical antipsychotic. Within a few weeks, the patient again became psychotic. Perphenazine was prescribed and within a day he became febrile, mute, and rigid. He was hospitalized, the diagnosis of a neuroleptic malignant syndrome was made, and he was transferred to a tertiary care medical facility.

Antipsychotic medications were discontinued and he was treated with large doses of bromocriptine and dantrolene. Repetitive motor movements erroneously prompted the diagnosis of epilepsy, so anticonvulsants were administered. Lorazepam, prescribed in low doses, controlled infrequent agitation. He remained mute and rigid and required total nursing care. After a few weeks, he was unable to stand; his hands and legs were in a rigid, immobile posture. A gastrostomy was done to permit feeding. He developed pulmonary and bladder infections requiring antibiotics.

After he had been in intensive medical care for four months, a visiting consultant recommended lorazepam at high doses. When the daily dose was increased to 12 mg, the patient responded to commands and smiled at his parents, though he remained mute. ECT was recommended, but the hospital did not have this facility available, so he was transferred to one that did. When his mother was signing the consent for ECT on behalf of her son, she recalled that he had a similar episode of rigidity, mutism, and psychosis when he was 16 years of age. He had responded well to ECT.

Lorazepam was reduced to 6 mg/day and bilateral ECT was begun. After four treatments, he recognized his parents, vocalized, smiled, was less rigid, and took oral feedings. By the ninth treatment, he was verbally responsive, but the four months of rigidity and forced bed rest had left him with limb contractures and such badly impaired movement that he was unable to stand or to use his hands to feed himself. Both catatonia and psychosis were relieved. After 22 ECT, he was transferred to a rehabilitation center and four months later he was again able to walk, use his hands, and care for himself.

Comment: This patient's ordeal was prolonged by several clinical missteps. Persisting in a failed clinical trial with bromocriptine and dantrolene did him no service. Generally, if an acutely ill patient has not improved substantially with 7 to 10 days of treatment, that treatment needs to be reconsidered and probably changed. Catatonic features interfering with general medical health, even catatonic features attributed to antipsychotic drugs, improve substantially within several days when properly treated. For this patient, inadequate nursing care allowed contractures to develop. The unavailability of ECT at a tertiary care hospital was indefensible, not only as a necessary treatment for psychiatric disorders, but for the lack of opportunity for the professional staff and residents-in-training to learn about its merits and appropriate use.

A long-ill catatonic patient with joint contractures was successfully and safely treated with ECT.[5]

Stupor

Stupor has long been recognized as evidence of a psychiatric and neurologic illness. Until the 1830s, stupor was thought to represent a numbing or failure of sensation. It was next seen as evidence of melancholia and as a severe inhibition of movement related to catatonia. During the 20th Century, stupor was associated with brain stem lesions, infectious disorders (e.g., encephalitis lethargica), and normal pressure hydrocephalus. Stupor as a reflection of brain dysfunction was re-enforced by animal studies.[6]

In stupor, patients remain persistently unresponsive, with durations measured in hours, days, or longer. They seem unaware of the happenings around them. It is occasionally difficult to distinguish stupor from mutism without stupor. An early description characterized patients in catatonic stupor as:

taciturn, sparing of words; they may stop in the middle of a word or sentence and may gradually cease talking entirely (mutism). Sometimes they lisp softly some unintelligible words or phrases; they may carry on whispered conversations with themselves ... they are generally uninfluenced by environmental stimuli.[7]

Stupor occurs without other catatonic features. When there is no clear metabolic, pharmacologic, or neurologic explanation for it, a stupor may reflect the psychomotor retardation of a severe depression. In the 19th Century, stupor was described under the term *melancholia attonita,* a term used by Kahlbaum to encompass the symptom complex of stupor, mutism, and immobility. Von Economo described stupor as the third most common feature in his descriptions of encephalitis lethargica.[8]

A recent review of 25 patients in stupor found 10 to have a depressive syndrome, four a catatonic syndrome, and 10 with brain pathology. Twelve of the patients were successfully treated with ECT.[9]

Patients in stupor may suddenly become energized. The excitement is intense and may last an hour or two, simulating manic excitement. Such periods of energy usually reflect an underlying manic-depressive illness, as the patient fluctuates between stupor and excitement.

Patient 2.2   A 40-year-old man was hospitalized with a three-day history of depressed mood and psychotic thoughts. His speech was slow and slurred, and his utterances few. Within an hour of admission, he was mute and stuporous, analgesic to painful stimuli. A urine toxicology examination was negative. Lying in bed, he could be postured, consistent with waxy flexibility. Once postured, he remained in that position for several minutes before returning to an initial position. Two hours later, he suddenly stood and began singing and tap-dancing back and forth along the hallway. When he came to the nurses' station, he tap-danced in place, joking with aides and nurses. Then he tap-danced away. His excitement lasted for an hour, following which he again became stuporous, rigid, and mute. This cycle was repeated over several days.

Comment: This patient suffered from a rapidly fluctuating manic-depressive illness with catatonia. The pattern met criteria for a mixed mood state, and he responded to treatment of his mood disorder.

Excitement

In the early descriptions, catatonic patients talked incessantly, especially when in "the stage of exaltation."[10] They become impulsive and stereotypic with sudden outbursts of talking, singing, dancing, and removing their clothes.[11] Excited states are associated with the risks of exhaustion, dehydration, and injury (Aronson and Thompson, 1950). Today, such patients are likely to

be considered to be suffering from mania. Less common than "catatonic excitement" in a manic-depressive illness, is the catatonic patient who suddenly
and unexpectedly erupts from catalepsy.

Patient 2.3 A 19-year-old slight woman was hospitalized for mutism. She sat motionless for prolonged periods, disinterested in her surroundings, although she appeared alert. Automatic obedience and posturing were observed. Her general medical health was good
and she was afebrile. During the day, she was placed in a chair near the nurses' station
where she could "*see what was going on.*" She refused to eat, and was fed by hand, like
feeding a child. She ate and moved slowly, but was not stiff.

On the second day, suddenly and without warning, she leaped from her chair and
grabbed the throat of a passing activities-therapist, severely damaging the therapist's
thyroid. Catatonia resolved with bilateral ECT, but the patient remained avolitional, emotionally shallow, and suspicious. Her underlying condition was schizophrenia.

Unexpected violence with injuries to hospital personnel is most often
caused by young persons with drug-induced psychoses and by older demented persons. The first days of hospitalization, when staff members are least
familiar with their patients are the most difficult management period. The
next vignette exemplifies a patient in catatonic excitement.

Patient 2.4 A 28-year-old man was hospitalized for repeatedly accosting passersby. He shouted
rapid-fire comments and questions at them, making reference to vague dangers in the
world. In the hospital, he talked incessantly, disrupted meetings, turned light switches
on and off, and pulled the fire-alarm. He mimicked the movements of the nurses and
repeated what he heard. He resisted all attempts at restraint with equal force. Sedation
left him with slurred speech and ataxia, but excitement continued. When restrained in
a chair, he dragged the chair about the unit, speaking to whomever he met, his voice
reduced to a croaking whisper. He refused to eat or to drink and became dehydrated.

Excitement, echopraxia, echolalia, and negativism were signs of an exacerbated manic-
depressive illness. Emergency bilateral ECT on two successive days quickly ameliorated
the excited behavior and catatonic features. Additional ECT resolved the mania. (Antipsychotic medicines were not given to the patient to avoid inducing MC/NMS.[12])

Catatonic patients often make odd sounds of barking or sniffing or they
act like an animal.

Patient 2.5 A 33-year-old man was brought to the hospital by the police for acting as if he were
a wild animal. He would drop to all fours, growl and scurry along the street, roaring,
snapping, and biting at passersby. Dressed in pajamas and placed in bed in the hospital,

he became mute and immobile. He refused food and liquids. His eyes followed the examiner's movements. He was afebrile, insensitive to moderate pain, and his limbs could be postured after initial resistance.

During a conversation by his bedside, he suddenly roared, and jumped out of bed as if to attack the examiner, who reflexively raised his hands in a defensive posture, accidentally touching the patient's raised arm. The patient immediately froze into this new posture (automatic obedience). No one was injured.

Catatonic patients speak and move about.

Patient 2.6   A 38-year-old man was hospitalized for acute mania. On the unit, he was moving constantly, intruding on meetings and hallway conversations. He spoke rapidly. His mood was elevated and he described grandiose plans. When he conversed with the examiner, he was asked if he would mind if the examiner moved his arms *"just to make sure you're in good shape."* The patient consented. The examiner then grasped the patient's hand and swung his arm horizontally from side to side. The patient resisted this swing with equal and opposite pressure (Gegenhalten). The examiner then raised his right arm and then both his arms above his head. The patient did the same, despite instructions that it was not necessary to do so and he should not do it (echopraxia). Throughout the examination, the patient continued to converse. When the examination was over, the patient (arms still above his head) followed the examiner down the hallway trying to maintain the conversation. Lithium carbonate treatment resolved both his mania and catatonic features.

Features demonstrated in examination

Negativism, waxy flexibility, and automatic obedience are features that are demonstrated during the examination. Several rating scales to evaluate the signs and severity of catatonia have been developed in the past decade (see Chapter 5). Appendix I contains a representative rating scale developed at the State University of New York at Stony Brook.[13] The scale is modeled after those devised to evaluate the psychopathologies of depression, anxiety, mania, and psychosis, and the motor syndromes of Parkinsonism and tardive dyskinesia. The Stony Brook scale details methods of systematic examination and the scoring of items, providing measures of changes in the severity and pattern of the illness.

Stereotypy is the presentation of repetitive, awkward or stiff movements that appear to be senseless. The movements may be complex, taking the form of rituals or compulsive behaviors. Self-mutilation may occur, with patients biting, striking, burning, or gouging their skin.

Mannerisms often accompany stereotypes and may be incorporated into a seemingly goal-directed action but done in an exaggerated, distinct, or strange way. Catatonic stereotypes and mannerisms should be suspected when obsessive and compulsive features are observed in a psychotic patient.

Patient 2.7 A 63-year-old woman with recurrent hospitalizations for depression since age 26 years was hospitalized with depressed mood, slow speech, suicidal thoughts, rigidity, and posturing. Her illness progressed over many weeks despite many medications. She developed a deep vein thrombosis and survived an embolus to a lung. In her fifth week of illness, she assumed a fetal position, and was mute thereafter except for outbursts of repetitive expletives "*s–t, s–t, s–t*" when she was disturbed. The expletives were repeated in the fashion commonly described in patients with the Gilles de la Tourette syndrome.

On the 58th day of hospital care, her treatment was changed to lorazepam at 6 mg/day. On the 61st day, bilateral ECT was begun. After the second treatment, she slowly answered questions, stood, walked, ate, and went to the bathroom by herself for the first time in many weeks. The expletives were much less frequent. After the third treatment, the expletives were no longer present, and she was oriented for time, date, and place. She walked and spoke spontaneously, but rigidity and posturing were manifest.

The day after the fifth treatment, the signs of catatonia were gone. She was no longer depressed, smiled spontaneously, cared for herself, and remarked that she had "*been in a dream*" for many weeks. She accepted another treatment, and then, after a day at home, refused further ECT. She was discharged to the care of her son with maintenance medications of lithium, thiothixene, and olanzapine, the medications that she had been receiving in the months before this episode. Examinations one month, five months, and one year later found her without signs of catatonia or depression. She was caring for herself in her son's home when she relapsed with blank staring, mutism, negativism, and rigidity. She was hospitalized quickly. A high dose benzodiazepine trial brought no relief. A course of six ECT resolved the syndrome and she returned home.[14]

Echophenomena are the spontaneous mimicry of the examiner's movements (echopraxia) or repetition of his statements (echolalia). The examiner's posture is mirrored. Raising an arm over the head is imitated, the patient raising his right arm as the examiner raises his left. Patients do not know why they make these movements and they usually give a silly or inadequate reason for it, denying their illness (anosognosia).

Speech-prompt catatonia, or more specifically speech-promptness, is a variant of echolalia. The patient does not speak spontaneously, but answers questions by either repeating the examiner's questions or by answering with an automatic "*I don't know*," or with a "*yes*" or "*no*," often in contradictory ways. The question "*Do you like ice cream?*" is answered "*I don't know.*" The question "*You do like ice cream, don't you?*" with a "*yes*." And, "*You don't like ice cream, do you?*" is answered with a "*no*." Leonhard considered this a verbal form of automatic obedience (Leonhard, 1979). An example, described by Ungvari and Rankin (1990), is abstracted.[15]

Patient 2.8   A 26-year-old woman was committed for psychiatric evaluation because of unusual and asocial behavior accompanied by restricted communication. She did not comply with simple requests and acted oddly. For example, she watered the concrete walk instead of the flowers. Over the previous few years she had taken less and less care of her appearance and personal hygiene, abandoning normal social conventions in behavior, sometimes eating food with her fingers from the kitchen floor. Verbal spontaneity was decreased. In the year before admission, she would disappear into the woods without adequate clothing or food, and bring home dead animals. Collecting garbage in her room was another unexplained ritual.

Psychiatric examination demonstrated a fit, slim woman who sat isolated on the treatment unit, gazing with a blank, puppet-like facial expression, displaying a half-smile. Her gait was rigid and ungraceful with head and trunk tilted forward, shoulders partially lifted, arms symmetric and mildly flexed. She was tense and abrupt in her movements.

She did not initiate conversation or utter words spontaneously. When approached, however, she replied to every question with short, simple words or sentences as "*I don't know*" or "*It's all right.*" The prompted short responses were associated with aimless acts of mechanical tidiness and garbage collecting, done without an affective accompaniment and without explanation.

Neither behavioral care, intramuscular diazepam (10 mg) challenge, nor intravenous administration of sodium amobarbital improved her condition. She remained ill and hospitalized for at least a year. At three-year follow-up examination, she was unchanged.

Patients with echophenomena exhibit other *stimulus-bound* features. They are compelled to touch, pick up, or use objects such as turning light switches on or off, pulling fire alarms, taking other patient's possessions left in the open, or going into another person's room and lying on their bed. These behaviors are described as *utilization behavior*. In a test for stimulus-bound behavior, the patient is instructed: "*When I touch my nose, I want you to touch your chest."* Despite understanding the instruction, patients will touch their nose, mirroring the examiner's movement.

When echolalia is severe, obtaining a history of the illness and completing the behavior examination is difficult because the patient repeats questions and answers no further. Administering a benzodiazepine or a barbiturate in a low dose often resolves such behavior. Another maneuver is to use a third party to get the information, as illustrated in the following.

Patient 2.9 A 27-year-old marine was admitted to a Naval Hospital because he refused to do his assigned work after his surroundings and co-workers became unfamiliar. He stopped speaking. In the admitting area of the hospital, he sat calmly. He was afebrile, and demonstrated automatic obedience, but did not posture.

The examiner sat diagonally to the patient, rather than face to face. Each question was repeated with the same question (e.g., *"How old are you?" "How old are you?"*). The patient mimicked the examiner's movements. The patient's manner was smug, and his attitude silly. A third person joined the group and faced the examiner. Instead of asking the patient, *"How old are you?"* the examiner asked the third person (who was instructed not to respond), *"How old do you think the man sitting here is?"* The stimulus bound patient interrupted these exchanges with answers to the questions. The full examination was conducted this way.

In this examination, the examiner sat transverse to the patient. Directly facing the patient may be perceived as aggressive and anxiety-provoking, encouraging negativism and mutism. A dramatic example of an unusual examination position in evaluating a catatonic patient follows.

Patient 2.10 A 40-year-old man was brought to the Emergency Room (ER) after he was found wandering, seemingly confused, and making little sense when he spoke. In the ER, he knelt on the floor, pressed his forehead to the ground, and put one hand on the floor and the other on top of his head. He did not respond to questions or requests by the ER staff, and could not be moved out of his posture.

A psychiatrist got down on the floor beside the patient, mimicking his posture. The patient answered the psychiatrist's questions, although his speech was slow and he did not elaborate on his answers. He was delusional and was experiencing several first rank symptoms.

Ambitendency is another stimulus bound phenomenon. The examiner offers a hand, as if to shake hands, and firmly tells the patient *"Don't shake my hand. I don't want you to shake it."* The two conflicting signals result in the patient raising his hand as if to shake hands, lightly touching the examiner's hand but not grasping it, or moving his hand back and forth, as if he cannot make up his mind.

Catalepsy refers to the maintenance of postures for long periods without movement. Most often, patients remain in a sitting or standing posture, moving little. Some postures are dramatic, like *psychological pillow*, in which the supine patient lies with head and shoulders raised as if resting on a pillow, and resists any effort to lower the head. This behavior was seen in *Patient 2.7* and persisted for three days during the course of her treatment. Some patients will not only hold their head and shoulders off the bed but their legs as well, doing so for many minutes. *Schnauzkrampf*, in which the lips are puckered in an exaggerated kiss, is another dramatic posture. Other patients have kept the upper and lower parts of the body twisted in opposite directions, squatting on haunches with arms extended as if doing deep knee-bends, and sitting with arms and legs extended as if falling into the chair.

Cataleptic patients can be placed into new postures. The examiner tells the patient that he is concerned about his health and that he needs to make sure the patient's general medical health is "*O.K.*" He then checks out the patient's arms. As the examiner manipulates the arm, he may feel an initial resistance soon followed by a slow release, as if he were bending a warm candle. This phenomenon is termed *waxy flexibility.*

Some non-posturing patients instructed to resist the examiner's manipulations show catatonic phenomena. The patient is told to grab the arm of his chair or his bedspread tightly and is then told not to let the examiner lift his arm. With light pressure under his arm, the examiner seeks to raise the patient's arm, while simultaneously telling the patient "*Don't let me do this.*" *Automatic obedience* is the term applied when the patient is unable to resist a light touch despite understanding the instruction to resist. Once the limb is raised, the new posture may be maintained for a long period, or the arm lowered slowly. It is useful to test both arms, because unilateral catalepsy and automatic obedience can occur from contralateral brain lesions.

After testing for automatic obedience, the *grasp reflex* and *negativism* are tested. To test for the grasp reflex, the examiner places his index and middle fingers firmly on the patient's palm, to see if the patient tightly grasps the fingers. For negativism, the examiner takes the patient's hand and arm and moves the patient's arm horizontally back and forth, with varying degrees of force. A patient with negativism will resist these manipulations with a pressure equal to that of the examiner.

Social and interpersonal negativism is a response similar but opposite in intensity to the actions of others. These forms of negativism are seen in the ways patients interact with the unit staff or respond to unit rules. Attempts to induce patients to dress, to wash, or to eat may be met with stubborn resistance and tensing of every muscle. Such patients refuse any request, or do the opposite of what is asked. They lie under their bed and not on it, or they sleep under the mattress not on it, or go to another patient's bed. When a staff member attempts to feed them, they clench their teeth like a child in a tantrum. They retain urine and feces, refusing to evacuate bowels and bladder when placed on a toilet, and then soil themselves. Such behaviors are examples of negativism, not "bad" behavior.[16]

Mute and immobile patients may not respond to painful stimuli, exhibiting generalized and often severe analgesia. Testing with pinpricks is part of the neurologic examination, and when done properly, demonstrating analgesia in the mute, immobile patient is consistent with the diagnosis of catatonia.

Catatonic spectrum behaviors

The above signs are the most commonly identified catatonic behaviors. But many more subtle behaviors have been considered part of the catatonic spectrum. The behaviors listed in Table 2.2 suggest the presence of other, more specific, features of catatonia. These are often described as mannerisms and some authors consider them as core catatonic signs. Their appearance should stimulate a detailed examination, particularly if their appearance is of recent onset. By themselves, even in clusters of a few suggestive signs, these behaviors are not sufficient evidence of catatonia. Many are examples of obsessive and compulsive rituals and mannerisms, particularly when they have been present for months or years.

Table 2.2 Catatonic spectrum behaviors

Tiptoe walking, skipping, hopping

Repeating questions instead of answering

Manneristic hand or finger movements not typically dyskinetic

Inconspicuous repetitive actions, such as making clicking sounds before or
    after speaking; automatically tapping or touching objects or body parts;
    tongue chewing, licking; lip smacking; pouting; teeth clicking; grimacing;
    frowning; squeezing shut or opening eyes wide

Oddities of speech, such as progressively less volume until speech is an almost
    inaudible mumble (prosectic speech); using a foreign accent not typical for
    the patient; speaking like a robot or like a child learning to read; speaking
    without the use of word contractions (e.g., "*I am not going to the store because
    I can not do it*" rather than using "I'm" and "*can't*")

Holding head in odd positions

Rocking, shoulder shrugging, sniffing and wrinkling of nose, opening eyes wide
    and then squeezing them shut

Rituals, such as tapping the dishes or eating utensils in a specific order before
    eating; tapping buttons before buttoning a shirt

ENDNOTES

1 Kahlbaum, 1874; translated by Mora, 1973: 3.

2 Rogers (1991: 336) lists many motor behaviors that he sees among patients with
    catatonia: *disorder of posture, including flexion of the head, trunk, and limbs, persis-
    tence of postures, peculiar postures and extension postures; disorder of tone, including
    rigidity, stiffness and resistance to passive movement; disorder of motor performance,
    including decreased activity, motionlessness, decreased responsiveness and difficulty ini-
    tiating; disorder of activity, including general overactivity, outbursts, destructiveness, self-
    mutilation and stripping; abnormal movements of trunk and limbs, including jerking,
    tics, choreiform twitching, spasms, cramps, seizures, convulsive-like disorder, stereo-
    typed activity, gyration and tremors; abnormal facial movements, including choreiform,
    twitching and peculiar movements, spasms, cramps and contorted movements, and ex-
    pressionless, flaccid or fixed expression; abnormal eye movements and fixity of gaze;
    abnormal gait including halting, slow and stiff gaits; and abnormal speech production
    including mutism, decreased speech, slow speech, delay in answering, increased speech,
    outbursts of speech and swearing, abnormal volume and timbre of speech, unintelligible
    speech and speech restricted to sounds or lip movements.*

3 Kahlbaum, 1874, 1973; Kraepelin, 1896, 1903; Bleuler, 1950; Jaspers et al., 1963.

4 McCall et al., 1995; Fink and Francis, 1996; Arnone et al., 2002.

5 Mashimo et al., 1995.

6 Berrios, 1996a.

7 Hinsie, 1932b.

8 Von Economo, 1931; Plum and Posner, 1980; Berrios, 1981; Johnson, 1984; Benegal et al., 1992.

9 Johnson, 1984.

10 Kahlbaum, 1973.

11 Kraepelin, 1903, 1921, 1971.

12 Gelenberg and Mandel, 1977; Hermesh et al., 1989a,b, 1992; Bräunig et al., 1995a.

13 Bush et al., 1996a,b.

14 Trivedi et al., in press.

15 See also Ungvari et al., 1995.

16 Bakewell, 1815, cited in Hunter and Macalpine, 1982: 705–710.

3

The many faces of catatonia

Plurality should not be assumed without necessity. (All other things being equal, the simplest solution is usually the correct one.)

William of Occam[1]

Introduction

For over two centuries, the manifestations of catatonia have been given individual names as one author after another identified features that they considered unique. Whether each form is a distinct entity or a variation of a common pathophysiology is not clear. The differences in approach reflect personal attitudes, with the authors divided into "splitters" or "lumpers." We are among the "lumpers." The clinical conditions with a prominence of the classic catatonia motor signs in patients with disorders in mood and thought, and that respond to anticonvulsant and sedative treatments, reflect a common endophenotype. Despite the variation in overt forms, we think it useful to approach these diverse disorders as sharing a common brain pathophysiology.

Syphilis offers an analogy. A spirochaete infection is the common pathology with the clinical diversity depending on the organ that is involved and the severity and duration of the infection. The expressions of syphilis are so varied that the disorder has been called "the great imitator." The different forms respond to the same treatments, however, strengthening our belief in a common pathology (see Quetel, 1990). In like fashion, we see the different expressions of catatonia as due to a common brain pathophysiology. The etiologies differ, but the commonalities in expression of motor signs and the response to treatment brings these threads together.

In this chapter we first present an overview of the different overt forms of catatonia and the conditions associated with it (Table 3.1). We then describe

Table 3.1 The catatonia syndromes

	Eponyms
Retarded catatonia	Kahlbaum syndrome
Benign stupor	
Excited catatonia	Manic excitement
Delirious mania	Manic delirium
	Bell's mania
Oneiroid state	*Onirisme*
	Oneirophrenia
Malignant catatonia (MC)	Lethal catatonia
	Pernicious catatonia
	Acute fulminating psychosis
Neuroleptic malignant syndrome (NMS)	NMS; MC/NMS
	Syndrom malin
	Neuroleptic induced catatonia
Toxic serotonin syndrome (TSS)	TSS; Serotonin syndrome
Periodic catatonia	
Mixed affective state	Rapid cycling mania
Primary akinetic mutism	Apallic syndrome
	Stiff man syndrome
	Locked-in syndrome

the conditions and the features of catatonia that suggest these syndromes to reflect the same pathophysiology.

The main syndromes of catatonia are characterized by the presence of the cardinal motor signs in their history and presentation (Table 2.2). The signs may be transient, but when two or more features persist for more than an hour, catatonia becomes a highly probable syndromal diagnosis. Two principal varieties are a retarded form and a less frequent excited form. The course of the illness is either benign or malignant.

Subtypes of catatonia

Retarded catatonia

For the retarded forms of catatonia, some authors use the term *Kahlbaum syndrome* (or *KS*).[2] The patients are so poorly responsive as to be in stupor.

Such states include *benign stupor*, although this condition may be fatal when the patients develop systemic infections or pulmonary or cerebral emboli. In recent classifications, when catatonia appears in patients with a mood disorder, a specifier of catatonia may be added to the primary diagnosis.[3] When the signs appear in patients with schizophrenia, the catatonic subtype is diagnosed.

Stupor, a difficult term to define, is a clinical syndrome of akinesis and mutism, with preservation of awareness. There is a profound lack of responsiveness and apparent impairment of consciousness. Speech and spontaneous movement are absent or reduced to a minimum, and the patient is inaccessible to external stimuli. This state is contrasted with that of coma, in which the eyes are shut, even in response to strong arousal stimuli, do not resist passive opening, do not appear watchful, and the movements in response to stimulation are not purposeful.[4] A *delirious stupor* is usually a stupor of sudden onset without an obvious general medical explanation (e.g., infection). In the literature of the first half of the 20th Century, when patients recovered from prolonged periods of stupor that were associated with severe depressive illnesses, the term benign stupor was applied to contrast these patients with those who went on to the persistent "malignant" illness of dementia praecox.[5] Patients in benign stupor exhibit mutism, negativism, posturing, and rigidity. A pseudo-dementia of severe depression has been described, and in patients who meet the criteria, catatonia is a frequent feature.[6]

In his studies of encephalitis lethargica, von Economo (1931) described many patients in *catatonic stupor*. From time to time, patients in stupor have been shown to have abnormal electrographic seizure activity, and *nonconvulsive status epilepticus (NCSE)* has been identified as a cause for some catatonia.[7]

Excited catatonia

Acute excited states with prominent catatonic features have been described. These have been termed *excited catatonia, catatonic excitement, delirious mania*, and *manic delirium*. The conditions are characterized by excessive motor activity associated with disorganized speech, disorientation, confusion, and confabulation. In delirious mania (manic delirium) the catatonic features are usually obvious. If not, they can be demonstrated by careful examination, suggesting that the conditions are identical to those identified as catatonic excitement (excited catatonia).[8] These states are commonly seen in patients with manic-depressive illnesses and in acute toxic states.

A recurrent problem in this tradition has been distinguishing catatonic excitement from manic excitement. One assumption is that catatonic excitement is sudden in onset, at times purposeless, and of short duration. Manic excitement, in contrast, is said to occur within a manic mood state, often has a purpose, and may last for days or weeks. The observation that so many catatonic patients have an underlying or accompanying mania further confuses the issue (see Chapter 4).

The notion that catatonic excitement differs from manic excitement derives from Kahlbaum and Bleuler. Kahlbaum offers a description of mania in catatonia – i.e., catatonic excitement.[9]

Mania is common . . . cases without a trace of mania are less common than cases where the presence of mania, rage, frenzy, excitation . . . was noted (*page 31*) . . . the stage of mania or exaltation (*page 33*) . . . histrionic exaltation, sometimes more in the form of tragic-religious extasy . . . expansive mood which permeates all speech, actions and gestures, in many patients this pathetic mood, typical of catatonia, is expressed in the form of constant declamations and recitations accomplished by lively gesticulations . . . obvious megalomania . . . continuous recitation of poetry (*page 34*) . . . transient conditions of excitation and sudden, short-lived joy . . . simple mania (*page 84*) . . . and prolonged excitement or 'catatonia gravis' (*page 85*).

Bleuler described catatonic excitement.[10]

The hyperkinetic cases (as the term suggests) are constantly in motion without really doing anything (pressure of activity, "flight of activity" as Fuhrman called it). They clamber about, move around, shake the branches of trees in the garden, hop over beds, bang on the table twenty times, and then the wall; they bend the knees, jump, strike, break, twist their arms into impossible positions between the radiator and the wall, totally unconcerned about the burns which they receive. They cry, sing, verbigerate, laugh, curse, scream, and spit all over the room. They grimace, showing sadness, happiness or horror.

From these and other early descriptions of catatonic excitement, and from our own clinical experience, we cannot distinguish catatonic excitement from the excited states of manic-depressive illness. We have concluded, therefore, that without a systematic comparison study that has yet to be done, it is most parsimonious to consider these states the same condition, providing a single framework for delirious mania and catatonic excitement.

Malignant catatonia

The course of the illness, as benign or malignant, is another dimension in characterizing catatonia. *Malignant* or *pernicious* or *lethal catatonia*, or an *acute fulminant psychosis* is identified when the disorder is acute in onset, systemically devastating, and associated with fever and autonomic instability.[11] When inadequately treated, death may ensue.[12] Patients in these states may be retarded and in stupor, or excited.

Much attention has recently been paid to a neurotoxic state, known as the *neuroleptic malignant syndrome (NMS), neuroleptic induced catatonia*, or *syndrom malin*. It achieved prominence by its association with antipsychotic drugs, but the syndrome was described before these drugs were developed. It has also been described with drugs outside this class.[13] Some authors consider NMS to be a distinct disorder, but its clinical characteristics, course, and response to treatment are indistinguishable from malignant catatonia. It is very likely that NMS and malignant catatonia (MC) reflect the same pathophysiology, differing only in that the precipitant in NMS is an antipsychotic medicine.[14]

A **toxic serotonin syndrome** (*serotonin syndrome, TSS*) has recently been described as a risk of treatments that affect brain serotonin systems.[15] The signs are very similar to those of MC/NMS, the principal difference being the inciting agents and the prominence of gastrointestinal symptoms. Its descriptive characteristics are still poorly defined, but TSS is sufficiently like MC in its signs and response to treatment to consider it a subtype of malignant catatonia.[16]

Periodic catatonia

When catatonic signs wax and wane in a recurrent behavior disorder, it is labeled *periodic catatonia*.[17] When the shift in main symptoms in patients with a manic-depressive illness is rapid, in the order of minutes or days, the syndrome is labeled a *mixed affective state* or *rapid cycling mania*. These patients often exhibit prominent signs of catatonia.[18]

Primary akinetic mutism

In neurologic texts, a persistent state of mutism and rigidity has been variously labeled as *akinetic mutism, apallic syndrome, coma vigil*, or as a *stupor of unknown etiology.* Brain stem lesions have been identified in some patients.[19] Individual akinetic states have been described as *stiff-man syndrome* and *locked-in syndrome.*[20] The relation of these syndromes to primary akinetic mutism is unclear. The descriptions, however, are sufficiently like those of catatonic stupor to encourage neurologists to apply tests for catatonia, and even trials of the treatments for catatonia, in the hope that the instances may be therapeutically responsive.

From time to time, descriptions of psychopathologic entities surface with catatonia as a feature. One such is the term "cycloid psychosis," an eponym proposed by Leonhard to denominate syndromes of an endogenous nature and psychotic severity.[21] He subdivided the condition into at least three subtypes. The hyperkinetic-akinetic-motility psychosis subtype includes catatonic features, but the overall descriptions do not warrant inclusion as a catatonia subtype.[22] As we read the typical descriptions of patients with cycloid psychoses, the descriptions best fit the manic-depressive disorders.[23] An optimal integration of the classification of the description of these patients within DSM classifications is yet to be found.[24]

Retarded catatonia (*Kahlbaum syndrome*)

The term *Kahlbaum syndrome* or *KS* has been used for the most common syndrome of retarded catatonia, usually benign, with a favorable prognosis. The catatonic state was described by Kahlbaum as one *"in which the patient remains entirely motionless, without speaking, and with a rigid, mask-like facies, the eyes focused at a distance; he seems devoid of any will to move or react to any stimuli; there may be a fully developed 'waxen' flexibility, as in cataleptic states, or only indications, distinct, nevertheless, of this striking phenomenon. The general impression conveyed by such patients is one of profound mental anguish, or an immobility induced by severe mental shock; it has been classified either among states of depression (which explains the term atonic melancholia) or among the conditions of feeble-mindedness (stupor or dementia stupida)... Once the clinical signs are manifest, they tend to persist, although in some patients they appear for relatively short periods and then tend to recur..."*[25] A description of one of his depressed patients is summarized.[26]

Patient 3.1   A 27-year-old country-school teacher suffered moods of depression and irritability, occasionally acting unfairly to his pupils, for which he was reprimanded. He developed
choreiform facial 'tics' and jerking spastic movements of the extremities. He was admitted to the hospital, but no medical condition was found to explain the uncontrollable
jerking movements. He was seen to stand alone, upright, and motionless in a corner
for half an hour at a time, gesticulating with his arms. He was mute, appearing deep in
thought, isolating himself and taking no part in ward activities.

He responded to questions, slowly, softly, but accurately. When pressed for details of
his thoughts, the choreiform movements increased. If pushed or induced to change his
position, he resisted. Pinpricks elicited grimacing but no withdrawal. For long periods,
he did not feed himself, and had to be dressed and undressed. Attacks of muscle spasms
occurred several times a day, each lasting for many minutes. The illness was progressive.[27]

After about nine months, he became more animated, embraced a medical orderly,
laughing and weeping intermittently, but such an episode lasted only a few days. After
16 months he began to speak, and to write letters home. His facial expressions became
more animated but for the following two years, he was reluctant to speak, and participated intermittently in ward activities and in self-care. After more than three years, he
was sent home for lack of room at the hospital.

Kahlbaum described the catatonic patient as first going through a prodrome stage of melancholia, followed by impairment of thought and convulsive choreiform movements that limited his ability to carry out voluntary
movements. He described the patient as an example of "atonic melancholia."

The sudden onset of a behavior disorder with mutism, negativism, posturing, and rigidity is a common description of catatonia (see Chapter 2).
We take the presence of two or more signs for an hour or longer or are reproducible on two or more occasions as sufficient for the diagnosis. Rating
scales offer systematic methods of examination that facilitate the identification of catatonia. The rapid reduction or the full relief of the signs after an
intravenous dose of amobarbital or lorazepam is a positive test for catatonia.
Absence of the response, however, does not rule out catatonia because at least
20% of patients do not respond to such a challenge.[28]

Malignant catatonia

Since 1849 clinicians have described an acute onset, fulminating psychotic
and delirious illness, often with hyperthermia, that resulted in death in about

half the patients.[29] In 1934, Stauder described the sudden onset of intense excitement, delirium, high fever, and catalepsy in three patients previously in good general medical health.[30] Each was a young adult with a family history of psychiatric illness. In a matter of minutes, each went from "well" to extreme excitement and psychosis. Each was acrocyanotic and during the days of the illness each injured himself by slamming repeatedly into the ground or walls. All three died. He termed the syndrome *tödliche katatonie* (fatal catatonia).

The condition has been described often and each writer has given it a different name. The names include *Bell's mania, pernicious catatonia, lethal catatonia, malignant catatonia, manic delirium, delirious mania, syndrom malign, acute or fulminating psychosis, fatal catatonia, mortal catatonia, catatonic delirious state, hypertoxic schizophrenia, drug-induced hyperthermic catatonia, confusocatatonia, delirium acutum, delire aigu,* and *exhaustion syndrome.* The condition has a better prognosis today, so that the term *malignant catatonia* is in common use.

Patients posture and exhibit stereotypes, are episodically mute, rigid, and stuporous, and occasionally excited. They are febrile and autonomically unstable, with tachycardia, tachypnea, and hypertension. Behavior fluctuates dramatically, often changing from moment to moment. Speech is disorganized and thoughts delusional. They refuse food and liquids. Prior to the use of somatic treatments, they either recovered spontaneously or died from physiologic collapse, cardiac arrest, or infection within a few weeks. One of many examples follows.[31]

Patient 3.2 A 61-year-old woman was admitted to the psychiatric ward of a general hospital in cardiac decompensation with cor pulmonale, tachycardia, atrial fibrillation, respiratory insufficiency, and obesity. She became severely depressed and stuporous. Two weeks earlier, she had been successfully treated for a similar cardiac condition. The present episode was one of many hospitalizations for depression that had responded to antidepressant medications, but on three occasions she had required ECT.

She was rigid, severely dyspneic at rest, and tachycardic (120–180 bpm) with atrial fibrillation. She was treated with digoxin, verapamil, furosemide, and euphyllin for cardiac failure and fluvoxamin and perphenazine in low doses for her depressive condition. Within five days, her condition deteriorated and she was transferred to an intensive care unit of the hospital. She required intubation. Two days later, she became febrile, cataleptic, and hypertensive. A general medical cause could not be found for her fever and catalepsy, and the diagnosis of malignant catatonia with stupor was made.

Bitemporal ECT was begun and after the first treatment, both heart rate and temperature were reduced. A second treatment 12 hours later elicited a normal sinus rhythm. She was extubated, began to speak, and ate on her own. She improved progressively. Further treatment consisted of perphenazine alone, and after ten days she was discharged to her home, no longer depressed or catatonic.

Patients with malignant catatonia *look* as if they have an infectious disease, and infectious encephalopathy is often suggested as the diagnosis and followed by extensive neurologic assessments.[32] A specific infectious process, however, is rarely documented (see also *Patient 3.11*). *Patient 3.3* did not have an infectious disease, and was considered to suffering from a coma of unknown etiology.

Patient 3.3   A 24-year-old woman was brought to the emergency room of a community hospital by a co-worker who reported that she had appeared confused for two days, insisting that a guardian angel had told her that she was "the chosen one." The patient's speech was rambling, repeating words without meaning. She was afebrile. Haloperidol (5 mg) was given intravenously and she was admitted to the hospital medical service.

The next day, she was confused. Her speech and movements were slow and she exhibited catalepsy and waxy flexibility. Later that day, jerky uncontrolled movements and frothing of the mouth were observed, an epileptic seizure was inferred, and phenytoin was prescribed. That day she became mute and exhibited "flapping movements of her extremities." She was again given intramuscular haloperidol (5 mg).

Within six hours, she became febrile (102 °F) with leucocytosis, slow respirations, and facial cyanosis. Acute respiratory acidosis and hypoxia were diagnosed and she was intubated to assure ventilation. Heart rate slowed to 30 bpm followed by cardiac asystole. Atropine and dopamine were given. A post-intubation chest X-ray showed subcutaneous emphysema and right-sided pneumothorax. A chest tube was placed, and she was transferred to the tertiary care medical center.

The patient remained comatose, her breathing assisted by ventilator, and she was treated for sepsis. Antiepileptic medicines were continued as repeated EEG (electroencephalogram) examinations showed slow waves. All neurologic and general medical assessments failed to show an identifiable etiology for her condition. She was sustained by extensive nursing care.

Three months after admission, a psychiatric consultant found her to be in stupor, cataleptic, tremulous, cachectic, febrile and sweating with a rapid heart rate. A test dose of intravenous lorazepam (1 mg) elicited eye-opening, attempted response to commands, with head-nodding and hand movements in response to questions. A diagnosis of malignant catatonia was made.

Lorazepam dosages were increased to 14 mg/day as the anti-epileptic medicines were reduced. She remained mute, immobile, negativistic, febrile, sweating, with tachycardia and hypertension. A course of bitemporal ECT was begun with consent from her mother and fiancé. After the third treatment, her fever resolved, respiratory and heart rates normalized, and she was extubated. After the eighth treatment, she talked rationally, walked with assistance, and fed herself. After 15 ECT, she was discharged to a physical rehabilitation center and returned to her home four weeks later. At follow-up at two months, her illness had resolved and she planned a return to work.

An exception to the usual failure to document an infectious etiology is the report of the autopsy findings in a patient whose pathology was consistent with lymphocytic meningoencephalitis during an eastern equine encephalitis outbreak.[33] That patient's course also meets criteria for malignant and excited catatonia. Six ECT were given in four days with only transient alteration of behavior.

A review of the psychiatric manifestations in 108 patients with acute viral encephalitis finds delusions (54%), hallucinations (44%), mutism (21%), catalepsy (16%), perseveration (9%), and perplexity, negativism, echolalia, and grimacing (1% to 4% each).[34] When the diagnosis is properly made, treatment with antibiotic and antiviral agents can moderate the illness and the catatonia.

MC is usually of sudden onset, becoming rapidly severe and even fatal within a few days. The prognosis is poor unless the syndrome is aggressively treated, and ECT is described as the life-saving measure in numerous reports.[35] ECT was dramatically effective in a patient with an onset of malignant catatonia associated with the administration of haloperidol.[36]

Patient 3.4 A 38-year-old man with a 21-year history of manic-depressive illness entered the VA Medical Center in Philadelphia with a recurrence of mania. His speech was moderately pressured, his activity level increased, and he was euphoric and intrusive, shopping excessively at the hospital canteen. Haloperidol (10 mg daily) was prescribed on admission and then discontinued on day 7. Lithium (300 mg, three times daily) was started on day 8. His condition improved progressively until hospital day 18 when he abruptly became confused and agitated, developed an oral temperature of 100.5 °F with diaphoresis, tachycardia, and tachypnea. Catatonic features included stereotypes, repeated phrases, echolalia, and echopraxia. Muscle tone, however, was normal. The serum lithium level was 0.9 mEq/l. On hospital day 21, thioridazine (50 mg) was started but was stopped, after two doses were ineffective. Lithium therapy was stopped.

By hospital day 25, the patient was delirious. His speech was pressured, with incoherent chatter alternating with aggressive and hostile verbal outbursts. He twisted his bedclothes around his arms and head, thrashing from side to side, counting backwards and forwards, and responding inconsistently to questions. He required four-point restraints, was delusional, and appeared to be responding to hallucinations.

On hospital day 27, his oral temperature rose to 102.6 °F with severe autonomic dysfunction and catatonic features. At this point, an underlying general medical disorder was presumed present and he was transferred to the Medical Intensive Care Unit.

Spiking fevers, profuse diaphoresis, tachycardia, and tachypnea continued. Leukocytosis ranged to 18,200 wbc/mm^3. Serum creatine phosphokinase peaked at 10,900 IU/l. [Extensive laboratory tests revealed no specific disorder. Temperature elevations ranged from 102 °F to 104 °F. He was calmed by large doses of amobarbital.] Failure to identify a medical illness as the etiology of the disorder pointed toward the diagnosis of MC in the context of mania.

Treatment with bilateral ECT was initiated on hospital day 55. Ten seizures of adequate duration were elicited in three weeks. His body temperature returned to normal after the first treatment. Agitation, confusion, hallucinations, delusions, and catatonia disappeared. Chlorpromazine was started on day 87. The pressure of speech ceased and he was appropriately behaved. He was discharged on hospital day 117 on maintenance lithium therapy and remained at full remission at 18-month follow-up.

Another example of malignant catatonia is a patient acutely ill with lupus erythematosus and complex partial seizures who developed MC following the administration of antipsychotic medicines to control agitation.[37]

Patient 3.5   A 25-year-old, married woman was admitted with an acute onset of hyperactivity, insomnia, inappropriate mood, delusional thinking, and perceptual changes. She reported a three-year history of lupus erythematosus with malar rash, photosensitivity, discoid skin lesions, leucopenia, pleuritis, oral mucosal lesions, and a positive antinuclear antibody titer (1:2560; speckled pattern).

One month prior to admission she experienced transient aphasia and right-arm paresthesiae and weakness. Computerized tomography (CT) of the head demonstrated moderate diffuse atrophy, mild cerebellar volume loss, and a region of ischemia in the left internal capsule. A test for anticardiolipin antibodies was positive and she was treated with prednisone (20 mg, oral) three times daily. The neurologic signs improved.

Three weeks later she became excited and was admitted to the psychiatric ER. Intramuscular haloperidol (2 mg) was administered. A few hours later, facial grimacing, flailing movements, and failure to respond to questions led physicians to request an EEG that showed generalized slowing with a spike and slow-wave dysrhythmia. Cerebrospinal fluid (CSF) was normal. A repeat CT and a brain MRI (magnetic resonance imaging) showed diffuse atrophy. A seizure disorder was diagnosed and phenytoin prescribed.

She was belligerent and uncooperative, delirious, reporting auditory hallucinations and delusional thoughts. She received two additional intramuscular doses of haloperidol (2 mg) which were mildly sedating, but she remained delusional. Intravenous methylprednisone (100 mg every 8 h) was begun, without improvement. Plasmapheresis was performed for three exchanges without a change in her behavior.

On day 7 she exhibited negativism and mutism, alternating with agitation. After two additional doses of haloperidol, she became rigid, with increased pulse rate (110 bpm), elevated blood pressure (134/102), tachypnea (24/min), fever (99.5 °F), and severe sweating. Serum creatine phosphokinase was 175 IU/l. A test dose of intravenous lorazepam (1 mg) improved vigilance, elicited eye-opening with slow responses to questions and obedience to simple commands.

During the next three weeks her condition deteriorated. On day 28, she began an ECT trial. For each of seven bilateral ECT, a second induction at maximum currents was required. The catatonic symptoms improved and because of continuing difficulty in the induction of seizures, the course was discontinued. In the ensuing weeks, she exhibited periods of excitement and stupor. A repeat EEG was normal and the anticonvulsants were discontinued. Her CSF showed IgG anti-neuronal antibodies in high titer. Cyclophosphamide, an experimental treatment for lupus erythematosus, was begun.

On day 59, a second course of bilateral ECT was begun. These seizure inductions were considered adequate. The autonomic and catatonic signs resolved rapidly, and the psychotic thoughts more slowly, until none could be elicited. On day 100, after 10 ECT, she was discharged to her home for further physical rehabilitation. At follow-up two months after discharge, she was without psychiatric signs, improving in weight and able to care for her child. Cyclophosphamide treatment continued for one year when repeat CSF examinations showed no antineuronal antibodies. She was asymptomatic.

Comment: The story of this patient illustrates the ER use of intramuscular antipsychotic drugs leading to near disastrous consequences. It also illustrates the futility of going from one medicine to another, despite poor responses. Her catatonia was complicated by central nervous system lupus, complex partial seizures, and the multiple medications that had been prescribed. Even the recognition of catatonia was insufficient to trigger its proper treatment in a timely fashion. And, once ECT was agreed to, a satisfactory seizure was difficult to elicit requiring multiple inductions with bilateral electrode placements and electric charges to the maximum output of the ECT device (100 mC). The high seizure threshold was probably related to her extensive treatment with anticonvulsant drugs and lorazepam. Flumazenil had not yet been developed as a benzodiazepine antagonist for use with ECT in such patients. Reports of the non-response of patients to ECT occasionally appear in similar contexts. These reports probably reflect the high seizure thresholds of patients treated with high doses of anticonvulsant and sedative drugs. For an effective treatment course, each seizure needs to be monitored by EEG criteria for efficacy.[38]

The incidence of MC is not well defined, since most occurrences are sporadic. In a systematic review of the experience at the Mannheim Mental Health Institute for the six year period ending in June 1981, 656 patients were diagnosed as schizophrenic, with the catatonic type in 4%.[39] Ten patients were diagnosed with malignant catatonia. Two died, five recovered with ECT, and three recovered with antipsychotic medications.

Recognizing MC in a timely fashion and applying effective treatment is still difficult, however, and reports find 10–20% of patients with MC die.[40] The long-term outcome of those that survive is unclear. The acute course, if recognized, lasts a few days to several weeks. Memory and other cognitive difficulties, persistent motor features, and cerebellar degeneration have been anecdotally reported, but in the few follow-up studies, the surviving patients return to their pre-MC level of functioning.[41]

Neuroleptic malignant syndrome variant of malignant catatonia

A *syndrom malin*, the acute onset of fever, autonomic instability, rigidity, and changes in mood and alertness, was described soon after the introduction of antipsychotic drugs.[42] In 1980 the syndrome was labeled *neuroleptic malignant syndrome* (NMS), and this term was quickly accepted.[43] The syndrome was occasionally fatal, with a mortality rate of 25% before 1984 that decreased to 12% by 1989.[44] Patients exhibited many signs of catatonia but the systemic manifestations dominated the sporadic descriptions. Excited manic patients seemed to be at particular risk, probably because they were often dehydrated and received high doses of more than one antipsychotic drug at a time. Among laboratory test findings were elevated serum creatine phosphokinase (CPK) levels, low serum iron levels, and leucocytosis. A low serum iron has been reported during the acute phase of the illness in many patients with NMS and catatonia, especially the more severe forms of excited catatonia and MC. It resolves with recovery.[45]

A patient with MC/NMS was treated in 1984 at University Hospital at Stony Brook (New York, USA). The treatment was tentative, and the prolonged hospital course would probably not occur today using our present treatments.[46]

Patient 3.6 A 45-year-old woman with a history of manic-depressive illness and hypertension was hospitalized with depressed mood of one-month's duration. In prior episodes, she had received antidepressants, lithium, and ECT. On admission, she was excited, her behavior was unpredictable, and her thought and speech confused. Two doses of haloperidol were administered. Although her excitement lessened, she became grandiose, garrulous, and paced continuously. Lithium carbonate was prescribed and the next day fluphenazine hydrochloride (5 mg four times daily) added.

Within 48 hours she exhibited bilateral cogwheel rigidity, which improved with intramuscular diphenhydramine. The next day, she became tremulous, had persistent cogwheel, and her temperature rose to 100 °F. Because of concern for neurotoxicity, both lithium and fluphenazine were discontinued. Her condition worsened, as she became mute, tremulous, and rigid. Her blood pressure and heart rate increased, temperature rose to 103.5 °F, white cell count was elevated to 13,400 wbc/mm^3, and CPK was 486 IU/l.

NMS was diagnosed. Intravenous diazepam (5 mg) was slowly administered. Within one minute she became responsive, no longer mute, and both cogwheel and tremor disappeared. Four hours later, her blood pressure, heart rate, and temperature were improving.

Intravenous lorazepam (2 mg) was prescribed twice daily but the autonomic and motor signs recurred. Lorazepam was discontinued and after ruling out pneumonia, meningitis, and thyroid or other metabolic disturbances, intravenous dantrolene was prescribed at doses of 50 to 60 mg every six hours. Over the next week, the motor and autonomic signs gradually resolved, and dantrolene dosing was tapered and discontinued. She remained depressed, however, and a course of bitemporal ECT fully resolved her condition. She returned home 68 days after admission.

About 1% of patients treated with antipsychotic drugs develop the severe form of MC/NMS, usually within the first two weeks of exposure.[47] One reported patient had similar responses to three different antipsychotic drugs.[48] More men than women are affected (3:2), but male patients typically receive higher drug doses, and this may explain their increased risk.[49] Persons under age 20 and over age 65 are under-represented in the reported cases, probably as a result of practitioners limiting their use of antipsychotic drugs in these age groups. The same syndrome has been reported to occur when patients are given carbamazepine or valproic acid, and after the rapid

Table 3.2 Clinical features of MC/NMS

Fever
Muscle rigidity
Dyskinesia
Posturing, waxy flexibility, catalepsy, mutism
Dysarthria, dysphagia, sialorrhea
Altered consciousness; when severe, appears as stupor or coma
Autonomic instability: lability of blood pressure, tachycardia,
vasoconstriction, diaphoresis (a "greasy" sweat)

MC: malignant catatonia; NMS: neuroleptic malignant syndrome.

withdrawal of levodopa, amantadine, or benzodiazepines (see Chapter 7). Table 3.2 summarizes the principal features of MC/NMS.

Because NMS occurred in response to antipsychotic drugs whose mode of action was assumed to be dopamine (D_2) blockade, dopamine agonists such as bromocriptine and *l*-dopa were recommended for treatment. The muscle weakness and fever seemed similar to the signs in malignant hyperthermia, and for its relief, dantrolene was recommended. The regimen of withdrawal of antipsychotic drugs and prescribing dopamine agonists and dantrolene quickly became the main treatment for NMS.[50]

The MC/NMS syndrome, however, was described before the introduction of antipsychotic drugs (Chapter 1). It is induced by other drugs, limiting the usefulness of the term itself (Table 3.3). Although suppressed dopamine activity may be a neurotransmitter of a final common pathway, the fact that non-dopaminergic drugs also elicit MC/NMS argues that the singularity of dopamine in the syndrome's genesis is too limited. A dysregulated sympathetic nervous system hyperactivity may be another basis for the syndrome, arising from acute severe stress and psychosis.[51]

Many authors have tried to distinguish NMS and MC. Some argue that the degree of rigidity, the time of onset or the presence of fever, and the degree of abnormality of laboratory tests differentiate the two conditions.[52] But studies seeking to differentiate NMS and MC have not been successful.[53]

Others have also concluded that NMS is not a distinct entity, but an example of malignant catatonia triggered by exposure to antipsychotic medicines.[54] Most recently, Carroll and Taylor (1997) reviewed University of Iowa hospital records of nine patients with NMS and 17 with malignant catatonia admitted

Table 3.3 Drugs associated with MC/NMS

Antipsychotic drugs of all types and potencies, both typical and atypical
Abrupt withdrawal of antipsychotic drugs, or benzodiazepines
Antidepressant drugs combined with antipsychotic drugs
Disulfiram intoxication
Corticosteroid intoxication
Phencyclidine intoxication
Metoclopramide
Anticholinergic and antihistamine toxicity and abrupt withdrawal
Lithium combined with phenelzine
Phenelzine combined with dothiepin
Clozapine withdrawal
Levodopa, amantadine, or bromocriptine abrupt withdrawal
Carbamazepine and valproic acid
Tetrabenazine and alpha-methyltyrosine combined
Cocaine intoxication
Cyclobenzaprine

over an eight-year period. They could find no differences in clinical features and concluded that the separation was invalid.

The treatment response, either to ECT or to benzodiazepines, is similar for NMS and MC. In the report of the patient with MC cited as *Patient 3.4*, Mann et al. (1990) summarized the then published experience with ECT in 27 patients with NMS. Of these, 20 patients recovered, three had a partial response, and four did poorly with ECT. The four patients with poor responses developed cardiac irregularities limiting their course of treatments. Other reviews find similar treatment efficacy rates.[55] Such clinical experience compels the conclusion that ECT is effective for patients with either NMS or MC, and that their outcomes are indistinguishable in speed or efficacy of response.

Are patients with NMS relieved by the administration of benzodiazepines, as is predicted in the view that NMS is MC triggered by an antipsychotic medicine? While screening patients for catatonia, investigators in a six-month prospective study identified three of 15 (20%) catatonic patients who also met criteria for NMS.[56] These responded to benzodiazepine treatments as did the other catatonic patients identified in the study.

Table 3.4 Abnormal laboratory findings in MC/NMS

Proteinuria
Myoglobinuria
Diffuse EEG slowing
Leukocytosis (10,000 to 25,000 per ml)
Thrombocytosis
Abnormal electrolytes (low calcium, low magnesium, high potassium)
Elevated liver function enzymes (SGOT, SGPT, and on occasion increased bilirubin)
Low serum iron
Very high serum CPK
High LDH

SGOT: serum glutamic oxaloacetic transaminase; SGPT: serum glutamic pyruvic transaminase CPK: creatine phosphokinase; LDH: lactose dehydrogenase.

In another investigation, the records of patients diagnosed with NMS on psychiatric consultation were retrospectively identified.[57] NMS was diagnosed by the presence of rigidity, fever, and autonomic signs. Sixteen patients met DSM-IV criteria for NMS and 11 met more stringent research criteria for NMS. Fifteen of the 16 patients had two or more motor signs of catatonia. One patient exhibited catatonia before the autonomic signs of NMS were recorded. The features of NMS and of catatonia were strongly correlated. Each patient received benzodiazepines (mainly lorazepam) with prompt resolution of the NMS symptoms. None received dopamine agonists or dantrolene. The authors concluded that benzodiazepines are effective in treating NMS.

NMS and MC are also indistinguishable by laboratory testing. Serum CPK levels, normally under 100 IU/l, often exceed 1000 IU/l in both syndromes. White blood cell counts are elevated. Metabolic acidosis and hypoxia develop. MRI findings are usually normal. EEG may show diffuse slowing, or a high frequency low voltage record. CSF and other investigations for a fever of unknown origin are unhelpful. Table 3.4 summarizes the laboratory findings in MC/NMS.

Extrapyramidal motor signs are found in 60% of patients with MC/NMS before fever develops. In 8% of patients, fever occurs first, but the sequence of events does not distinguish NMS from MC.[58]

In summary, the features of NMS and MC are indistinguishable. Before the complete NMS syndrome is expressed, signs of catatonia are typically found. The effective treatments for NMS are the same as those for MC, and the evidence for a specific efficacy for dopamine agonists and dantrolene is weak (Chapter 7). We prefer to consider a patient with the clinical features highlighted in Table 3.2 to have MC/NMS.[59] We conclude that NMS is an example of MC, precipitated by exposure to high potency antipsychotic drugs.[60]

Whether or not NMS and MC are the same syndrome with different triggers, or separate pathophysiologic conditions, they are life threatening. Prevention remains the best strategy. The risk factors and early signs described in the literature are listed in Table 3.5. When the risks are present, antipsychotic drugs and other triggers (e.g., sudden withdrawal of dopamine agonists)

Table 3.5 Clinical risk factors and early signs of MC/NMS

Risk factors	Early signs
• Dehydration (clinical signs or laboratory findings); electrolyte imbalance	• Rapidly developed extrapyramidal signs of rigidity, tremor, dyskinesia to low or modest doses of an antipsychotic
• Exposure to high ambient temperatures	• Mania with fever
• Substantial agitation or excitement	• Any catatonic feature developing within 24 hours of initial antipsychotic administration
• Thyrotoxicosis	• Autonomic instability developing within 24 hours of initial antipsychotic administration
• Catatonic features, past or present	
• Tardive dyskinesia, akathisia, or other basal ganglia disorder, extrapyramidal side-effects from medication, previous episode of NMS	• Sialorrhea developing within 24 hours of initial antipsychotic administration
• Receiving a high potency antipsychotic or two or more antipsychotic drugs	
• Receiving a high potency antipsychotic with an antidepressant or mood stabilizer	
• Receiving IM antipsychotic or depot antipsychotic	
• Recent alcohol abuse with liver dysfunction	

IM: intramuscular.

should be avoided. The early signs should encourage the discontinuation of antipsychotic drugs.

Delirious mania, excited catatonia, and oneiroid state

For more than two centuries, clinicians have described the acute onset of agitated and excited, dreamy or delirious states with associated motor signs. These conditions have been given many names: delirious mania, manic delirium, Bell's mania, and catatonic excitement. The French term *onirisme* and the translated terms *oneiroid state*, *oneirophrenia*, and *oneiroid syndrome* are favored by some authors for the dreamy, stuporous state.[61] We prefer the term *delirious mania*.[62]

The syndrome has received little attention in the psychiatric literature. Bell (1849), in a 13-year chart review of 1700 admissions to the McLean Hospital in Boston, USA, described 40 patients, of whom three-quarters died. Bonner and Kent (1936) described catatonia and delirious mania as overlapping syndromes. Goodwin and Jamison (1990), in an extensive review of manic-depressive illness, offer few citations, referring to the original description by Bell, a commentary by Kraepelin (1913), a report of three patients by Bond (1980), and a summary in the textbook edited by Mayer-Gross et al. (1960). More recent citations are found in Carlson and Goodwin (1973), Taylor and Abrams (1977), Klerman (1981), and Fink (1999b).

The outstanding feature of a delirious mania is a nightmarish, dream-like, derealization within an altered sensorium. The change in perception is profound, frightening the subject and leading to restlessness, agitation, and thrashing about. Patients harm themselves and others. Stereotypy, grimacing, posturing, echolalia, and echopraxia are common. Negativism and automatic obedience are almost always present. Patients sleep poorly, are unable to recall their recent experiences, or the names of objects or numbers given to them, and are disoriented. They confabulate, often with fantastic stories. The onset develops rapidly, within a few hours or a few days. Fever, rapid heart rate, elevated blood pressure, and rapid breathing are prominent. Patients hide in small spaces, close the doors and blinds on windows, and remove their clothes and run nude from their home. Garrulousness, flights of ideas, and rambling speech alternate with mutism.

The acute onset leads clinicians to search for a toxic or general medical cause such as drug intoxication and seizure disorder. When speech becomes incomprehensible, schizophrenia is considered. When grandiosity and delusional ideation dominate the picture, mania is more easily recognized. When delirium is the main feature, a full neurologic evaluation, including extensive brain imaging procedures, is usually done. Regardless of presumed cause, the presence of the complex syndrome of mania and delirium, with or without obvious catatonia, justifies the syndromal diagnosis of delirious mania. When stupor without a clear etiology dominates the picture, the diagnosis of oneirophrenia is made. Catatonic features, however, will be found if looked for.

Patient 3.7 A 17-year-old adolescent boy developed an acute confusional delirium after a week-end of partying. For two weeks he refused to go to school, slept and ate little, and closeted himself in his room, listening to rock music. At times, he became excited and shouted at his parents, and after three weeks they brought him to a community hospital. He was unclean, continuously talking, singing, and beating rhythms with his hands. Sedation with oral lorazepam proved inadequate and restraints were used. After two doses of haloperidol, he developed fever, rigidity, elevated blood pressure, and a rapid heart rate. Haloperidol was withdrawn and he was treated with intravenous fluids and dantrolene. The febrile reaction was muted but he remained psychotic and manic and was transferred to an academic tertiary care psychiatric unit.

On admission, he was restless and confused, with slurred and disorganized speech. Consciousness waxed and waned. He told of having strange powers; that his parents, who accompanied him and were present, were not his real parents; and that he had been selected for a spectacularly successful career in finance. For minutes at a time, he stared past the interviewer, not answering questions. Although he seemed oriented to time, place, and person, he could not recall the names of three objects after five minutes. His ability to do simple numerical calculations was poor and he was unaware of notable current events. His temperature, heart rate, and blood pressure were normal.

He was given lorazepam and clonazepam, followed by chlorpromazine and lithium. His behavior warranted restraint and sedation with injections of lorazepam and droperidol. He was seen to be suffering from an acute delirious mania.

ECT was recommended. The parents agreed and despite his excitement, the patient signed consent. All medications except lithium were discontinued. On the fourth hospital day, he was given bitemporal ECT, an adequate seizure was induced, and recovery was uneventful. Within an hour, he was rational and oriented, neither overactive nor delusional, and no longer in need of restraint. Later that afternoon, however, he relapsed to his manic state and after each of the next two treatments he followed the same pattern. After the fourth treatment his thoughts, mood, and affect were appropriate, his delusional ideas had disappeared, his self-care was normal, and he remained well. He was discharged after the sixth treatment with a prescription for biweekly outpatient ECT and continuation treatment with lithium. He received four additional treatments. He returned to school, and quickly made up the work that he had missed. Lithium therapy was sustained for four months and then discontinued. He was discharged from the clinic as recovered, and was well at two month follow-up.

Delirious mania is a frightening condition that typically leads the emergency-room physician to prescribe injections of antipsychotic medicines. The antipsychotic usually prescribed is haloperidol. More than 50% of the reported patients with MC/NMS were exposed to haloperidol.[63] Such intervention, especially when patients are dehydrated and have an electrolyte imbalance, is likely to induce malignant catatonia. Intravenous or intramuscular benzodiazepines are effective alternatives to sedate the patient, allowing the examination for the common causes of delirium.

Because many patients with delirious mania are suffering from manic-depressive illness, reports of prior episodes of mood disorder or a family history of mood disorder are often elicited. It is also useful to obtain serum levels of mood stabilizing drugs to rule out intoxication.

A patient with delirious mania, one of three reported patients, is described by Bond (1980):

Patient 3.8   A 44-year-old executive had been functioning well under increasing business pressures for several weeks before he attended a celebration party at his company. He became excited and hyperactive, talked loudly, swore, and acted "wild." He offered lavish gifts to his co-workers to make them *"feel better."* His personality and behavior were distinctly changed from his usual manner. That night, he slept poorly, awakened in tears, and was preoccupied with religious themes including messages from God *"to love everyone and live forever."*

On admission to the hospital, he was hyperactive and delusional with rapid speech and flights of ideas. Except for tachycardia of 120 bpm, his medical examination and laboratory tests were normal. Over the next two days he became lethargic and disoriented. He talked of "racing thoughts," religious delusions, and described visual and auditory hallucinations. Psychomotor retardation alternated with stereotyped pacing and restlessness. He was treated with haloperidol and chlorpromazine. (This experience was reported at a time before the risks of antipsychotic medicines in similar instances had been defined.)

On the fourth day, he was coherent, lucid, and oriented. He reported that his recent episode was *"like a nightmare,"* a horrible experience, although he remembered few specific details of his behavior. Medications were discontinued and he was discharged within nine days. Three years later, he remained free of symptoms.

A delirious mania can also be part of a general medical illness, not directly related to a history of a psychiatric illness. It can be so severe as to warrant anesthesia with intubation and mechanical ventilation for its control.[64]

Patient 3.9 A 38-year-old married businessman was admitted to hospital in an acute excited delir-ium of a few weeks duration. His heart and breathing rates were rapid, and his temper-ature was 100.3 °F. He required physical restraint and he was treated with intravenous haloperidol, lorazepam, and midazolam, with little effect. He continued to thrash un-controllably despite restraints, was diaphoretic and flushed, and incontinent of urine and feces. He was thought to have taken an overdose of first generation antidepressants and treated with activated charcoal. All efforts to reduce the delirium failed and he was paralyzed and intubated for his protection.

Six years before, he had developed peripheral neuropathy of unknown etiology and after years of fruitless treatment was enrolled in an experimental treatment program with a non-opioid analgesic delivered continuously through an intrathecal catheter from an implanted infusion pump in the abdominal wall. The treatment relieved his pain and he was able to return to work. At one point, increasing dosage and refreshing the medication in the pump led to fleeting memory lapses and involuntary slow muscle twitches, most apparent as he was falling asleep.

He remained anesthetized with propofol and cisatracurium, intubated, and ventilated in the hospital intensive care unit for two and a half weeks. All medications were discon-tinued except methadone so as to avoid precipitating opioid withdrawal. The intrathecal pump for ziconotide was switched off. He remained febrile, anemic, and with a mild leucocytosis. The EEG showed diffuse slowing without focal seizure activity.

Four attempts to wean the patient from the ventilator failed. On each occasion he exhibited such severe agitation that once he fractured two toes although he was immo-bilized with four-point leather restraints. He was treated with haloperidol to a maximum dose of 25 mg/h and valproate was added. Cogwheel rigidity and muscle twitches were prominent.

On day 17 he spiked fever of 104 °F, right lower lobe consolidation with bilateral pleu-ral effusion was diagnosed, and was treated with antibiotics. CPK was elevated on admission and remained persistently so.

On days 19, 20, and 21, with consent of the patient's wife, he was treated with bifrontal ECT on a daily basis. On day 21, he was weaned from neuromuscular paralysis. He showed no signs of psychomotor agitation and was successfully extubated. Post-extubation, he exhibited delirium, dysarthria, and disorientation to place and time. Three days later, the delirium had resolved. He remained dysarthric and ataxic, with persistent involuntary muscle twitches. He described his mood as very anxious although his affect was flat. He had no recollection of ever having the pump inserted or of the events of his illness. One month later he returned to work on a part-time basis, and three months after that he was back at work full-time.

The oneiroid syndrome, a dream-like state often associated with stupor or with excitement, is described in the European literature.[65] In a monograph titled *Oneirophrenia: The Confusional State*, Meduna (1950) described six patients with the syndrome that he compared to the descriptions of similar patients by Kahlbaum. His patients were successfully treated with ECT.

Patient 3.10 An 18-year-old boy, one of several children, an honor student and athlete, just graduated from high school. Without any visible cause, he became nervous, with difficulty in concentration. On an occasion he failed to understand his father's instruction about the family's car, left it somewhere, and could not recall whether he had put it into the garage or left it in the street. He was undecided, hesitant, and irritable. That night, he left for a "formal" dance, and returned at 9 a.m., giving such a confused account of what had occurred that his mother thought he was drunk. His girl friend reported that he had not had any alcohol, but that he had appeared strange and confused.

He talked continuously, night and day. His speech was not comprehensible. He was apprehensive, fearful, and hid when people came to the house lest they should kill him. He feared that the police were out to get him. On the fourth day, he was mute and catatonic. Progressively, he refused food, was negativistic, grimaced, and postured, with waxy flexibility and echopraxia. When mutism lifted, his confusional state came to the surface. He thought he had hand grenades in his pockets, and that his father had lost his legs. He failed to recognize his parents.

He was treated with ECT and was discharged, symptomatically improved, with confusion and catatonic signs relieved. Eighteen days later, however, he relapsed and was again confused, clouded, puzzled, disoriented, apprehensive with mutism and negativism. He responded to a second course of treatment and six weeks later was discharged as well.

Comment: The predominance of confusion, apprehension, fear, hallucinations, and feelings that the events were unreal suggested to Meduna that the patient was suffering from an independent perceptual disorder of unreality, similar to Kahlbaum's catatonia. Among many studies, Meduna reported that the glucose tolerance test was abnormal when the patient was ill, but normal when he recovered.

The treatment of such acute deliria with ECT is an uncommon application of the treatment, but one that is effective.[66]

Not all patients with delirious mania are successfully diagnosed and treated. In another acutely ill patient with a severe delirium and signs of catatonia, the administration of large doses of haloperidol led to a transfer to a university neurologic service and extensive testing.

Patient 3.11 A 35-year-old single woman was admitted by the police to the Emergency Room of an academic medical center. She had been running, naked and screaming, down city streets. On admission, she was calm for some moments and then became agitated, warranting physical restraint and injections of lorazepam and haloperidol. Soon after admission, she ran down the hall, tore off her gown, and tried to grab a trauma patient. She provided minimal history, saying that she had "*freaked out,*" that her boy-friend had left her a few days earlier after an eight-year friendship, and that she had used diet pills for about three weeks. She had not been able to sleep for three days, unable to go to work or eat, crying much of the time. For 13 years she had been employed in one position and had no history of a previous psychiatric disorder.

On admission to the hospital Psychiatric Service and for the next few days, she was uncooperative, agitated, and often screaming. She could not be directed. On the second day, she attempted to tear down the door to her room, fracturing two fingers. She responded calmly, but her behavior and consciousness fluctuated wildly. She appeared depressed, occasionally answered questions, and denied suicidal ideation, hallucinations, or disordered thoughts. At times, she spoke loudly to God, insisting that he answer her. Her behavior fluctuated from stupor and mutism to overactivity, screaming, and agitation, requiring physical and chemical restraint, the latter including haloperidol to 60 mg/day and lorazepam to 12 mg/day.

A diagnosis of delirium was made and neurologic consultation requested. Lumbar puncture, CSF examination, CT scan, MRI, and EEG were done. None explained her condition. On the eighth day she was transferred to the Neurology Service for further work-up. Lumbar punctures were repeated and after the first, were found to be "bloody." She was treated with intravenous acyclovir for a presumed viral encephalitis.

By the second week, she was described as "catatonic," refused to answer questions, staring and posturing with "waxy positions of her hands in the air" and "arching of the back and head, turning to the left." She was "alert with a blank stare;" and "her behavior is waxing and waning."

To sedate her for an EEG, MRI, and lumbar puncture, she was given intravenous lorazepam (2 mg) on three occasions. Within 10 minutes of each injection, she was alert, cooperative, and friendly, asking where she was and what was being done. After one such session, she spoke calmly to her brother and on another occasion to her mother and friends. Within an hour, however, she relapsed to her stuporous state.

Psychiatric consultations recommended ECT. The neurologists and internists, however, saw her as too ill for this treatment, refusing 'to clear' her for ECT. For three weeks, she became progressively less alert, requiring parenteral feeding and total nursing care. During one such gastric feeding, on hospital day 45, the gastric tube was badly placed, and an aspiration pneumonia and death ensued.

Comment: The psychiatrist described the catatonia and recommended the appropriate treatment. The request for a medical or neurologic consultant 'to clear' a patient for ECT misunderstood the purpose of such consultations for a patient for whom ECT was being considered, and interfered with the patient's proper care. The decision to administer ECT is always made by the treating psychiatrist, just as the decision to operate is always made by the treating surgeon.[67] The advice from an internist is often requested to optimize the patient's medical condition before exposure to anesthesia. It is not a request for permission.

Mixed affective states

Many authors describe the rapid changes in mood with brief periods of depression during an episode of mania as a mixed affective state (MAS). Patients who have four or more episodes annually ("rapid cyclers") may be most prone to MAS. Many causes are considered in shifts from mania to depression and vice versa, with the administration of antidepressant drugs a frequent precipitant. Interestingly, ECT is a rare precipitant of mania. Patients with MAS are difficult to treat with medications and polypharmacy often results.[68]

Mixed affective states may approach delirious mania in intensity as patients shift from one mood to another within seconds. Euphoria or irritability occur and lithium or an anticonvulsant is prescribed. Within hours, a patient shifts to an agitated depression and an antidepressant is added. The next day the patient is excited and hallucinating, and an antipsychotic medicine is also prescribed. Modest sedation followed by ECT may be the more prudent treatment. It is rapidly effective.

Such rapid mood shifts are seen in the following vignettes. A 45-year-old woman in manic excitement ran angrily screaming down the hallway with the professional staff in pursuit. The patient turned a corner into a solarium, saw "the beautiful day outside," realized that she was "locked up" and burst into tears, re-appearing around the corner (almost crashing into the staff members) in what appeared to be profound melancholia with apprehensive whining, tearless crying, and hand-wringing.

A middle-aged manic man was declaiming in a flight-of-ideas while standing on a chair, as if an orator. Another patient angrily slapped him and told him to "shut-up." The manic excitement evaporated and he remained despondent and weepy the remainder of the day. The following day he decorated himself in a suit of newspaper and once again orated.

Catatonia is commonly found among patients with manic-depressive illness, but we lack evidence of the incidence of catatonia among patients with MAS.[69] A few reports of patients with MAS refer to ECT, but it is usually with a note as to its efficacy. Berman and Wolpert (1987) describe an 18-year-old woman who developed a refractory manic-depressive psychosis after initiation of treatment with trimipramine. A complete remission was obtained after a course of six ECT.

In the treatment of 20 therapy-resistant manic-depressive patients, resistant to lithium carbonate or carbamazepine, ECT given *en bloc* (daily) for five to ten sessions or every other day resulted in remissions of the illness that allowed further management with lithium therapy. MAS remitted in three of eight patients.[70]

It is not clear from the available data whether MAS is a subtype of delirious mania or a defined entity as considered by some researchers in manic-depressive disorders. Further study of MAS is needed to clarify the incidence of catatonia and the response to anti-catatonic treatments to break up the acute MAS episodes, but also to allow further management with conventional anti-manic treatments. We consider it likely that MAS is a variant of delirious mania and that catatonic features will commonly be found in this group of patients.

Periodic catatonia

Kraepelin described a condition of periodic excitement and catatonic features alternating with normalcy.[71]

At shorter or longer intervals, often every few weeks, sometimes only every few years, there occur sudden, confused states of excitement . . . After very slight warning signs – groundless laughter, glazed eyes, restless wandering – the patient from one day to the next, often in the middle of the night, becomes violently excited. Sometimes this may be limited to increased irritability, mood swings, restlessness and pressure of talk, but usually the condition gradually worsens, and may reach acute mania, accompanied often by delusions and hallucinations. There is a sudden fall in weight . . . The excitement often lasts only a few days or weeks and is then interrupted by a few days of calm . . .

The period of calm usually begins as suddenly as the phase of excitement . . . Recovery is instantaneous, though the patient is noticeably quiet, indifferent and dull and . . . does not have full insight into the nature of his illness . . . A small number of cases eventually come to fluctuate regularly, over decades, between short periods of severe excitement and intervals of calm.

Reading this description today suggests that this patient was probably suffering from partial complex epilepsy.

Gjessing also reports that Kraepelin identified one patient as suffering from periodic catatonia and that Kraepelin then quotes Bleuler.[72]

Bleuler (1911) also mentions "periodic cases . . . This name is applicable mostly to those psychoses in which acute attacks follow the typical, recurrent manic-depressive pattern. In most such cases the residual symptoms are, to begin with, slight . . . In some cases the periodic phases may be very short, and sometimes they occur with disconcerting regularity, such as I have never seen in manic-depressive illness.

Gjessing described patients to be in stupor alternating with excitement, waxing and waning for years without evident deterioration.[73] They exhibited periods of mutism, posturing, negativism, rigidity, echophenomena, and stereotypy. Although considered a benign illness, about 3% of his patients had a more malignant form that was incorporated into the dementia praecox concept. Labeled *periodic catatonia*, the disorder was characterized by dramatic remissions and relapses of varying duration, with rapid shifts in the main features. In 1938, he suggested that the condition resulted from a cyclic nitrogen imbalance. He treated patients with thyroid extract. Following is an abstract of his Patient A_1.[74]

Patient 3.12 A 22-year-old Danish electrician showed changes in mood and thought for many months until, on his way home from work one day, he suddenly hallucinated fantastic experiences. Catastrophic feelings of terror and anxiety dominated his thoughts. On admission to the psychiatric hospital, he was dazed and disoriented, had difficulty conversing, his answers coming slowly after prolonged intervals. He felt anxious as if he was "threatened by some sort of annihilation" and he thought he was dead and rotten. He was mostly quiet, withdrawn, and occupied with aimless writing or drawing. At times he would remain staring and motionless in bed in a twilight state. On a few occasions he absconded from the hospital, only to return spontaneously.

For five years he exhibited stupor of 1- to 32-day periods alternating with periods of excitement. The attacks would begin at night. In the evening he would be his normal, cheerful self but next morning he would be half-sitting up in bed, pale, motionless, with an oily face, staring with widely dilated pupils. He was mute, with a strong flow of thick, ropy saliva. Feeding was a problem and was limited to a liquid diet. He would not urinate spontaneously and had to be catheterized. After a week the stupor eased into a twilight state and he was able to feed and toilet himself. The stupor would end as dramatically as it had begun as he would suddenly awaken, be cheerful, and crow for joy like a cock. He would seek out the nurse and ask the date and day of the week, look in the drawer for any letters, and immediately after breakfast, he would eagerly set about answering them. His mood was contented and happy, and he was talkative. He would again spend his time writing, singing, and working with photographic equipment. The euphoria would last, with a few swings towards excitement or dullness, until the next stupor phase.

Comment: We do not know the basis for the catatonia exhibited by this patient. Gjessing assumed that he was observing a discrete disease rather than a syndrome. But with the sudden onsets and resolution of features, anxiety, twilight states, and catatonia, a seizure disorder would be high on the list of differential diagnoses.[75]

Gjessing undertook detailed studies of motor activity, fluid intake and output, basal metabolic rate, weight, and biochemical measures of blood and urine of his patients. He observed his patients through repeated episodes for 22 years. He identified systematic metabolic changes with the changes in behavior. He attempted treatment with thyroid extract, iodine, and massive doses of nucleic acid, concluding that thyroid extracts were compensatory, controlling the functional disturbances but not curing the disorder. He described his patients to exhibit regular rhythms of two phases, an interval and a reaction phase, with the reversal occurring suddenly. The change in phase was first seen in measures of autonomic activity. The fluctuations in nitrogen balance and residual nitrogen occurred with the same durations as the autonomic phases, although with a time lag. Thyroid hormone controlled the functional disturbances, both the somatic and the psychologic. Another report finds oral dessicated thyroid hormone and intramuscular reserpine to relieve a patient with periodic catatonia.[76] Gjessing's report is among the first systematic studies of a psychiatric disorder from a biologic perspective with laboratory technology.

Similar vignettes of patients with periodic catatonia are found among Leonhard's descriptions of his patients.[77] Strongly influenced by Leonhard's nosology, the German researchers Stöber, Beckmann, Pfuhlmann and their co-workers at the University of Würzburg classify periodic catatonia as a separate *cycloid psychosis* unrelated to manic-depressive illness or to schizophrenia.[78] Two clinical forms of catatonia are described. *Systematic catatonia* is a form with insidious onset and a progressive chronic course without remissions. (Leonard's term is "systemic" catatonia.) Patients respond poorly to antipsychotic drugs and are seen as pharmacotherapy resistant. The Würzburg researchers find the relatives of these patients to be at great risk for schizophrenia, suggesting a genetic component to the etiology of this disorder. *Periodic catatonia*, by contrast, is considered recurrent, exhibiting a typical "bipolar" course with prominent grimacing, stereotypes, impulsive actions, aggressivity, and negativism, alternating with stupor, posturing, mutism, and waxy flexibility.[79] Their preferred treatment for periodic catatonia, however, is consistent with the consensus guidelines of a trial with benzodiazepines followed, if unsuccessful, with ECT.[80]

These German researchers rely on Leonhard's classification of the psychoses. It is unfamiliar to most U.S. psychiatrists, markedly different from DSM classifications, and not used in other German psychiatric research centers. It offers subtypes of conditions we consider to be clinically homogeneous. The validity of Leonhard's system is unknown (but so is the validity of a substantial part of the DSM). An early criticism of Leonhard's system was its unreliability; however, its average inter-rater reliability co-efficient of 0.8 was recently reported, well within the reliabilities of DSM diagnoses.[81]

The Würzburg researchers support their ideas of two forms of catatonia with family studies, in which they show that the first-degree relatives of patients with periodic catatonia are at substantial risk for the syndrome. In family studies of 139 probands and 543 first-degree relatives, the age corrected morbidity for systematic catatonia was 4.6%, and for periodic catatonia 26.9%. More parents than siblings were affected. Patterns of anticipation occurred, with the age of onset in probands earlier than the onset in their parents.[82]

Although not a study limited to periodic catatonia, additional support for a genetic basis for patients with the catatonic form of schizophrenia comes from long-term Croatian studies. A Croatian register of hospitalized mentally ill individuals admitted in 1962–1971 was examined in follow-up in rolling assessments to 1990–91. Of 402 schizophrenic patients, 59 were identified as meeting criteria for schizophrenia, catatonic type by ICD-8 criteria.[83] The family histories were positive for psychosis in 44.1% of the catatonic schizophrenic patients compared with 20.1% of the non-catatonic schizophrenic patients.[84] It is important to note, however, that ICD-8 criteria were used and by modern standards, many of these patients would be diagnosed as suffering from a manic-depressive illness.

Certainly, clinicians in the U.S. would likely diagnose patients with periodic catatonia as manic-depressive disorder or schizo-affective-mania. As mood disorders are highly familial and have a high prevalence of catatonia, the syndrome demarcated as periodic catatonia may be a form of catatonia that is a frequent expression of manic-depressive illness.[85] "Systematic" catatonia, by contrast, would likely be diagnosed by U.S. clinicians as schizophrenia, catatonic subtype. The "two catatonias" theory is best understood as two underlying illnesses, mood disorder and schizophrenia, with catatonia a manifestation of each, just as delusions occur in each condition.

Stöber and his co-workers present the history of four families with periodic catatonia. The description of the syndrome in three members in one family illustrates the murky diagnostic implications of periodic catatonia. The patient summary is abstracted from their report of Family B.[86]

Patient 3.13 An 18-year-old woman begins a course of illness with an acute episode of aimless excitement, bodily twitches, and unprovoked giggling. Later she lies in bed without movement, staring blankly. The episodes of excitement and immobility alternate. She expresses ideas of reference. A year later she has a second episode of excitement with lively, jerky movements, stereotyped repetition of words, and persecutory ideas. In a third admission, she again exhibits abrupt, jerky movements, often remaining in uncomfortable positions. When the acute symptoms remit, she is left with diffuse muscle weakness and poverty of movement.

Her mother was first diagnosed as mentally ill at 24 years-of-age after attempting suicide. She appeared stuporous, negativistic, with delusions of persecution. Later she became excited, her facial expressions were distorted, and she giggled groundlessly. She suffered 10 catatonic attacks with stupor and excitation, posturing, grimacing, stereotyped repetition of words and laughter. During an examination at age 58, she showed residual effects of jerky and clumsy body and facial movements, reduction in drive, and apathy.

The grandfather became acutely psychotic at 65 years-of-age. On admission, he was agitated, jumped around the ward excitedly, waving his arms with stereotyped yells. He expressed ideas of reference. He had two subsequent admissions, once in an immobile stuporous state and the second when he was excited and hallucinating. Remissions from each episode were rapid.

Toxic serotonin syndrome

A toxic serotonin syndrome (TSS) is described in patients exposed to a rapid increase in a selective serotonin reuptake inhibitor (SSRI) or when an SSRI is combined with other agents that affect the brain's serotonin system (e.g., monoamine oxidase inhibitors).[87] Patients are restless and sleep poorly. The sensorium is altered, the skin flushed, and the patient complains of sweating, tremor, shivering, lethargy, salivation, nausea, diarrhea, and abdominal pain. Temperature and blood pressure are elevated, tendon reflexes are hyperactive, movements ataxic, and myoclonus appears. The "big picture" is of an MC/NMS syndrome with gastrointestinal symptoms. Although most patients respond rapidly to withdrawal of the offending medicines and supportive care, ECT has also been used successfully.[88]

Patient 3.14 A 59-year-old married woman with a 21-year history of psychiatric disorder and three prior hospitalizations for agitation, mood swings, and psychosis was admitted to an academic in-patient psychiatric unit. She had acute behavioral and motor function changes following the addition of a single 25 mg dose of nortriptyline to a regimen of *l*-dopa and trazodone.

Her life course was marked by episodes of depressed mood and psychosis, complicated by insulin dependent diabetes. Three years earlier, a severe episode of grandiosity, agitation, auditory hallucinations, mutism, and rigidity failed to improve with thiothixene combined with either imipramine or fluoxetine, but resolved after a course of ECT. Thereafter, she intermittently exhibited depressive mood, thought disorder, and catatonia that was treated with antipsychotic and antidepressant drugs, with limited benefit. She developed tremors, the antipsychotic medicines were discontinued, and *l*-dopa prescribed. One week later, to relieve her depressive mood, trazodone (150 mg twice daily) was begun. She developed urinary incontinence leading the therapist to discontinue trazodone abruptly and to prescribe nortriptyline.

Within five hours of the administration of the first dose of 25 mg nortriptyline, she became fearful, tremulous, sweating, and incontinent of urine. Blood sugar was 159 mg%, pulse rate 125 bpm, and blood pressure elevated to 160/110 mm Hg (usually 140/75). On a call to her physician, she was advised to withhold further medications, including *l*-dopa and nortriptyline. The systemic signs persisted with waxing and waning of motor restlessness, rigidity, and tremors. Four days later, she became tremulous, confused and reported episodes of explosive diarrhea.

At the psychiatric emergency room, she was mute, rigid, tremulous, tachycardic, sweating, and hypertensive. The initial examination appeared to be consistent with a neurotoxic syndrome, a single dose of 1mg lorazepam was administered, without benefit. On admission to the psychiatric unit, she was afebrile, depressed, oriented, drowsy, and described auditory hallucinations. Her posture was rigid and she did not obey simple commands. CT scan, EEG, thyroid function tests, and blood studies were within normal limits. CPK was 92 IU/l (24–195 normal). ECG was normal with resting heart rate of 92 bpm. Fluctuating elevated blood glucose measurements were treated without difficulty using glipizide and insulin.

TSS was diagnosed, all medications were withdrawn, and lorazepam (1 mg every six hours) prescribed. She remained depressed and psychotic. In view of the severity of her condition, and complex history of medication treatment failures, a course of bilateral ECT was begun. A day after the first treatment, motor rigidity, mutism, and negativism became more prominent and additional lorazepam was prescribed. The afternoon of her second ECT, motor rigidity and mutism were gone, she was more interactive and responsive, denied hallucinations, and attended unit activities. Three additional treatments resolved the psychosis, depressed mood, agitation, and motor and vegetative signs.

Lorazepam was prescribed as continuation treatment. In a follow-up visit three months later, she was neither depressed nor psychotic. When she failed to take the prescribed doses of lorazepam, however, she became mute, withdrawn, inattentive, and inactive – signs that were relieved by increasing the dosage of lorazepam.

Although the full-blown TSS is infrequently recognized, milder forms occur in patients who receive SSRI antidepressant medicines. The incidence and severity rises with the use of polypharmacy, but virtually every medicine that increases levels of central nervous system serotonin has been implicated. Laboratory findings include leukocytosis, rhabdomyolysis with elevated CPK, myoglobinuria and renal failure. Hyponatremia, hypomagnesemia and hypercalcemia are also reported. Although none of these laboratory features of TSS are as common as the laboratory features that characterize MC/NMS, the pattern is remarkably similar to that syndrome.[89]

The overlap of the diagnosis of TSS and NMS is reported in a review of the calls to the NMS Information Service, an expert referral service.[90] Of 28 records meeting general criteria for NMS, 22 (79%) simultaneously met criteria for TSS,[91] and 25 (89%) met criteria for NMS.[92] The authors conclude that the two syndromes are conditions allied with catatonia.

Benign stupor

The term "benign stupor" was applied to severely depressed and delusional patients who became mute, withdrawn, stared, and postured. Detailed descriptions are provided by Hoch (1921) and the description of a teenager with alternating stupor, mania, and catatonia is abstracted. The description of her syndrome also meets criteria for periodic catatonia.

Patient 3.15 A 15-year-old girl was brought to the New York State Psychiatric Institute in 1907 with a three-week history of changed behavior, lately marked by mutism, staring fixedly into space, and failing to feed or dress herself. Three weeks earlier she had returned home from work claiming that a girl in the shop had made remarks about her red hair. She wanted to change her position, but continued to work at the same location until six days before admission when she refused to go to work or to go out of her home because "everybody was looking at her." She cried often, stating that "*Oh, I wish I were dead – nobody likes me – I wish I were dead and with my father*" (dead). Four days before admission she was febrile, became immobile, lay in bed, did not speak, eat, or drink.

For five months she remained in stupor – inactive, mute, staring vacantly, often not even blinking, so that her conjunctiva became dry. She did not swallow but held her saliva; did not react to pin pricks or to feinting motions before her eyes. She retained her urine, wetting and soiling the bed, maintained awkward postures, and was usually stiff, offering resistance to movement. She was tube-fed at first, but later would swallow when spoon-fed. During the first month, the stupor was interrupted for short periods by a little freer action: she walked to a chair, sat down, smiled and fanned herself very naturally when a fan was given to her, but she did not speak. During this period she did not menstruate, was periodically febrile to 103 °F with a moderate leucocytosis and tachycardia. She became emaciated.

After five months, she was seen to be smiling and then weeping, began to talk a little to the nurses, though not to the doctors. She ate excessively, gaining 30 pounds in two months. For the next two months she was apathetic, sluggish, but neat in her self-care. She exhibited no mood except when the examiner asked her to put out her tongue so that he could stick a pin in it, and then she blushed and hid her face. (Kraepelin's test for automatic obedience.) When questions were asked, she sometimes answered promptly and in normal voice, while at other times she remained silent despite repeated questions. She was oriented. When asked about her personal experience, she remained mute. When, however, questions were posed in a fashion that they could be answered by "yes" or "no," she answered promptly.

In the eighth month of her illness, the apathy cleared, and she was bright, active, smiled, and talked freely. She recalled the experience noted in the introductory description but was amnesic for much of her stay at the Institute. After returning home, she became elated and talkative, conversing with strangers in the street. She told her mother that she was now 16 years of age and wanted "a fellow." She was returned to the hospital for an additional two months during which time she was elated and talkative. She recovered spontaneously.

She had a second attack of stupor with immobility, mutism, catalepsy, and rigidity two years later and was treated at another hospital. She made an excellent recovery. After two years, she again felt "queer," "nervous," "depressed," and became sleepless. She thought that she was dying and that her father's picture was talking and calling to her. "Then I lost my speech." After recovery from this episode, she willingly came to be examined in response to a letter and was quite open about giving information.

Patients with prolonged stupor of indeterminate etiology are found in many long-stay neurologic services.[93] The medical and neurologic assessment of such patients is extensive and often without specific findings of either a structural or infectious cause. It is probable that some patients are suffering from a catatonic stupor. Considering the diagnosis and offering treatment trials should be a consideration when the etiology is poorly defined and the response to intervention insufficient.[94]

Primary akinetic mutism

Diverse neurologic syndromes have in common the acute onset of stupor, immobility, rigidity, and inability to undertake voluntary movement except for movements of the eyes. These are labeled *akinetic mutism, apallic syndrome*, and *coma vigil*.

Akinetic mutism was described as a consequence of brainstem or diencephalic neurologic pathology.[95] Patients are mute, negativistic, and stuporous. Onset is usually acute. They lie immobile and rigid, but their eyes follow the examiner's movements. The sleep–wake cycle is disturbed, emotional responses to stimulation are blunted, and the Babinski and other abnormal reflexes are elicited. The syndrome has been associated with orbitomesial frontal lobe trauma, third ventricle tumor, bilateral anterior cerebral artery and anterior cingulate lesions, and lesions of the caudal hypothalamus. Descriptions of coma vigil and apallic syndrome are similar and hardly distinguishable.

When a careful neurologic assessment fails to reveal a structural cause for the syndrome, primary akinetic mutism needs to be considered and the patient challenged with an intravenous benzodiazepine or barbiturate. Primary akinetic mutism, described by Bleuler, is a form of catatonia. The patient who behaved like a "wild animal" (*Patient 2.5*) in Chapter 2 exhibited akinetic mutism when first seen on the physicians' rounds.

ENDNOTES

1 William of Occam (*aka* Okham): Occam's Razor. *Oxford English Dictionary*, 2nd edition.
2 Magrinat et al., 1983; Barnes et al., 1986; Peralta et al., 1997; Carroll, 2001.
3 American Psychiatric Association, 1994, DSM-IV
4 Lishman, 1978.
5 Hoch, 1921.
6 *Patient 4.4.* Bright-Long and Fink, 1993.
7 Trimble, 1978, 1991; Bear, 1986; Lim et al., 1986; Louis and Pflaster, 1995; Cocito and Primavera, 1996; Miyata et al., 1997; Kanemoto et al., 1999.
8 Bell, 1849; Kraepelin, 1921; Bonner and Kent, 1936; Carlson and Goodwin, 1973; Taylor and Abrams, 1977; Bond, 1980; Klerman, 1981; Berman and Wolpert, 1987; Goodwin and Jamison, 1990; Bräunig et al., 1998, 1999; Fink, 1999b.
9 Kahlbaum, 1973: 29; and others noted.
10 Bleuler, 1950: 213.
11 Adland, 1947; Arnold, 1949; Arnold and Stepan, 1952; Huber, 1954; Mann et al., 1986, 1990; Ahuja and Nehru, 1990; Ferro et al., 1991; White, 1992; Philbrick and Rummans, 1994; Fricchione et al., 2000.
12 Arnold and Stepan, 1952; Philbrick and Rummans, 1994.
13 Gelenberg, 1976, 1977; Caroff, 1980; Fricchione, 1985; Lazarus et al., 1989; Caroff and Mann, 1993. Table 3.3.
14 Fricchione, 1985; Mann et al., 1990; White, 1992; Fink, 1996a, 1997b; Bush et al., 1996a,b; Carroll and Taylor, 1997.
15 Insel et al., 1982; Sternbach, 1991; Fink, 1996b; Keck and Arnold, 2000.
16 Fink, 1996b; Keck and Arnold, 2000.
17 Lindsay, 1948; Minde 1966; Gjessing, 1974, 1976; Stöber et al., 1995, 2000b, 2001; Kinrys and Logan, 2001.
18 Bräunig, 1991.
19 Cairns et al., 1941; Cairns, 1952; Cravioto et al., 1960; Klee, 1961; Sours, 1962; Segarra and Angelo, 1970; Dalle Ore et al., 1977; Lishman, 1978.
20 Blum and Jankovic, 1991; Barker et al., 1998; Bauer et al., 1979.
21 Leonhard, 1942a,b, 1961, 1979; Berrios and Porter, 1995.

22 Perris, 1995.

23 Brockington et al., 1982a,b.

24 American Psychiatric Association, 1994, DSM-IV

25 Kahlbaum, 1973: 8–9.

26 Kahlbaum, 1874; translated by Mora, 1973: 9–14; description is that of Patient Benjamin L.

27 In assessing the causes of the condition Kahlbaum writes: "*No hereditary factors are present. The main etiological factor seems to be weakening of the nervous system due to onanism; this assumption is borne out to some extent by the patient's downcast, hesitant gaze, his sallow complexion, and his entire confidence-lacking demeanor.*"

28 McCall et al., 1992; Bush et al., 1996a.

29 Bell, 1849.

30 Stauder, 1934.

31 Geretsegger and Rochowanski, 1987.

32 Trigo et al., 2001.

33 Penn et al., 1972.

34 Also Carroll et al., 1994, and Caroff et al., 1998; Caroff et al., 2001.

35 Arnold and Stepan, 1952; Geretsegger and Rochawanski, 1987; Weller et al., 1992; Philbrick and Rummans, 1994; van Dael, 2001.

36 Mann et al., 1990.

37 Fricchione et al., 1990.

38 Abrams 1997; Fink, 1999a.

39 Häfner and Kasper, 1982.

40 Arnold and Stepan, 1952; Tolsma, 1967; Peele and von Loetzen, 1973; Regestein et al., 1977.

41 Koponen et al., 1991.

42 Delay and Deniker, 1968.

43 Caroff, 1980. The syndrome was described but not labeled by Kinross-Wright, 1958: 62–70; Delay and Deniker, 1968; Meltzer, 1973.

44 Lazarus et al., 1989; Shalev et al., 1989; Spiess-Kiefer, 1989.

45 Rosebush and Mazurek, 1991a; Raja et al., 1994; Lee, 1998; Peralta et al., 1999.

46 Greenberg and Gujavarty, 1985.

47 Pope et al., 1986; Keck et al., 1989; Rosebush et al., 1990; Spivak et al., 1990; Rosebush and Mazurek, 1991a; Osman and Khurasani, 1994; Berardi et al., 1998.

48 Lavie et al., 1986.

49 Lazarus et al., 1989.

50 Lazarus et al., 1989.

51 Guerrera, 1999.

52 Pearlman, 1986; Pope et al., 1986; Addonizio et al., 1987; Castillo et al., 1989; Rosenberg and Green, 1989; Fink, 1992c; Woodbury and Woodbury, 1992; Caroff

and Mann, 1993; Revuelta et al., 1994; Blumer, 1997; Peralta et al., 1997; Caroff et al., 1998a; Mathews and Aderibigbe, 1999; Biancosino et al., 2001.

53 Fricchione, 1985; Chandler, 1991; Carroll and Taylor, 1997; Fricchione et al., 2000; Koch et al., 2000; Carroll et al., 2001.

54 Rosebush et al., 1990; Ahuja and Nehru, 1990; White, 1992; Philbrick and Rummans, 1994; Fink, 1996a; Pavlovsky et al., 2001.

55 Hermesh et al., 1987; Davis et al. (1991); Schott et al., 1992; Troller and Sachdev, 1999.

56 Bush et al., 1996b.

57 Koch et al., 2000; Francis et al., 2000.

58 Mann et al., 1986.

59 Many authors have reviewed the diagnosis and treatment of NMS. Selected reports are those by Kurlan et al., 1984; Levenson, 1985; Pearlman, 1986; Addonizio et al., 1987; Rosebush and Stewart, 1989; Lazarus et al., 1989; Keck et al., 1991; Caroff et al., 1991; White, 1992; Blumer, 1997; Assion et al., 1998; Pelonero et al., 1998; Fricchione et al., 1997, 2000.

60 At a symposium at the American Psychiatric Association in May, 2000, investigators of NMS and MC concluded that the two syndromes were one syndrome, to be treated the same. The participants and discussants included B. Carroll, M. Fink, A. Francis, D. Healy, S.C. Mann, C.A. Pearlman, G. Petrides, P. Rosebush, and D.A.C. White. (Fink, 2000b).

61 Regis, 1901; Meduna, 1950; Kapstan et al., 2000.

62 Fink, 1999b.

63 Shalev and Munitz, 1986.

64 Dr. George Petrides (personal communication). The experimental medication was ziconotide, a non-opioid analgesic (Levin et al., 2002). Another patient developed severe delirium post gastrectomy, was treated with haloperidol, developed MC/NMS, and was relieved by ECT (13 ECT in 6 days) (Masuda et al., in press).

65 Mayer-Gross, 1924; Meduna, 1950; Kapstan et al., 2000.

66 Kramp and Bolwig, 1981; Strömgren, 1997; Fink, 1999a, b; Malur et al., 2000.

67 American Psychiatric Association, 1990, 2001; Fink, 1999a.

68 Kilzieh and Akiskal, 1999.

69 Abrams and Taylor, 1976, 1977; Bräunig, 1991.

70 Mosolov and Moshchevitin, 1990.

71 Kraepelin, 1913. Quoted by Gjessing, 1976: 1.

72 Kraepelin, 1921.

73 Gjessing 1938, 1974, 1976.

74 Gjessing: 1976: 11–18.

75 Minde 1966; Lindsay, 1948.

76 Komori et al., 1997.

77 Leonhard, 1942a,b, 1979, 1995.

78 Stöber et al., 1995; Beckmann et al., 1996; Pfuhlmann and Stöber, 2001.

79 Stöber et al., 1995; Beckmann et al., 1996; Pfuhlmann and Stöber, 2001.

80 Ungvari et al., 1994b, 2001a.

81 Pfuhlmann et al., 1997.

82 Stöber et al., 2000a, 2000b, 2001; Stöber, 2001; Meyer et al., 2001.

83 World Health Organization. Internationale Klassifikation der Krankheiten, 8th revision, 1967. Published 1968, Basel: Kruger.

84 Mimica et al., 2001.

85 Looper and Milroy, 1997.

86 Stöber et al., 1995: 140.

87 Insel et al., 1982; Sternbach, 1991; Fink, 1996b; Carbone, 2000; Mason et al., 2000; Keck and Arnold, 2000; Carroll et al., 2001.

88 Fink, 1996b.

89 Keck and Arnold, 2000.

90 Carroll et al., 2001.

91 Hegerl et al., 1998.

92 Hynes and Vickar, 1996.

93 Spear et al., 1997.

94 Swartz and Galang, 2001.

95 Cairns et al., 1941; Cairns, 1952; Cravioto et al., 1960; Klee, 1961; Sours, 1962; Dalle Ore et al., 1977; Lishman, 1978.

4

The differential diagnosis of catatonia

According to an old story, there are three different types of baseball umpires. The first says: "I call them [balls and strikes] as they are"; the second says: "I call them as I see them"; and the third says: "What I call them is what they become."

Frederick Grinnell, 1992

Catatonic features are observed in many psychiatric conditions. Primary catatonia, in which a person has the syndrome and no evidence of another disorder, is a hypothesized condition, but is not established.[1] The clinical challenge is to recognize catatonia and the condition that causes it. In this chapter, we describe the differential diagnosis of disorders that underlie the expression of catatonia, and syndromes that simulate and may be mistaken for it.

"*The duck principle*" is a fundamental tenet of diagnosis: if it looks, walks, and quacks like a duck, it is a duck. The tenet is applicable to the diagnosis of catatonia. If a patient exhibits catatonic features, it is best to consider the patient as having catatonia. If features seem isolated from a clear underlying cause or are inconclusive, catatonic features can be temporarily relieved with an intravenous sedative, such as lorazepam or amobarbital. An intravenous injection of 1–2 mg lorazepam (0.5 mg/ml) or up to 500 mg amobarbital (50 mg/ml) over two minutes should relieve mutism, posturing, and rigidity. (At this rate of injection, laryngospasm is not a problem.) During the injection, talk to the patient, even if he is mute. The relaxation of posture, increased speech, fewer mannerisms, and response to commands confirm the presence of catatonia.

Once the diagnosis is established, etiology is the next consideration. The most likely cause is a mood disorder. Exposure or withdrawal of psychoactive medicines, especially antipsychotic drugs, is another common cause. A neurologic disorder or a general medical condition must also be considered.

Table 4.1 Laboratory findings in catatonia

Increased CPK

Low serum iron

Increased CSF homovanillic acid

Frontal slowing on EEG that may be intermittent; features wax and wane

Increased size of lateral ventricle or cerebellar atrophy on brain imaging

Decreased sensory motor cortex functioning and altered laterality on functional MRI and SPECT

Cognitive problems in attention, and motor and visuo-spatial functioning

CPK: creatine phosphokinase; CSF: cerebrospinal fluid; EEG: electroencephalogram; MRI: magnetic resonance imaging; SPECT: single photon emission computed tomography.

Some illnesses may be identified by specific laboratory tests, but catatonia secondary to mood disorder or a non-affective psychosis has no pathognomonic laboratory signs.

Laboratory tests and catatonia

Many efforts have been made to use objective laboratory tests to diagnose psychiatric states and disorders, but only the EEG (to confirm a diagnosis of epilepsy or delirium) and tests for infection (syphilis) and endocrinopathy are in widespread use. No laboratory test specifically defines catatonia (Table 4.1). The body's reactions to the stresses of malignant catatonia in its many forms are fever, hypertension, tachycardia, tachypnea, leucocytosis, elevated CPK, and decreased serum iron, but these signs do not indicate an etiology.

Electroencephalography

The recording of the human EEG by Hans Berger in 1929 stimulated hope that these electrical measurements would, like the electrocardiogram for the heart, provide a direct examination of the brain's control of behavior.[2] Many researchers sought avidly for a relationship of EEG patterns to psychiatric diagnosis, but no specific EEG abnormalities were discerned, either in patients with schizophrenia, manic-depressive illness, nor any of the primary

psychotic disorders.[3] Diffuse slowing has been reported in patients in catatonic stupor. Frequencies are similar to those described for delirium, with the
EEG showing a lower percentage of alpha activity, frequent periods of symmetric, bilateral theta, or almost flat records filled with beta frequencies.[4]
But the EEG patterns accompanying stupor from other causes are highly
variable and not related to either the severity or the duration of stupor.[5]
When the above patterns were examined prospectively for a connection to
catatonia, however, the predictions failed.[6] In one report of a patient in
catatonic stupor associated with hyperparathyroidism, the EEG frequencies
slowed during stupor and normalized following parathyroid surgery with
relief from high calcium levels.[7]

Some authors have sought to relate catatonia to the presence of a dys-
rhythmic EEG consistent with non-convulsive status epilepticus. When these
patients were treated with intravenous phenytoin or lorazepam and the EEG
signs resolved, so did the catatonia.[8]

The EEG was recorded in eight patients with catatonia.[9] Seven exhibited
low voltage fast records, with a mean frequency of 16–18 Hz. In six patients,
intravenous lorazepam resolved catatonia. The amplitudes of EEG rhythms
increased, rhythmicity improved to a more regular, homogeneous rhythm,
and alpha frequencies were enhanced. In two patients, catatonia did not
resolve with lorazepam, and they were treated with ECT. The relief of their
catatonia was accompanied by slowing of dominant frequencies to theta
rhythms of high amplitude, seen clearly on the day after ECT treatments
4 and 5. One week later, the EEG was dominated by well-modulated alpha
frequencies. These changes in interseizure EEG patterns are the same as those
recorded in depressed patients without catatonia treated with ECT.[10]

The amobarbital sedation threshold is an EEG method for assessing
arousal.[11] In this procedure, a solution of amobarbital sodium is injected
intravenously at 0.5 mg/kg/40 seconds. The EEG is examined for the development of rhythmic beta activity or the eyes are examined for the development of nystagmus.[12] The sedation threshold is defined as the number
of milliliters of solution that first elicited EEG beta-frequency-spindling or
nystagmus. In patients with schizophrenia and those with severe anxiety, the
EEG beta response occurs slowly, requiring 6–10 ml doses to the criterion
(a "high" sedation threshold). Depressed patients, those with catatonia, and
those with structural brain syndromes quickly exhibit EEG beta frequencies

and nystagmus with 2–4 ml doses ("low" sedation threshold). When amobarbital was administered to catatonic patients, their low sedation threshold was accompanied by the transient resolution of catatonia.

The scalp-recorded EEG studies in catatonia are few. We find no reports of studies of other electrophysiologic measures, such as averaged evoked potentials or magnetoencephalography, of patients in catatonia.

Although EEG instrumentation has improved much, the interest and facilities for EEG recording have shifted from psychiatry to neurology services making EEG investigations of patients with psychiatric illnesses difficult and expensive. Catatonia is often not recognized so that the study of the relationship with catatonia is today hardly commented upon.

In summary, we find no direct connection between EEG measures and catatonia. Catatonic patients may show normal EEG patterns, or the abnormal EEG patterns associated with a medical or neurologic illness. When they are treated with medications or with ECT, the EEG shows the changes commonly associated with the signatures of the medicines or ECT, but little that is related to catatonia.[13]

Neuroendocrine tests

The discovery of the neuroendocrine systems of the brain is a relatively new feature of neuroscience. The hypothalamus, anterior and posterior pituitary, and pineal glands of the brain produce hormones that modulate almost all of the body's physiology, either directly or indirectly, by feed-back mechanisms with other endocrine glands.[14] Although the association between abnormalities of the neuroendocrine system and disturbances in mood, affect, thought, and cognition is well documented, the relationships with the motor system are less well studied. We find little in the neuroendocrine literature that connects with catatonia.

The dexamethasone suppression test (DST) is a widely studied clinical test of the integrity of the neuroendocrine system.[15] The DST is grossly abnormal (i.e., cortisol blood levels are not suppressed by a dexamethasone dose) in patients with mood disorders. It is correlated with weight loss and starvation. Elevated cortisol is the body's attempt to redress an imbalance that comes from loss of body tissue.

Greden and Carroll (1979) described a 67-year-old woman who became psychotically depressed with negativism, mutism, staring, and rigid posture.

Weight loss was severe and the DST was abnormal. After two ECT, catatonia resolved, and after four ECT she was improving rapidly. On follow-up several weeks later, she was well, had gained weight, and a single serum cortisol determination at 4 p.m. was elevated. She soon relapsed, was re-admitted showing catatonia and an abnormal DST. Catatonia and depression improved and the DST normalized with seven ECT. Lithium and imipramine were prescribed as continuation treatments and she remained well at the 20-month follow-up. The authors consider the DST as a test of an underlying mood disorder in catatonic patients. Reports of neuroendocrine studies in catatonia are sparse, however, and do not suggest that the available measures of neuroendocrine functions are of specific diagnostic value.[16]

Other laboratory tests

Increased CPK is a common feature of a severe motor syndrome. Excited manic patients and those who receive frequent intramuscular injections exhibit elevated levels. Numerous authors have commented on the association of a low serum iron in patients with MC and with NMS.[17] The finding is considered non-specific, as it occurs in many acute illnesses.[18] Antipsychotic drugs, however, are weak chelating agents for iron and facilitate iron to enter tissue cells. Iron metabolism dysregulation has been implicated in some movement disorders, so although a likely reflection of acuity rather than a specific catatonic pathophysiology, low serum iron may increase the risk for catatonia. The combination of an elevated serum CPK and low serum iron in a psychiatric patient should be a warning of an MC/NMS response to antipsychotic drugs.

Conditions in which catatonia is expressed

Catatonia is commonly expressed in patients with mood disorders (mania and depressive states), psychosis, drug intoxication and withdrawal, structural neurologic conditions, and abnormal metabolic states. It is also found in patients with epilepsy, Parkinson disease, and pervasive developmental disorder. It needs to be distinguished from the behaviors that mark obsessive–compulsive conditions.

Mania

Catatonia is found in about 15% of manic episodes of manic-depressive illness. Catatonic signs, like psychotic features during a manic episode, relate to severity, but their presence does not affect the prognosis when appropriate treatments are applied. Whenever the clinical picture meets the classic criteria of mania with euphoria, infectious mood, flight of ideas, grandiosity, and pressured speech, the co-occurrence of catatonia requires no specific intervention. It responds to active anti-manic treatments.

A diagnostic problem arises, however, when catatonia occurs in an irritable, psychotic, manic patient, or when the affect state is mixed, shifting to and from mania, depression, and catatonia, or when the patient is "stuck" between mania and depression, appearing emotionally blunted. Such patients may be classified as suffering from schizophrenia and are unsuccessfully treated with antipsychotic drugs alone. Behaviors that might be mistaken for schizophrenia occurring during manic episodes are:

- a woman put a pile of ashes on her head to counteract the cosmic rays controlling her mind;
- a woman placed furniture in strategic places throughout her home so that she could hop from one to another, like stepping on stones to cross a stream, to avoid touching the floor which would result in danger to her children;
- a man dressed in black leather clothes attacked buildings on Fifth Avenue in New York City to defend society from a powerful conspiracy.

Each patient responded to lithium treatment and their "bizarre" behavior resolved with their mania.

When a manic patient is psychotic, irritable, and cataleptic, the recognition of mania may be difficult. A useful clinical aphorism is: "*When you scratch a catatonic, you most often are tickling a manic.*" Half the patients with catatonia suffer from manic-depressive illness. For hospitalized patients, regardless of the number or strangeness of psychotic features, the likelihood of mania increases with the more words that the patient utters, the more often he interrupts conversations, the more rapidly he speaks, the more activities in which he engages, the more moods he expresses, the more clothes he has on, and the more clothes that he takes off. Table 4.2 offers guides to identify mania with catatonia.

Clinicians associate catatonia with schizophrenia, the result of teaching based on the DSM classification system that links these conditions. Although

Table 4.2 Identifying manic patients with catatonia

Hospitalized manic patients are most often irritable, not euphoric

The combination of hyperactivity, pressured speech, and altered mood identifies a manic patient

Among psychotic patients, manic patients are most likely to have more than one generation of psychiatrically ill relatives

Although 30–50% of manic patients become chronically ill and may become avolitional regarding job and family, most retain full emotional expression

Although some schizophrenic patients experience an early depressive episode, depression late in the course of an illness in a patient with periodic psychoses likely reflects a manic-depressive illness

Prior to their first episode of psychosis, schizophrenic patients are frequently schizoid, whereas manic patients are normal or have soft manic spectrum behavior (cyclothymic, dysthymic, irritable)

DSM-IV recognizes catatonia as a specifier for mania in the same fashion that it recognizes melancholia as a specifier of depression, patients with catatonia are most likely to be diagnosed as schizophrenia, catatonic type (295.20).[19] Nevertheless, the link between catatonia and mania is strong and well documented. A catatonic patient is more likely to be suffering from a manic-depressive illness than any other disorder. This association would be no surprise to Kahlbaum (1973: 26),

We have come to recognize that *in most cases* the disease (meaning catatonia) manifests itself in the first stages with an easily recognizable clinical picture of melancholia; very often the stage of melancholia is preceded by *true manic states*, which cannot be regarded merely as outbursts of despair, described as raptus melancholicum because in addition these patients pass through definite and unmistakable attacks of mania, they present the typical signs of heightened total reaction of the psyche, accompanied by signs of increased self-expression and self-awareness. [Stress is ours].

Early 20th Century writers were familiar with the relationship between mania and catatonia. Kraepelin reported that nearly 50% of catatonic attacks begin with a depressive episode. Such patients were most likely to recover. In *Manic-Depressive Illness and Paranoia*, he described catatonic features that are likely to be seen in a manic episode.[20] Similarly, Bleuler observed that:

As a rule, catatonic symptoms mix with the manic and the melancholic conditions, in some instances to such a marked degree that the catatonic symptoms dominate the clinical picture and one can speak of a manic or a melancholic catatonia.

Yet, both manic and melancholic catatonic patients were included in the dementia praecox (schizophrenia) category by these authors.[21]

The American psychiatrist George Kirby was the first to explicitly state that catatonic symptoms were consistent with classic manic-depressive illness (Kirby, 1913):

We have also shown that marked catatonic syndromes may appear in otherwise typical manic-depressive cases. In some cases a catatonic attack apparently replaces the depression in a circular psychosis. In cases showing both manic and catatonic phases the manic-depressive features have the greater prognostic significance. There can be little doubt that Kraepelin over-valued catatonic manifestations as evidence of a deteriorating psychosis and that many of these cases have served to unduly swell the dementia praecox group.

Reports throughout the 20th Century link manic-depressive illness and catatonia. Of 700 manic-depressive patients, Lange (1922) found 25% to have several or more catatonic features. Bonner and Kent (1936) prospectively compared 100 consecutive patients diagnosed with manic excitement with 100 diagnosed with catatonic excitement. The two groups had overlapping features with 10% of the manic patients exhibiting several catatonic features. In a retrospective analysis of hospital records, Morrison (1974a,b) found that 20% of the catatonic patients to be ill with a mood disorder. Similarly, Abrams and Taylor (1976) found 39 of 55 catatonic patients (70%) to have a mood disorder (mostly mania). In another study (Taylor and Abrams, 1977), 34 of 120 manic patients (28%) had two or more catatonic signs during a hospital admission for mania. Bräunig et al. (1998) studied 61 hospitalized manic patients and found 19 (31%) to meet criteria for catatonia. These authors concluded that manic patients with catatonia had a more severe form of mania, but were similar in all other clinical ways to manic patients without catatonia. In an earlier report, Bräunig (1991) described a patient with a rapid 48-hour cycle of mood and catatonic features. Northoff and his co-workers (1999b) could also find no differences in catatonia rating scale scores or sub-scores between catatonic patients with schizophrenia and those with mood disorder, supporting catatonia as a syndrome, not a disease, and not synonymous with schizophrenia.

Most recently, Krüger and Bräunig (2000b) examined 99 manic patients for catatonic features, finding 27% to meet DSM-IV criteria for catatonia. Verbigeration, stereotypy, immobility, mutism, and grimacing were the most common features. When manic patients who were not catatonic were compared to those who were, those without catatonia were more likely to abuse street drugs and have impulse control problems when not manic. The differences were attributed to severity of illness.

Given these experiences, what prevents clinicians from more readily recognizing the manic features of catatonia? Fein and McGrath (1990) reported that of 12 patients with catatonia, eight were initially diagnosed as schizophrenic, but at a two-year follow-up, eight of the 12 were re-diagnosed as manic-depressive. All responded to lithium. The misdiagnoses were attributed to the failure to recognize the fluctuating presentations of mania (manic patients are not always manic-like during an episode), misidentifying the stuporous states of catatonia as emotional blunting, and assuming catatonic signs to represent schizophrenia.

Some clinicians interpret the mutism, negativism, and slow reduced movements in a patient with catatonia as emotional blunting and as signs of schizophrenia. The liberal use of antipsychotic medicines for any psychotic patient results in drug-induced parkinsonian features of mask-like facies, monotone speech, and reduced gestures, leading to the conclusion, occasionally mistaken, that the patient is emotionally blunted and therefore suffering from schizophrenia.[22] In young adults, the typical years of onset of schizophrenia, the challenge is great to distinguish emotional blunting of schizophrenia from the motor signs of catatonia or those that are drug-induced. It is also true, however, that some patients with catatonia are suffering from schizophrenia making the distinction between emotional blunting and catatonia important. Catatonia needs treatment before antipsychotic drugs are applied for schizophrenia.

The following vignette illustrates catatonia amid a manic episode.

Patient 4.1   A 23-year-old man in a euphoric-manic state with delusions and hallucinations was hospitalized. His excitement increased and he was sedated with sodium amobarbital. He was quiet for an hour but did not sleep. When examined again, he stood at attention in the middle of the room peering intently out the window. He commented in rapid-fire fashion at movements occurring in the scene outside. He could not be interrupted and his speech at first seemed unintelligible, but when followed carefully, it was seen to be

Table 4.3 Mania and catatonia

Author/Year	Mania	% Catatonia
Lange, 1922	700	25
Bonner and Kent, 1936	100	10
Taylor and Abrams, 1977	120	28
Bräunig et al., 1998	61	31
Krüger and Bräunig, 2000a	99	27

Author/Year	Catatonia	% Mania
Morrison, 1973	200	20
Abrams and Taylor, 1976	55	70
Fein and McGrath, 1990	12	66

a running commentary of the events outside. Otherwise, he did not move. He resisted efforts to move his limbs, but then waxy flexibility set in and he could be postured. His rapid speech continued. Sedation relieved the catatonia and lithium resolved the mania.

Various systematic studies report a strong link between mania and catatonia (Table 4.3). These studies show that among hospitalized manic patients, a quarter will meet criteria for catatonia, and that among catatonic patients, more than half will meet criteria for manic-depressive illness.

Catatonia in manic-depressive illness typically takes one of three forms: catatonia wholly replaces the mood episode; the mood episode fluctuates between depression, mania, and catatonia; and, catatonic features occur simultaneously with the mood features, with the mood features predominant. *Patient 4.1* fits the last pattern.

The speech of *Patient 4.1* was unintelligible, almost to the point of word salad, until the key to his associations was found. Then, though clearly based on distractible associations to visual cues, it became a running commentary of real events outside his window. Psychosis, unintelligible speech (Bleuler defined it as looseness of associations), and catatonic features should not be interpreted automatically as signifying schizophrenia, particularly when mood symptoms are present.

Patient 4.2   A 48-year-old man with a long history of psychotic episodes was re-hospitalized because he had become mute and stuporous. He sat in a chair for hours without moving or paying attention to events around him. He moved slowly and occasionally froze in the middle of a motor sequence. Getting up to urinate, he moved slowly to the bathroom doorway, stopped just before it, and stood still until he soiled himself. He exhibited automatic obedience and could briefly be postured, his limbs then slowly returning to their original position.

In two previous severe suicide attempts, he had been psychotically depressed, often becoming irritable and violent, expressing grandiose delusions and rapid pressured speech. The nursing staff were fearful of him, even in his stuporous state.

Throughout the years of his illness, he had been diagnosed as suffering from paranoid schizophrenia. On this admission, he was re-diagnosed as suffering from a manic-depressive illness with catatonia. ECT resolved the catatonia, and he was discharged to the community with a prescription for lithium. He was said to be a "new person," pleasant and soft spoken, intelligent and potentially high functioning. (We do not know if this man had catatonic features during his other illnesses.)

Mania with prominent catatonic features is described next.[23]

Patient 4.3   A 25-year-old musician was hospitalized with a two-week history of overactivity, insomnia, and excitement following his return from an exhausting working trip overseas. His condition worsened rapidly as he became agitated, intrusive, screaming continuously. His speech was incoherent. For many minutes he was mute, staring, and rigid. He was dehydrated, febrile (102 °F), and tachycardic (150 bpm). He was disoriented for time, date, and place, unable to recall numbers or objects shown to him, and could not do simple calculations.

He was treated with lorazepam to 8 mg/day and with parenteral fluids. The delirious syndrome resolved, but he remained disoriented, grandiose as to his wealth and his power to help others. At other times, he spoke in word salad.

After being in restraints continuously for four days, permission for ECT was obtained from his wife. Because of his excited state, the first bilateral ECT was given with ketamine anesthesia. A successful EEG seizure of 83 seconds was induced, despite the high doses of lorazepam. That afternoon, he spoke clearly and responsively for a few hours, was approximately oriented for place and date, but then relapsed to a delirious state again. Two additional treatments were given on successive days, and after the third treatment, he was lucid, oriented, cooperative, and followed directions in the afternoon and evening. Restraints were no longer necessary and he fed himself. ECT continued and he was discharged in remission to the care of his family and returned to work.

He remained well for four years, when he was again hospitalized because of insomnia, restlessness, grandiosity, flights of ideas, poor appetite, confusion, and disorientation. Again, the symptoms developed after he returned from an overseas trip. He had worked around the clock to complete his work by a deadline, and had resorted to repeated doses of amphetamines.

Treatment with fluphenazine was started. Periods of excitement and delirium became less intense. On the 12th hospital day, bilateral ECT with ketamine anesthesia was again given. Six hours later, he exhibited fever, rigidity, sweating, tachycardia, tachypnea, and an elevated serum CPK. Medication was discontinued, parenteral fluids were administered, and he was sedated with lorazepam. The toxic signs resolved rapidly, and four days later, on the 16th hospital day, ECT was re-instated. After four additional treatments, delirium, mania, and catatonic signs resolved. He was fully oriented, and was discharged to his family to continue weekly outpatient ECT. He resumed his work and returned for three additional treatments, after which he was discharged.

Comment: The patient was suffering from a recurrent delirious mania. In both episodes, his catatonia resolved with ECT. The first treatment in the second episode was followed by a neurotoxic syndrome that responded to withdrawal of fluphenazine and treatment with lorazepam. He was treated in the early 1990s, before we recognized the merit of resolving NMS with ECT. Our present practice would be to continue ECT.

Ketamine is administered intramuscularly, and is useful in patients in whom it is difficult to establish an intravenous line. The dosages are 0.5–1.0 mg/kg. Ketamine is pro-convulsant, does not raise seizure thresholds, and as a consequence, enhances seizure duration. It is not used regularly as the duration of its action is variable, and on rare occasions, may be associated with a transient delirious state after the treatment.

Depression

The second most likely condition underlying catatonia is depression, particularly melancholia. Catatonia in depressed patients is typically associated with profound psychomotor retardation, occasionally progressing to stupor. Patients are mute and cataleptic (mundane positions are most common). When they speak, they sound robotic or overly formal (e.g., "I can not" rather than "I can't"). The tone of voice is altered. They show automatic obedience, and less frequently, waxy flexibility and echophenomena. Rather than being stimulus-bound like manic patients, they seem unaware of surrounding activity. After recovery, however, they are able to clearly describe events that occurred during the episode.

Depressed catatonic patients stop eating and drinking, lose weight, and become dehydrated and incontinent. If they express psychotic thoughts and are given an antipsychotic medicine, they are at risk for developing MC/NMS.

Table 4.4 Identifying depression in young catatonic patients

Vegetative signs (problems with sleeping, eating, libido) take diagnostic precedence
  over psychotic features
Premorbid and inter-episode good functioning with active libido suggests depression
Comorbidity of bulimia or migraine suggests mood disorder
Winter episodes suggest mood disorder
A family history of mood disorder, suicide, or alcoholism suggests mood disorder
Depression is many times more likely at any age than is schizophrenia or other
  non-drug related psychoses

Table 4.5 Identifying depression in elderly catatonic patients

Vegetative signs (problems with sleep, eating, and libido different from age related
  problems) suggest depression unless a co-occurring general medical condition can
  account for them
Maximizing problems suggests depression; minimizing problems and denial of illness
  (anosognosia) suggests dementia
A history of mood disorder before age 50 suggests the episode in later life is also one of
  depression
A family history of mood disorder or suicide suggests depression; a family history of
  progressive Alzheimer-like disease suggests a dementia secondary to structural
  abnormality
The most common single cause of reversible dementia is depression. In persons under
  age 70, depression is four times more common than a dementia caused by a
  progressive degenerative brain process

They doze, but rarely exhibit adequate periods of stage-3 or stage-4 deep sleep. The younger patient is often misdiagnosed as schizophrenic, while the elderly patient is seen as demented. Guidelines to identify the young catatonic patient who is depressed are presented in Table 4.4. Because first-episode depression is now occurring at a younger age than years ago, an early depressive-like psychosis is statistically more likely to be the onset of a mood disorder than the onset of schizophrenia.

Guidelines for identifying depression in the elderly catatonic patient are cited in Table 4.5. These patients are usually cognitively impaired and may appear demented. "Pseudodementia" is a form of dementia that results from the cognitive impairments of depression that exaggerate the cognitive decline commonly seen in the elderly. Depressive illnesses in patients over age 45 years respond very well to treatment, indeed more so than the depressive disorders of patients from 18 to 45 years of age (90% versus 70%, respectively).[24]

Catatonic features are infrequently reported in patients with Alzheimer's disease, making its appearance more likely due to a depressive mood disorder. A neurologic or metabolic disorder other than an Alzheimer's type of dementia also warrants consideration.

The signs and symptoms of patients with depressive stupor and those with depressive mood disorder with catatonia overlap. A depressive stupor is dominated by profound bradykinesia and bradyphrenia. There is no clear pathophysiological distinction between a depressive stupor and a depressive mood disorder with catatonia. The nihilistic delusion of being dead in *Patient 4.4* is identified as Cotard's syndrome, a syndrome that is associated with non-dominant parietal lobe lesions and also found in patients with psychotic depression.[25] In one description of the syndrome in a 15-year-old girl, the authors concluded that the illness was an example of malignant catatonia that resolved with ECT.[26]

Patient 4.4, hospitalized with pseudodementia, had been misdiagnosed as suffering from a structural dementia. She responded to ECT and was maintained in the community for many years with continuation ECT. When her behavior was identified as an example of catatonia, lorazepam treatment was prescribed and was equally effective.[27]

Patient 4.4   A 58-year-old woman was referred for evaluation of her altered behavior and to confirm the diagnosis of Alzheimer's disease made nine years earlier. She stared aimlessly, postured with her arms wrapped about herself, and with a rhythmic motion of the right arm and leg engaged in masturbation, oblivious to others in the room. She was perplexed and anxious as she touched paintings on the wall, picked up magazines to glance at them momentarily and then quickly discarded them. Her speech was slow and halting. When asked the year, she said it was 1976, the year she became ill (actual year was 1985). She did not complete serial-sevens beyond "93, 86…" She spelled w-o-r-l-d forwards but it became d-o-g when asked to do so backwards.

Sixteen years earlier, at age 42, she had become withdrawn and non-communicative, lost weight, and failed to care for herself or her family. She was treated with an unspecified antipsychotic medicine and then with ECT, with relief of her symptoms. At age 47 she relapsed, became withdrawn and mute, underwent ECT again, and recovered. At age 49, she again became depressed, anorexic, sleepless, and withdrawn. She was treated with amitriptyline, responded rapidly, and then quickly relapsed becoming confused, wandered aimlessly, was mute, and withdrew from her family. A computed X-ray tomographic study of the head showed "cortical atrophy," a diagnosis of Alzheimer's disease was made by a consulting neurologist. The family was advised that further intervention was useless. For the next nine years she was cared for at home by her husband and five daughters. She became emaciated, weighing only 75 pounds. Incontinent of both bladder and bowel, she wandered aimlessly around the house staring from the windows, grimacing frequently, and posturing for long hours.

On admission, a trial of nortriptyline was begun, and adequate plasma levels achieved. She improved, slept and ate better, and engaged in brief conversations. Haloperidol was added and the combined regimen continued for three weeks. She became continent and occasionally verbal, but quickly relapsed. ECT was recommended, and her husband consented. After the 5th bilateral ECT, she became alert, engaging, and communicative. She was amazed and puzzled to learn that it was 1985, and that her five daughters were grown. She insisted that the year was 1976 and that the grown women visiting her were not her daughters, who were much younger. After 13 treatments, she was verbal, friendly, well oriented (30/30 on the Mini-Mental State examination [MMSE]), and was able to care for herself. Nortriptyline was prescribed as maintenance treatment.

Four days later she was again withdrawn, minimally verbal, and referred for out-patient ECT. Through the remainder of 1985 she received 13 additional treatments, averaging one every six days. She cared for herself, cooked and cleaned for her family, and enjoyed her children and grandchildren.

Lithium carbonate was added, but she required ECT to sustain her remission. The return of her symptoms followed a typical course: her hands developed redness, the signs of Raynaud's phenomenon. She became hesitant and indecisive, and progressively worked and cooked less. She stood for minutes staring into space, answered questions hesitantly, with "I don't know." She did not dress herself, and appeared perplexed, postured, and performed poorly on the MMSE. At such times, ECT was re-instated, usually two or three treatments in a series, and she quickly recovered. This pattern was followed for nine years, with 9 to 19 treatments given each year.

In 1994, the syndrome was recognized as one of catatonia and her medicines were changed to lorazepam in doses from 3 to 8 mg per day. For the next six years, she has no longer required ECT, suffered no relapses, being maintained with lorazepam alone and various antidepressants.

Comment: This patient was in depressive stupor. The initial diagnosis of Alzheimer's Disease (AD) was premature. AD typically expresses itself when patients are in their mid-seventies.[28] In persons under age 70, depression is many times more common than AD. Persons with early onset AD typically have a strong family history of the illness, and they often exhibit muscle rigidity and sensory aphasia. They show deficits in tempero-parietal functions of new learning, facial recognition, and motor-perceptual coordination. They complain of memory problems, experience motor car accidents, lose their way as they travel, and become easily confused. They do not show the vegetative signs of melancholia.

Melancholic patients, having experienced hypercortisolemia, may exhibit cortical atrophy on CT scans, making this test unhelpful in distinguishing AD from the pseudodementia of depression. Metabolic imaging methods (SPECT, PET, functional MRI) may be better instruments to demonstrate decreases in frontal lobe functioning rather than the tempero-parietal abnormalities seen in patients during the early stages of AD. Further, AD affects the enterorhinal cortex early, leading AD patients to have problems with odor identification.

Because it is often difficult to separate AD from the pseudodementia of depression, it is prudent for each patient with AD to have a detailed examination for depression. Even modest evidence of a mood disorder warrants therapeutic optimism and a treatment trial. Using a Hamilton Rating Scale for Depression may be useful to quantify the clinical impression and monitor the treatment effect. Antidepressants with anticholinergic properties are usually avoided because they are associated with worsening of the cognitive impairments of AD. When the depression/dementia is accompanied by psychotic features, ECT offers the safest treatment choice, both for the relief of depression and of the psychosis.

Non-affective psychosis

About 10% of patients with catatonia meet criteria for schizophrenia, especially when schizophrenia is rigorously defined.[29] "Rigorously defined" includes no past or present mania so that the schizoaffective diagnostic option is unlikely. Catalepsy, mannerisms, posturing, and mutism are traditionally associated with schizophrenia. In addition, the schizophrenic patient exhibits chronic avolition and poor emotional expression during and after an exacerbation of psychosis. As the prognosis for patients with schizophrenia is generally poor, and the diagnosis commonly calls for extensive use of antipsychotic medications with their neurologic risks, it is clinically better to consider diagnoses with better prognoses whenever patients exhibit catatonia. We limit the diagnosis of schizophrenia to persons with a long-standing non-affective psychosis characterized by auditory hallucinations, delusions, avolition, and loss of emotional expression, that often have a premorbid history of neuro-motor, emotional, cognitive, or social problems beginning in childhood.

Although catatonia responds well to treatment, an underlying schizophrenia usually does not fully remit. The prolonged use of antipsychotic medications increases the risk of tardive dyskinesia. Tardive dyskinesia is debilitating (some patients cannot stand erect without leaning on walls). Because of its effects on pharyngeal and esophageal muscles, it interferes with swallowing, leading to aspiration pneumonia and to death. As with other basal ganglia disorders, tardive dyskinesia is associated with cognitive decline with frontal-lobe features, further reducing the long-term functioning of patients.[30]

Patient 4.5   A 21-year-old woman became progressively withdrawn over six months, remaining alone in her room, refusing to wash or to clean up after herself. Her speech became "disorganized", and she became increasingly less verbal. She pulled away from family members when they tried to interact. She showed little emotion toward or interest in the people or the activities occurring around her. She mumbled to herself, and sat or stood for long periods without moving, staring blankly into space. Her hands were held in front, in a twisted manneristic position. When examined, she resisted body manipulations with passive resistance.

The catatonic features resolved with bilateral ECT, but she remained avolitional without emotional expression and her conversational speech was without emotion (dysprosodic) and without elaboration or details. She showed no evidence of delusions or hallucinations, and denied having had these experiences. She did not return to her unskilled job.

The experience of a patient with schizophrenia, catatonic type illustrates the difficulties in treating the psychosis and managing the signs of catatonia.[31]

Patient 4.6   A 31-year-old man had been hospitalized 22 times for delusional thoughts, hallucinations, excitement, and the inability to care for himself, over a span of 13 years. He first became ill during his second year at college and improved partially with treatments that included antipsychotic, antidepressant, anticonvulsant, and sedative medications. During his third hospitalization at age 20, he responded to a course of ECT and returned to college for one semester. When the illness recurred, his psychiatrist concluded that ECT had failed and did not consider it again. Over the years, his parents sought the advice of many consultants, one of whom suggested that ECT be tried once more.

On admission he was tall, bearded, and unkempt, mumbling to himself, posturing in a crucifixion stance. Speech alternated between mutism and slow, hesitant responses to questions. He stated that he was Jesus Christ, that the Lord spoke often to him, and that he was bringing His message to the world. He was cooperative except for bathing or shaving. Psychological testing showed his intelligence quotient to be high; EEG and blood measures were normal. ECT was recommended. The risks and possible gains were explained to him and to his parents; all signed consent.

Medications were discontinued and a course of bilateral ECT begun. After the third treatment, he recognized his parents and asked after his sister. Mutism and posturing abated. The patient's psychotic symptoms persisted despite more than 18 treatments. On the day after the 23rd treatment, he showered, shaved his beard, and asked to visit a barber. He was alert, oriented, and said he had no delusional thoughts. When he was reminded of his statements about Jesus and God, he was surprised, though he did recall thinking of God. After a visit by his parents, he was puzzled by the date; he had lost track of the years during which his sister had graduated from college, married, and had two children.

Treatments were continued once a week, with fluphenazine also prescribed as mainte-nance treatment. As preparations were made for him to return to the community, he had to face his lack of social and work skills. Because he had read very little, it was difficult to see how he could return to college. He did not accept the suggestion of acquiring train-ing in manual skills and for many years, continued to be a resident in a state-sponsored adult home. He participated in group activities and cared for himself.

Bi-weekly continuation ECT inhibited his delusional thoughts and mutism. He re-mained amotivational, took no interest in his welfare, but followed requests and direc-tions. Periodically, mutism, posturing, and staring recurred. Lorazepam at high dosages failed to do more than suppress his catatonic signs. Modern atypical antipsychotic medicines were of little benefit. For more than 16 years, he has been given ECT at inter-vals of 10 to 14 days with lorazepam at 3–4 mg/day.

Comment: The patient had no past or present evidence of a mood disorder, and no specific cause for catatonia could be determined. He was diagnosed as suffering from schizophrenia. This experience indicates that catatonia responds to lorazepam or ECT regardless of its associated psychopathology. The long-term prognosis of catatonic patients, however, is based on the cause of the underlying disorder, not the presence of catatonia.

General medical conditions

Catatonia is a feature of many general medical conditions, the same condi-tions that are associated with delirium. It is often seen in patients suffering from metabolic, autoimmune, and endocrine disorders, infections, burns, and neurologic syndromes. The incidence of catatonia in a burn unit is estimated as more than three times that in a general hospital.[32] Patients with systemic lupus erythematosus are prone to develop catatonia.[33] An association between the syndrome of inappropriate antidiuretic hormone secretion (SIADH) and catatonia was relieved by ECT (see Anfinson and Cruse, 1996).

Acutely ill patients seen in medical and psychiatric emergency rooms often exhibit excitement or stupor with the motor signs of catatonia. An interesting example is the report of catatonia in 12 patients during an epidemic of typhoid fever.[34] After fever and other signs of infection had disappeared, catatonia persisted. The syndrome was distinct from typhoid delirium and had none of the characteristics of a mood disorder or schizophrenic illness. A patient in this series is described.

Patient 4.7   A 23-year-old man experienced high fever, insomnia, and withdrawal for one week. He was unkempt and exhibited posturing, waxy flexibility, and negativism, responding to questions only when questioned repeatedly. He was fully oriented, memory was intact, and he showed no evidence of depression or psychosis. His general medical examination was consistent with typhoid fever.

He was treated with chloramphenicol and betamethasone, and became afebrile. The psychiatric symptoms persisted for 10 days, and he was given six bilateral ECT in two weeks. The catatonia disappeared. Four weeks after admission he was communicative without any psychiatric abnormality. Six months later he was still asymptomatic.

A patient with typhoid fever, treated with ciprofloxacin, exhibited signs of catatonia. When ciprofloxacin was discontinued, and the patient treated with chloramphenicol, both the infection and the catatonia resolved. The authors suggest that catatonia was induced by ciprofloxacin, but it is more likely that catatonia developed as a result of typhoid fever alone.[35]

Another example of catatonic stupor was assumed to result from encephalitis lethargica.[36] The authors did not find evidence of infection, but they concluded that their diagnosis was supported by the sudden appearance of depression and catatonia in the absence of a history of schizophrenia, the similarity of the syndrome to that of patients described by von Economo, and concurrent reports of sporadic cases of encephalitis lethargica.

Patient 4.8   A 17-year-old man had a three-week history of an acute depressive illness with the somatic delusion that he had contracted typhoid fever and was infecting his family. He took an overdose of an antihistamine and was hospitalized. Three days later he was mute, akinetic, negativistic, and exhibited waxy flexibility. When he could be induced to move, he would 'freeze' in fixed postures. He was incontinent of urine and had low-grade fever. He was dehydrated and hypotensive. An EEG showed diffuse asynchronous delta and theta activity compatible with encephalopathy.

After rehydration with intravenous fluids and a course of 12 bilateral ECT, the catatonic signs disappeared and he improved. At discharge, he was amnestic for the illness. The EEG was normal. On a two-year follow-up, he exhibited no signs of psychiatric illness other than a lack of spontaneity and poverty of expression.

Comment: This episode, however, was likely stimulated by an overdose of an antihistamine. This is a better explanation than the authors' resort to a presumptive diagnosis of encephalitis from circumstantial evidence only. Histamine has been implicated in the induction of experimental catatonia and antihistamines ameliorate this effect.[37] The sudden withdrawal of antihistamines has elicited catatonia.[38] Antihistamines have been used to treat dyskinesia and histamine/antihistamine interactions are implicated in malignant catatonia and its relief.[39] The antihistamine overdose and its sudden withdrawal in *Patient 4.8* may explain the sudden appearance of MC/NMS. ECT elicits an increase in brain histamine, suggesting an explanation for its relief of the syndrome.[40]

Drug-induced (toxic) states

Antipsychotic drugs elicit catatonia, often in its malignant form. Exposure to the high potency and depot forms of antipsychotic drugs is most likely to do this, with MC/NMS occurring in up to 2% of exposures.[41] MC/NMS has a rapid onset and is severe in its expression. Many authors emphasize the risks in such instances, and encourage the prompt use of ECT.[42] Because antipsychotic drugs are widely used, the development of NMS is assumed to result only from the use of such drugs. Other conditions, however, induce or increase the likelihood of MC/NMS (Table 4.6). Because psychiatric patients are not immune to other diseases, we do not automatically assume that a sudden or recent behavioral change in a psychiatric patient is an exacerbation of the psychiatric illness or its treatments.

Benzodiazepine withdrawal, if done rapidly, may elicit catatonia.[43] The basis may be incompletely expressed seizures, similar to the episodes seen as an absence-status or nonconvulsive status epilepticus. Such patients are delirious, with fluctuating catatonic signs. Perseveration of speech, mannerisms, stereotypes, forced thinking and speech, and compulsive behaviors occur.

Table 4.6 Conditions associated with non-antipsychotic drug causes of MC/NMS[a]

Hypoparathyroidism, with resulting hypocalcemia
Infection (virus, HIV, typhoid fever)
Tumors (frontal-temporal brain lesions)
Stroke (involving anterior brain regions)
Traumatic brain injury (subdural frontoparietal hematoma)
Epilepsy (post-ictal immobility and NCSE)
Autoimmune disease (systemic lupus erythematosus)
Endocrinopathies (thyrotoxicosis, pheochromocytoma)
Heat stroke (in younger, excited male patients)
Toxins (strychnine, tetanus, staphylococcal, fluoride)
Poisonings (salicylates, inhalational anesthetics)

[a] *See also* Levinson and Simpson, 1986; Taylor, 1990; Carroll et al., 1994. NCSE: non-convulsive status epilepticus.

Anxiety is usually high. This form of catatonia may be associated with visuo-spatial disorientation, gait dyspraxia, and dysgraphia.[44]

Dopaminergic drug withdrawal also precipitates catatonia. The rapid withdrawal from L-dopa/carbidopa or amantadine may elicit a cataleptic state with rigidity, tremor, and waxy flexibility, and the signs of MC/NMS.[45] Patients receiving these medicines have severe basal ganglia disease and are at particular risk for developing catatonia.

Gabapentin withdrawal has also been associated with catatonia in a patient with bipolar illness. Catatonia resolved with lorazepam treatment.[46]

Opiates and opioids, in overdose, produce an immobility syndrome with rigidity and posturing. Temperature regulation is disturbed. The presumed mechanism for opiate induced catalepsy is an endorphin interaction in the dopaminergic systems.[47] Other signs of opiate intoxication (pinpoint pupils, cold skin, reduced bowel sounds) are usually present.

Illicit (Street) drugs.[48] Chronic stimulant use elicits stereotyped behaviors. Cocaine, mescaline, and LSD intoxication are risk factors for lethal catatonia.[49] *Phencyclidine (PCP)* induces an excited manic state accompanied by violence. Superficially, these patients look like non-drug related manic patients, but PCP intoxication is associated with nystagmus and ataxia.[50]

Patients may go in and out of cataleptic postures, and generalized analgesia is demonstrable. They may be violent, sustain physical trauma, and
appear unaware of their injuries. Chronic PCP users are repeatedly hospitalized for excitement. They exhibit flights of ideas and repetitive speech,
but unlike typical manic patients they use paraphasic phrases, private word
usage, jargon speech, and driveling. The combination of flight of ideas with
elements of formal thought disorder (the speech and language problems
observed in schizophrenia) is associated with drug-induced psychotic states
where excitement is the typical presentation. The patient with flight of ideas
is hyperverbal with distractible associations, jumping from topic to topic. In
Bleuler's (1950) illustration of looseness of associations, he gives examples
that are to be considered flights of ideas. Paraphasic phrases are approximate
word usage, as in "the thing you sit on" instead of the word "chair." Private
word usage is also paraphasic but it is so far removed from the construct that
it is not understandable, as in "the mechanism for stagnation" for "chair".
Terms like "jargon" and "driveling speech," the former used in neurology and
the latter in psychiatry, refer to the same phenomenon of strings of seemingly
meaningless phrases.[51] Although their emotional expression is spared, they
are typically avolitional other than in their drug-seeking behaviors.

Disulfiram has been associated with catatonia.[52] *Mescaline* and *psilocybin*
produce euphoric and dysphoric intoxications with catatonic features.
Patients appear in reverie or dream-like states. Stereotypes, perseveration,
posturing, and verbigeration are common. An example of a psilocybin-
induced catatonia follows.

Patient 4.9   A 19-year-old man used mushroom extracts on several occasions. One dose resulted in
hospitalization during which he was psychotic and manic. Following a new "dose" he
became terrified, despondent, and agitated, saying he was evil and needed to die. He
required restraints, was sedated with lorazepam, and hospitalized. The following morning he was no longer agitated, but appeared in a dream-like state. He could provide no
details about his life or his thoughts, spoke in cliches, and answered questions incompletely. He became echolalic. When released from restraints, he spent hours posturing
at attention in a continuous salute, or on both knees as if in prayer, or lying prone on the
floor with eyes open, staring at the ceiling. Lorazepam did not relieve his symptoms but
bilateral ECT did. After a course of treatment, his thinking remained vague but he was
able to return to his home.

Epilepsy

Partial complex seizures and the postictal states after partial complex and generalized seizures are accompanied by stereotypy of limbs, facial posturing, catalepsy, stupor, and mutism. Ipsilateral motor automatisms and contralateral dystonic posturing, unilateral to the seizure focus, occur.[53] Seizure foci in the prefrontal and supplementary motor areas, the basal ganglia, and the anterior temporal lobes are associated with catatonic signs. Because we do not find the basis for seizures in 70% of epileptic patients, and since 20% of epileptic patients have normal EEG recordings even with extensive monitoring, the differential diagnosis is difficult. In one report of 29 catatonic patients, four (13.8%) were diagnosed with epilepsy, 15 with a mood disorder, and eight with schizophrenia.[54] One "schizophrenic" patient was also diagnosed as having "dystonic seizures," and another as having childhood obsessive–compulsive disorder (OCD). Of the patients with seizures, the diagnoses included complex partial seizures, absence status epilepticus, and dystonic seizures (with a subcortical brain stem focus).

Compared to catatonia in mood and psychotic disorders, catatonia in seizure disorders is more likely to be of shorter duration (less than one hour) and more frequently recurrent. Sensations of unexplained warmth and fuzzy-headedness as if drunk, and the feeling as if one's head is stuffed or swollen (occurring with frontal foci), are reported. Psychosensory features such as *déjà vu*, *jamais vu*, dysmegalopsia, dysmorphopsia, olfactory or visual hallucinations, and brief intense emotional incontinence are occasional consequences. Dysmegalopsia and dysmorphopsia are perceptual distortions, the former of objects changing their size, the latter objects changing their shape. The patients report *"the world suddenly seems small, as if looking through the wrong end of a telescope;" "the pattern in the wallpaper gets bigger and then smaller;" "everything looks as if I am looking through a glass of water;"* or *"that it is reflected from a fun-house mirror."*

A history of paroxysmal "spells" with poor recall for the details of the spell, a family history of epilepsy or migraine, and a personal history of migraine also point to a seizure disorder. Table 4.7 displays the features of epilepsy to consider when evaluating a patient with catatonia. The more of these features, the more episodes, and the more atypical the psychiatric symptoms, the more likely a patient has epilepsy.

Table 4.7 Features of epilepsy[a]

Prodrome
Hours or days of unease, irritability, lack of focus in thought and behavior

Ictus
Often starts with a few-seconds' experience (aura) that may reflect the location of a
    focus; for *temporal lobes:* anxiety, olfactory hallucinations, intense memory
    experiences (*déjà vu, jamais vu,* visual distortions); for *frontal lobes:* warmth, head
    sensations, thinking changes; for *parietal lobes:* somatosensory experiences
Seizure is sudden in onset, paroxysmal (maximum features occur rapidly), of short
    duration (usually less than 60 seconds), associated with an alteration in arousal
    (partial complex), and some memory loss for the events during the episode

Post-ictal
Behavioral changes range from fatigue and irritability to rage, fugue states, psychosis

---

[a] See Taylor, 1999, chapter 10: 298–324.

About 40% of patients with severe and chronic forms of epilepsy are
likely to have personality changes described as "viscous" or "adhesive."[55]
They cling to one topic in conversation and may be persistent, pedantic, and
perseverate. They repeat themselves in great detail. Speech is circumstantial,
providing endless details about mundane events and thoughts. Some keep
copious notes and diaries, or become overly religious to the point where
it consumes their lives and interferes with their functioning in other areas
of life, despite having only superficial understanding of theology. They lose
interest in sex.

Petit mal status has also been associated with a psychosis with catatonic
features. The patients appear to be in a dream-like state, delusional and
hallucinating, with mutism and immobility. They respond poorly to verbal
commands, but do respond to light tactile cues. They grimace and maintain
positions into which they are placed, even when the positions are awkward.
Symptoms of depression and psychomotor slowing mask their epilepsy. The
EEG is usually abnormal, showing continuous bilateral symmetric and syn-
chronous three-per-second slow waves with intermingled spikes.

Patients in non-convulsive status epilepticus (NCSE) may exhibit catatonic
features in the absence of a full motor convulsion. They suffer prolonged confusion and delirium with stereotypes, repetitive speech, and echophenomena.

They may be delusional and hallucinate. The EEG shows diffuse high-voltage slowing with sharp waves, without well-defined seizure patterns. The level of arousal varies from mild lethargy to severe clouding. Patients may be mute or may speak continuously, with rambling speech or flights of ideas. Speech may be altered in tone or rhythm, or may consist of verbigeration, the morbid repetition of words, phrases, or sentences. Repetitive stereotypic phrases occur during speech, often toward the end of sentences such as "*I think I should leave doctor. I should leave, leave. I should leave.*"

Patient 4.10 A 46-year-old man was found wandering along a highway. He hardly spoke, and when he did, he mumbled and made little sense other than saying "*I don't know.*" When asked a question he commonly responded with "huh?" and looked dazed. On the psychiatric unit, he stood for long periods in the middle of the hallway slowly rubbing his head and face with both hands. When the staff tried to stop the rubbing he resisted with equal force, but neither spoke with them nor tried to evade them. EEG showed sharp spike and slow wave complexes. Both the abnormal EEG and his behavior were relieved by anticonvulsant treatment.

Patients with partial-complex or petit mal status epilepticus may exhibit catatonia. Their response to questions is altered, and may be mistaken for "hysteria" or as being factitious because the degree of vigilance is variable and they respond negatively when touched (stiffening), spoken to (tightly shutting their eyes which were previously open), or encouraged to eat (clamping their teeth). A search for seizure-related behaviors and EEG studies is part of the evaluation of a catatonic patient with altered arousal.[56]

When a seizure-like event is observed, drawing blood for serum prolactin levels 15–25 minutes later may provide evidence of a seizure.[57] A sharp rise in serum prolactin is considered evidence of a grand mal seizure.[58] Serum prolactin levels are also elevated in 60% of temporal lobe and 40% of frontal lobe epileptic patients following a seizure. Temporal lobe epileptic patients may also have reduced temporal lobe volume on MRI and hypometabolism on SPECT (single photon emission computed tomography) at the site of the focus.[59]

Catatonic patients with altered states of consciousness warrant an EEG to rule out NCSE or petit mal status. The EEG is recorded *before* administering a benzodiazepine as these drugs temporarily relieve catatonia. If a nonconvulsive, petit mal, or partial complex status epilepticus is identified, the patient is treated with the appropriate anticonvulsant. If there is no evidence of a seizure disorder, the patient is treated for catatonia. The following patient was in a partial complex status.

Patient 4.11 A 40-year-old woman was hospitalized after she was found wandering in the streets "dazed and confused." She moved slowly and paced the hallway with her hands held in front of her as if she were about to catch a ball. At times, she brought her hands to her face and at other times she would stand in a posture for many minutes. Her face was expressionless except for frequent blinking. She was mute much of the time, and occasionally she mumbled in a whisper. Passive resistance to movement was demonstrable. She refused food and liquids. An injection of sodium amobarbital did not relieve her symptoms. She would not cooperate with EEG studies. Catatonia of unknown etiology was diagnosed and she was treated with ECT. She fully recovered after the second treatment and said she suffered from epilepsy and that she had abruptly stopped her medication because she was becoming increasingly despondent about her future. Four more ECT relieved the depression. Phenytoin was then restarted. Prior medical records confirmed epilepsy with a fronto-temporal right-sided focus.

Epileptic disorders are common. The point prevalence in the U.S. is estimated to be about 1 in 200 persons. The lifetime risk is higher and epileptic patients are repeatedly hospitalized for psychiatric care. Many are not recognized as having epilepsy and are treated with antipsychotic drugs or are seen as depressed and treated with antidepressant drugs. The signs of catatonia in *Patient 4.11* saved her from such treatments. About 40% of epileptic patients become seriously depressed. The seizure threshold is raised by ECT in about half the patients treated. To assure adequate treatments in epileptic patients, increases in electrical energy to induce a seizure are frequently necessary.[60]

Ganser syndrome (pseudologica fantastica)

The syndrome of pseudologica fantastica (Ganser syndrome) is a "hysterical twilight condition" in which subjects give approximate answers to questions.[61] The answers are incorrect but they bear a relationship to the sense of the question, showing that appropriate concepts have been touched upon. For example, to the question "How many legs does a three-legged stool have?", the patient answers "Four."

Ganser described three prisoners awaiting trial who presented approximate answers, amnesia, confusion, and hallucinations.[62] The illnesses were suddenly relieved and the patients were amnestic for the experience. One patient was cataleptic, lying motionless in bed, staring fixedly at the ceiling, with posturing and waxy flexibility. A second exhibited widespread analgesia, rigidity, and staring. In a later collection of patients, Ganser described the syndrome in association with psychosis and central nervous system disease.[63]

Many authors consider the syndrome as a hysterical "pseudo-stupidity" occurring in prisoners.[64] Others find it among patients with neurologic disorders including NCSE.[65] In one report of five patients with the syndrome, one patient suffered a brief Ganser syndrome with psychosis, flaccid paralysis, and profound sensory loss.[66] The syndrome was relieved with amobarbital. Three days after the interview, the patient exhibited an excited catatonic illness requiring prolonged hospitalization; the illness was relieved by ECT.

These descriptions suggest that the syndrome of approximate answers may be a manifestation of catatonia, consistent with negativism, and patients with Ganser syndrome should be evaluated fully before labeling them as "hysterical" or malingering.

Other neurologic diseases[67]

Catatonia has been associated with many brain diseases that affect the motor system. Lesions or localized metabolic impairment of the frontal lobes, basal ganglia, cerebellum-pons, or parietal lobes elicit signs of catatonia. Neurologic conditions associated with catatonia are listed in Table 4.8. These should be considered when an older person, without a previous history of mood disorder, shows signs of catatonia. Neurologic conditions are also to be considered when the motor signs are unilateral, or when they are associated with focal neurologic features or isolated cognitive problems, suggestive of parietal lobe dysfunction (e.g., neglect, dyspraxia, dysgraphia). Neurologic conditions that elicit stupor, such as brainstem disease due to tumor, aneurysm, or traumatic injury, are particularly difficult to distinguish from a stupor associated with major depression. Stuporous catatonic patients who do not respond quickly to intravenous lorazepam, who exhibit focal or lateralized neurologic signs, or signs of increased intracranial pressure should have detailed neurologic assessments. Those who do respond to lorazepam with relief of stupor require further evaluation for psychiatric disease.

Metabolic disorders

Patients with a variety of metabolic disorders may exhibit catatonia (Table 4.9). As most persons with these conditions do not exhibit catatonia,

Table 4.8 Neurologic conditions associated with catatonia[a]

Encephalitis (particularly when limbic structures and temporal lobes are involved, as
   with herpes, encephalitis lethargica)
Postencephalitic states (particularly with parkinsonism)
Parkinsonism
Subacute sclerosing panencephalitis
Bilateral lesions of the globus pallidus
Bilateral infarction of the parietal lobes
Temporal lobe infarction
Thalamic lesions
Periventricular diffuse pinealoma
Anterior cerebral and anterior communicating artery aneurysms and hemorrhagic
   infarcts
Frontal lobe traumatic contusions, arteriovenous malformations, neoplasms
Primary frontal lobe degeneration
Traumatic hemorrhage in the region of the third ventricle
Subdural hematoma
General paresis
Tuberous sclerosis
Paraneoplastic encephalopathy
Multiple sclerosis (particularly the mid-life onset form which often affects the
   cerebellum)
Familial cerebellar-pontine atrophy
Epilepsy (particularly psychosensory)
Creutzfeldt–Jakob's disease
Alcohol degeneration and Wernicke's encephalopathy
AIDS related dementia and other white matter dementias
Narcolepsy

[a] *See also*: Pauleikhoff (1969); Gelenberg (1976); Johnson (1984); Hippius et al. (1987);
Rogers (1992); Taylor (1993, 1999); Fricchione et al. (1997); Joseph (1999); Ahuja
(2000a).

it is unlikely that the pathophysiology is based on the metabolic disorder
itself. Severe electrolyte imbalance or dehydration may be a factor in its expression. Once catatonia is recognized, however, a medical evaluation reveals
the etiology. The reversal of the pathology with medical treatment usually
relieves catatonia.

Table 4.9 Metabolic disorders that are associated with catatonia[a]

Diabetic ketoacidosis
Hyperthyroidism
Hypercalcemia from a parathyroid adenoma
Pellagra, vitamin B12 deficiency
Acute intermittent porphyria
Addison's disease
Cushing's disease
Syndrome of inappropriate antidiuretic hormone secretion (SIADH)
Hereditary coproporphyria, porphyria
Homocystinuria, uremia, glomerulonephritis
Hepatic dysfunction or encephalopathy
Thrombocytopenic purpura
Lupus erythematosus or other causes of arteritis
Infectious mononucleosis
Langerhans carcinoma
Tuberculosis
Typhoid
Malaria
Toxic states secondary to mescaline, amphetamine, phencyclidine, cortisone, disulfiram,
   aspirin, antipsychotic agents, illuminating gas, organic fluorides

[a] *See also*: Gjessing (1976); Fricchione (1985); Fricchione et al. (1990, 1997); Rogers (1992); Taylor (1993); Carroll et al. (1994); Ahuja (2000a).

Catatonia in adolescents and children

Catatonia occurs often in young persons with psychiatric and developmental disorders.[68] The range of primary diagnoses with which catatonia is associated is similar to that described in adults, but in addition, catatonia is reported in patients with the defined childhood disorders of autism, the Prader–Willi syndrome, and mental retardation. Young patients with NMS exhibit the same signs of catatonia as do adults.[69] But catatonia in adolescents may be difficult to recognize, and patients are then poorly treated until the proper diagnosis is made and effective treatments applied.[70]

Patient 4.12 A 17-year-old girl had three-weeks of "spells" of confusion, asking the same question again and again. She postured, was tearful, paced aimlessly, and told her parents that God commanded her to protect her father from harm. She protested his leaving the home. A pediatrician prescribed sertraline and her syndrome worsened. At a psychiatric hospital emergency room, she was excited and was given haloperidol, olanzapine, and lorazepam. Within 24 hours, she became mute, unresponsive, and stopped eating and drinking. Her temperature, heart rate, and blood pressure rose and for five days she received extensive neurologic and medical examinations. She withdrew from painful stimuli, resisted passive movement, and had decreased tone in her lower extremities. Her EEG showed diffuse slowing, attributed to medications or metabolic encephalopathy. A SPECT scan showed decreased activity in the right basal ganglia, left temporal lobe, and both parietal lobes.

After 12 days she was transferred to a university center where: "*She was mute and immobile, with rigid posturing, increased muscular tone, cog wheeling, and waxy flexibility. She was occasionally tremulous, displayed stereotypic movements of rolling over and bicycling her lower extremities, chewing, picking at her bed sheets, and whispering to her self.*"

A diagnosis of neuroleptic malignant syndrome was made and bromocriptine and lorazepam prescribed.[71] Fever, tachycardia, and hypertension improved, but mutism, perplexity, confusion, staring, echolalia, and echopraxia persisted. Her gait was "robot-like" and examination showed her limbs to be rigid with waxy flexibility. She was incontinent of urine and needed assistance with activities of daily living. The physical examination was otherwise normal.

After a week of many consultations, ECT was prescribed. "*Following the third ECT, the patient displayed marked improvement. She became oriented, had brighter affect, responded to questions…no detectable rigidity or cogwheeling…movements were fluent* (sic) *and less clumsy.…After the 7th ECT she was dramatically improved…*" The signs of catatonia, mood disorder, and psychosis resolved.

Numerous reports of catatonia in adolescents dot the literature. Dhossche and Bouman (1997a,b) summarized the diagnoses in 30 adolescents and children with catatonia described in the literature between 1966 and 1996. Eleven patients had been diagnosed as suffering from atypical or brief psychotic disorders, 10 had a neurologic or a general medical condition (epilepsy, drug intoxication, viral infection), six had a mood disorder, and three had schizophrenia. Of the patients with atypical psychoses, three were seen also to have a developmental disorder (two with infantile autism; one with mental retardation). Stupor or catalepsy (27/30), mutism (26/30), posturing/grimacing/stereotypy (16/30), echolalia or echopraxia (4/30), and excessive motor activity (4/30) were the catatonic features that met DSM-IV specifier criteria. The frequency of the catatonic features in adolescents was comparable to the frequencies in adults.

Cohen and his associates (1999) describe their personal experience with nine catatonic adolescent psychiatric patients. Six patients were classified as schizophrenic, one as schizophreniform, and two as bipolar depressed, with each responding to either benzodiazepines or ECT. Cohen et al. reviewed published reports finding data on 42 patients, with 20 (48%) suffering from a mood disorder, nine as bipolar depressed and 11 as unipolar depressed. Seven (17%) patients were suffering from schizophrenia. Among the neurologic etiologies, epilepsy was the most frequent. In a report presented at the 2001 Mac Keith conference from the same clinic, Flament added five catatonic patients, again reporting the efficacy of ECT.[72] The latest report from this group assessed the attitudes of patients and parents to their experiences with ECT after a mean of 4.5 years. Their attitudes were mostly positive and ECT was considered to have been helpful.[73]

In a retrospective study in a University-based inpatient service, catatonia was identified in six of 12 adolescents treated with ECT. Each benefited.[74] In another survey, consecutive patients attending a child psychiatric out-patient clinic during a four-month period were examined using a catatonia rating scale.[75] Of 62 patients with a psychiatric illness, 11 had two or more signs of catatonia. Eight of the 11 subjects had a diagnosis of mood disorder. The patients were first treated with lorazepam and antipsychotic medications for up to nine days. When relief was not obtained, ECT was administered to nine patients, with relief achieved in all within four ECT.

A clinical report by Kinrys and Logan (2001) describes a second episode of catatonia in an adolescent male diagnosed as suffering from bipolar disorder. He scored very high on a catatonia rating scale, responded transiently to intravenous lorazepam, and was successfully treated with six ECT. In summarizing the literature, the authors reported 43 examples of pediatric catatonia.

In a doctoral thesis, Garry Walter (2002) has completed a detailed review of the reports of ECT in young persons to the end of 1999, finding 194 reports with adequate information. The highest number (81) met criteria for manic episodes or bipolar disorder, with 62 (74%) remitting or improving markedly. At six-months follow-up for 35 patients, 26 (74%) were functioning well. Similar data for catatonia (27) and NMS (6) found 20 (74%) and four (67%) remitted.

Children and adolescents develop NMS. A 12-year-old boy developed fever, autonomic instability, and muscle rigidity in response to haloperidol.

He responded to withdrawal of haloperidol and treatment with lorazepam. Hynes and Vickar (1996) describe a 12-year-old boy who developed fever, autonomic instability, and muscle rigidity in response to haloperidol. They also summarize reports of 34 similar incidents of NMS among adolescents.[76] Another report that year (Zuddas et al., 1996) describes a 15-year-old girl with two episodes of catatonia and psychosis responding slowly to clobazam and risperidone therapy. The authors ascribe the improvement to the use of risperidone. This conclusion is criticized by Dhossche and Petrides (1997) who suggest that the improvement in catatonic signs was best explained by the use of clobazam. The suggestion that risperidone relieved catatonia is also inconsistent with many reports of the induction of MC/NMS by risperidone.[77]

Patients with childhood autism exhibit catatonia. Wing and Atwood (1987) divided their patients with autism into three descriptive groups.[78] In the *aloof* form, they found examples of mutism in half the sample, with echolalia, echopraxia, repetitiveness, stereotypy, facial grimacing, odd flapping movements, and insensitivity to pain as other characteristic features. In another review, Wing (1987) found the incidence of autism to be associated with mental retardation in half the patients, and a high incidence of epilepsy.

More recently, Wing and Shah (2000a,b) used a standardized catatonia rating scale to describe features of catatonia among 506 consecutive referrals in six years to a child communications social disorders program in the U.K. Of these, 30 children with autism (6%) met diagnostic criteria for catatonia.[79] It was not detected in those under age 15 years, but in those aged 15–50 years, catatonia was found in 17% of all referrals. Odd gait and posturing were the most common features (63%). Pathological inertia (difficulty starting movement or stopping once started) was the next most common. Twelve children were psychotic and seven excited. Four (13%) had epilepsy.

A retrospective literature review of the incidence of autism in reports from 1966 to 1997 found its incidence to be increasing.[80] It is unclear whether the increase is a change in psychopathology or increased recognition of the syndrome in young children and the inclusion of atypical cases.[81]

In a clinical report, catatonia was described in a 15-year-old boy with life-long features of autism.[82] The catatonic features did not resolve with clozapine alone but did resolve when lorazepam (2.5 mg three times a day) was added. Three patients with autistic disorder were also shown to have the catatonic features of mutism, echolalia/echopraxia, and stereotypy.[83]

A 14-year-old boy with a pre-existing history of autism exhibited stupor with mutism, akinesia, rigidity, waxy flexibility, posturing (including psychological pillow), facial grimacing, and involuntary movements of the upper extremities. While intravenous amobarbital elicited no benefit, intravenous zolpidem did. A course of ECT caused dramatic and sustained relief of the catatonia without a change in the symptoms of autism.[84]

The Prader–Willi syndrome (PWS) is a developmental disorder characterized by hypotonia, hypogonadism, excessive appetite and obesity, short stature, dysmorphic facies, self-injury, and mental retardation.[85] One report describes a 17-year-old adolescent boy with PWS who developed an acute onset of catatonia with stupor, staring, incontinence, mutism, rigidity, waxy flexibility, posturing, refusal to eat or drink, and disruption of the sleep-wake cycle. He failed to improve when treated with haloperidol but catatonia gradually resolved with lorazepam (4 mg/day). Persistent psychosis was then successfully treated with risperidone (6 mg/day).[86]

Motor disorders were systematically assessed in 236 patients in a hospital for the mentally handicapped.[87] Of the signs of catatonia, 48% exhibited psychological pillow, 40% echopraxia, 20% posturing, 6% passive resistance, and 4% repetitive speech. Many other movement problems were noted.

Reports of catatonia are also prominent in pre-pubescent children referred for ECT. An 11-year-old depressed boy with suicidal intent, exhibited catatonia and head banging. His illness remitted with ECT.[88] A 12-year-old girl with mania and catatonic features responded similarly.[89] Another pre-pubescent boy with depressive stupor, with a positive dexamethasone suppression test paralleling similar findings in adults, was successfully treated.[90] The successful treatment with ECT of an eight and a half year-old girl with major depression and catatonic symptoms was reported.[91]

What conclusions can be drawn from this literature? The signs of catatonia in the young are similar to those in other age groups. Further, catatonia is sufficiently frequent among children and adolescents that any young patient with motor symptoms should be formally assessed for it. When catatonia is found, the differential diagnosis in order of decreasing frequency is mood disorder, seizure disorder, developmental disorder and autism, and then schizophrenia. The same treatments for catatonia that are effective in adults have been found useful in pediatric patients.[92]

A caveat in treating adolescent depressed patients with ECT, however, is that clinical improvement and recovery may be slower than the rate of recovery in adults. Adolescent patients may require more treatments than that required by elderly patients. The prescription of a fixed number of treatments in an ECT course, using adult standards, is not recommended for young patients because discontinuing a course of ECT after the usual adult course of six to eight treatments is likely to be associated with an incomplete or a poor outcome. The number of treatments needed for a sustained effect may well be double the number in elderly adults.[93]

Special attention needs to be paid to persons with pervasive developmental disorders (PDD). As they often have language impairment and may be mute, the presence of mutism should not be deemed a sign of catatonia unless it is episodic. Other features, especially posturing, echolalia/echopraxia, and stereotypy need to be present. Catatonia should also be considered when adolescents have episodes of irritability and excitement followed by periods of mutism, catalepsy, and negativism. As young patients run the same risks for MC/NMS as adults, it is preferable to use alternative forms of sedation rather than antipsychotic drugs for disruptive behavior.[94]

Other syndromes with signs of catatonia have been described in young patients. British authors delineate a *pervasive refusal syndrome* (Lask et al., 1991). The patients are mute, withdrawn, apathetic, with a paucity of interactions. The syndrome is assumed to result from psychological trauma, and the treatment offered is individual and family psychotherapy. Graham and Foreman (1995) describe an 8-year old girl who stopped eating and drinking some weeks after a viral infection. She became withdrawn and mute, complained of muscle weakness, developed incontinence of urine and feces, and was unable to walk. She was treated with psychotherapy and family therapy for more than a year, after which she was discharged back to her family in partial remission. The records of the patients described by Lask et al. (1991) and Graham and Foreman (1995) meet our criteria for catatonia. The failure to treat the 8-year-old girl for catatonia, either with benzodiazepines or ECT, was criticized.[95]

A syndrome of *idiopathic recurrent stupor* (IRS) is described in patients who exhibit periodic stupor without toxic, metabolic, or structural brain damage. Some patients have exhibited fast 14 Hz background activity in the EEG. Administration of flumazenil resolves both the abnormalities in EEG and in behavior.[96] The relationship of IRS to the syndromes of catatonia, autism, myalgic encephalopathy, pervasive refusal syndrome, and varieties of mental retardation is a puzzle that now interests child and adolescent psychiatrists.[97] Regardless of their pathophysiologies, the presence of catatonia in patients with these syndromes warrants recognition as a treatable aspect of their disorders.

Conditions that may be mistaken for catatonia

Elective mutism, metabolic-induced stupor, Parkinson disease, obsessive–compulsive disorders, malignant hyperthermia, locked-in syndrome, and stiff-person syndrome are among conditions that may be difficult to distinguish from catatonia. These disorders warrant different treatments and their diagnostic separation from catatonia is necessary.

Mutism

Mutism alone is not sufficient to diagnose catatonia. At least one, and preferably two, motor features listed in Chapter 2 (Table 2.1) should also be present for the diagnosis of the syndrome. *Elective mutism* is the failure to speak and respond to questions, occurring as a singular feature. It is a conscious withholding of speech usually found in an otherwise vigilant person. Elective mutism is usually associated with a pre-existing personality disorder, environmental stress, or both. When these factors are identified and the stressors dealt with, mutism resolves.

Catatonic mutism may be fluctuating and variable in severity. Occasionally, a mute, nonspontaneous catatonic patient responds briefly when spoken to (speech-prompt catatonia) or exhibits echolalia. The mutism of catatonia or a psychotic disorder rarely occurs in isolation. Occasionally, delusional and suspicious patients refuse to speak because they distrust the examiner, have other suspicions, or are responding to command hallucinations. Such behavior is typically associated with irritability, failure to cooperate, or a history of chronic illness secondary to drug abuse or alcoholism. They have no other features of catatonia and their refusal to speak is unchanged with injections of lorazepam. Effective treatment of the psychosis also resolves mutism. Because catatonia is common among acutely hospitalized psychiatric patients

(Chapter 5), any mute psychiatric patient should be fully assessed for catatonia and challenged with a benzodiazepine.

A report (Altshuler et al., 1986) describing an experience with 22 psychiatric patients recently ill with mutism found five to have schizophrenia (four paranoid and one catatonic subtype), and 12 to have a mood disorder (two secondary to neurologic disease). Other etiologies included phencyclidine intoxication, cerebral stroke, and post-encephalitic parkinsonism.

Bradykinesia (slowing of movement) and *bradyphrenia* (slowing of cognition) can be so profound that they resemble mutism. A toxic sedative–hypnotic drug state or severe depression are the likely underlying conditions, and treating these states usually resolves this form of mutism.

Neurologic disorders may be associated with the patient's failure to speak. *Postictal mutism* may follow seizures of sudden onset, with paroxysmal and stereotyped motor movements and altered consciousness. The duration of the illness is short and the patient is amnestic for the event. The EEG is usually abnormal, consistent with a seizure disorder.

Mutism may follow a cerebrovascular stroke.[98] With brain-stem lesions, mutism is a dominant feature in the states labeled akinetic mutism, apallic syndrome, locked-in syndrome and others (see also Chapter 3). *Transcortical motor aphasia* is typically associated with an initial period of mutism without other motor changes. Such episodes are usually marked by a history of cardiovascular disease, sudden onset, and an initial episode late in life.

Stupor

Reduced arousal is consistent with catatonia, but like mutism, its appearance alone is insufficient to diagnose catatonia. Stupor occurs with melancholic depression, drug intoxications (sedative-hypnotics, opioids, and opiates), metabolic disorders, cerebrovascular stroke, post-seizure states, after traumatic brain injury, brain stem encephalitis, basilar aneurysms with pontine infarction, and brain tumors that effect the midbrain directly or by mass effects. A syndrome of idiopathic recurring stupor that resolves with the benzodiazepine antagonist flumazenil has been described.[99]

A careful history and a detailed general medical examination for associated features frequently reveal an explanation for the stupor. An EEG is usually normal in catatonic stupor, but a stupor may be associated with diffuse slowing of EEG frequencies, suggesting an encephalopathy. Malignant cata-tonia, however, is also associated with diffuse EEG slowing.[100]

Parkinson disease

About 2% of the total population and as much as 20% of persons over age 65 are affected by Parkinson disease (PD). Bradykinesia, rigidity, and resting tremor are the main features. About half the patients are depressed. The patients also complain of slowness of thinking and impaired mem-ory. About 15% of patients have a family history for PD, and about 30% develop dementia.[101] PD is distinguished from catatonia by the presence of tremor, pill-rolling finger movements, and short-stepping, shuffling gait disturbances. Typically PD patients do not posture bizarrely.

Akinetic parkinsonism closely resembles akinetic mutism.[102] The patient is rigid and mute, often with peculiar and abnormal postures. This condition usually follows years of illness with PD, and is typically accompanied by dementia. Diagnostic problems arise, however, when the patient is young, because early onset parkinsonism develops quickly with akinesia and mutism as the predominating features. Tremor and cogwheel rigidity are often absent. Drug screen will be negative and the EEG is typically normal. Sedative-hypnotics do not relieve the syndrome, but anticholinergic drugs have some benefit. A test dose of diluted benztropine mesylate (2 mg IV) may produce relief within 30 minutes.

Obsessive–compulsive disorder

In patients with catatonia, the repetitive nature of their stereotypes, grimac-ing, and tics brings the diagnosis of obsessive–compulsive disorder (OCD) into the differential diagnosis. At a time when the psychodynamic image of catatonia dominated psychiatric thinking, a patient with obsessive–compulsive features who also exhibited catatonic features was described in detail. Both catatonia and OCD were interpreted as psychologic defenses to internalized conflicts.[103]

A high incidence of catatonia is described among patients with bipolar disorder.[104] A 35% incidence of OCD features has been described among pa-tients with bipolar disorder, similar to the incidence among patients with unipolar depressive disorder.[105] The most parsimonious explanation for these findings is that the mannerisms and rituals of catatonic patients were misinterpreted as signs of OCD. Some patients, however, clearly suffer from both OCD and mania, an association warranting further study.[106]

The signs of OCD and of catatonia are also prominent in adolescents with autism. Among these patients, it is difficult to tease out and separate the OCD, catatonia, and autism.[107] When catatonia is identified among autistic patients, it may be prudent to offer clinical trials with the treatments for catatonia. The same difficulty may occur in patients with mental retardation who develop repetitive head-banging and self-mutilation. A clinical description finds one such patient responding to ECT.[108]

Gilles de la Tourette's disorder (GTD) is a disorder with prominent vocal and motor tics, echolalia, and echopraxia. The patients have signs of both OCD and of catatonia.[109] GTD typically has a childhood age-of-onset and a pre-eminence of vocalizations. GTD has been described in a patient with infantile autism.[110] In one depressed patient with catatonia, scatological vocalizations were prominent during her acute illness and disappeared when she responded to ECT (*Patient 2.7*). Efficacy for ECT in GTD has also been reported.[111] Here, again, the prominence of motor signs that are features of catatonia offers an alternative therapeutic approach to these patients that warrants wider consideration.

Although adult patients with OCD are aware of the inappropriateness of their ideas and actions, their symptoms are demanding and take on a life of their own. Obsessions about contamination (of themselves or others) are difficult to separate from delusions and depressive ruminations. The accompanying compulsions may become stereotypic and elaborately manneristic. OCD with elaborate mannerisms can be distinguished from catatonia in that the mannerisms and stereotypes occur daily for many years rather than in episodes. Checking, orderliness, and tics tend to be present in OCD and an anxious–fearful personality disorder usually predates the OCD behavior. A family history of OCD or tic disorder is often present. In patients with catatonia, a family history of mood disorders, particularly mania, is more likely. OCD has recently been associated with basal ganglia hypermetabolism on SPECT and PET (positron emission tomography), whereas catatonia is more often associated with hypometabolism.[112] Secondary OCD, due to basal ganglia lesions (particularly non-dominant), is often associated with manic-like episodes and the combination of mania and OCD may appear to be an episode of mania with catatonic signs. An MRI may reveal lesions as secondary to an ischemic stroke.[113]

Malignant hyperthermia

This syndrome is a rare autosomal-dominant genetic disorder in which the skeletal muscles respond to inhalation anesthetics and depolarizing muscle relaxants (succinylcholine) by hyper-metabolism, producing muscular rigidity and tremor, fever, and elevated CPK levels. About 70% of patients die when untreated. The diagnosis is confirmed with a muscle biopsy. When exposed to halothane and caffeine, the biopsy shows a characteristic reaction that is not seen in catatonic states. In early descriptions of NMS, the motor signs were seen to be similar to malignant hyperthermia and treatment with dantrolene was recommended.[114]

Stiff-person syndrome and locked-in syndrome

The stiff-person syndrome (SPS) is a rare condition of unknown etiology characterized by progressive symmetric rigidity of axial muscles with painful spasms precipitated by touch, passive stretching, startling noises, movement, and emotional stimuli.[115] The symptoms are relieved during sleep, general anesthesia, myoneural blockade, peripheral nerve blockade, and with benzodiazepines and with baclofen. Some patients exhibit increased cerebrospinal fluid antibodies against glutamic-acid-decarboxylase.

The locked-in syndrome (LIS) is characterized by total immobility except for vertical eye movements and blinking.[116] Cortical functions are spared. The syndrome is caused by an acute lesion in the ventral pons with both cerebral peduncles involved paralyzing the cranial nerves. Consciousness is preserved and is demonstrated by voluntary blinking in response to questions. Synonyms for LIS are *pseudo-coma* and the *de-afferented state.*

These two syndromes are reminiscent of descriptions of primary akinetic mutism and benign stupor.[117] We find no record of the use of benzodiazepines or ECT for these conditions. The signs of catatonia are sufficient, however, to consider benign stupor in the differential diagnosis and to administer a lorazepam or barbiturate challenge test in the evaluation of these patients. An improvement in response, even if transient, should encourage a treatment for catatonia.

ENDNOTES

1 Bush et al., 1996a.

2 Berger, 1929. Berger published 14 original reports between 1929 and his death in 1941. His major works on the EEG were translated by P. Gloor, 1969.

3 Davis and Davis, 1939; Hill and Parr, 1963.

4 Engel and Romano, 1944; Engel and Rosenbaum, 1945; Gjessing et al., 1967.

5 Walter, 1944.

6 Kennard et al., 1955; Kennard and Schwartzmann, 1957; Hill and Parr, 1963.

7 Cooper and Shapira, 1973.

8 Lim et al., 1986; Primavera et al., 1994; Louis and Pflaster, 1995; Cocito and Primavera, 1996.

9 Unpublished observations, 1994–96, SUNY at Stony Brook (New York).

10 Fink and Kahn, 1957; Fink, 1979.

11 Shagass, 1954; Fink, 1958.

12 Fink, 1958.

13 Fink, 1968, 1969, 1985.

14 Nemeroff and Loosen, 1987.

15 Carroll et al., 1981; American Psychiatric Association, 1987; Nelson and Davis, 1997.

16 Hall and Reis, 1983; Linkowski et al., 1984; McCall, 1989; Ferro et al., 1991.

17 Rosebush and Mazurek, 1991a; Weller and Kornhuber, 1992a; Ben-Shachar et al., 1993; Sachdev, 1993; Lee, 1998; Penatti et al., 1998; Wirshing et al., 1998; Peralta et al., 1999; Hofmann et al., 2000.

18 Rosebush and Mazurek, 1991a; Raja et al., 1994; Lee, 1998; Peralta et al., 1999.

19 American Psychiatric Association, 1994 DSM-IV.

20 Kraepelin, 1921, translated 1976.

21 Bleuler, 1950, p. 211; Kraepelin, 1971.

22 McKenna et al., 1994; Dhossche and Petrides, 1997.

23 Fink, 1999b.

24 O'Connor et al., 2001.

25 Hansen and Bolwig, 1988; Allen et al., 2000.

26 Cohen et al., 1997a,b.

27 Bright-Long and Fink, 1993. Following a fall in December 2001 in which she suffered a severe head trauma, she again exhibited a depressive pseudodementia syndrome and was hospitalized. Lorazepam, lithium, and risperidone medications, and parenteral feedings brought no relief. ECT was re-instated and within the course of six ECT she was able to return home.

28 Taylor, 1999, chapter 12; Fink 1999a.

29 Chandrasena, 1986.

30 Wade et al., 1987.

31 Fink (1999a), patient Hancock (p. 65–6).

32 Zarr and Nowak, 1990; Still et al., 1998.

33 Guze, 1967; Fricchione et al., 1990. See *Patient 3.5.*

34 Breakey and Kala, 1977; Case 2.

35 Akhtar and Ahmad, 1993.

36 Johnson and Lucey, 1987, Case 2. Also Hunter, 1973.

37 Chopra and Dandiya, 1974, 1975.

38 Good, 1976.

39 Neveu et al., 1973.

40 Turek and Hanlon, 1977; Zawilska and Nowak, 1986.

41 Mann et al., 1986, 1990; Philbrick and Rummans, 1994; Fricchione et al., 1997, 2000.

42 Arnold and Stepan, 1952; Tolsma, 1967; Geretsegger and Rochowanski, 1987; Philbrick and Rummans, 1994.

43 Modell, 1997; Zalsman et al., 1998; Deuschle and Lederbogen, 2001.

44 Fruensgaard 1976; Levy 1984; Hauser et al., 1989.

45 Hermesh et al., 1989b; Yamawoki and Ogawa, 1992.

46 Rosebush et al., 1999.

47 Ezrin-Waters et al., 1976.

48 Taylor, 1999: 379–409.

49 Kosten and Kleber, 1988.

50 McCarron et al., 1981; Taylor, 1999.

51 Taylor, 1999, chapter 3.

52 Fisher, 1989; Schmuecker et al., 1992.

53 Dupont et al., 1999.

54 Primavera et al., 1994.

55 Bear, 1986; Bolwig, 1986; Trimble, 1991.

56 Thompson and Greenhouse, 1968; Lugaresi et al., 1971; Weintraub, 1977; Yoshino et al., 1998; Kanemoto et al., 1999.

57 Swartz, 1985a,b.

58 Trimble, 1978.

59 Taylor, 1999.

60 Abrams, 1997; Fink et al., 1999.

61 Epstein, 1991.

62 Ganser, 1904.

63 Ganser and Shorter, 1965.

64 Wertham, 1949, cited in Whitlock, 1967.

65 Whitlock, 1967.

66 Lieberman, 1954.

67 Chapter 8. Also Taylor, 1990; Philbrick and Rummans, 1994; Ahuja, 2000a.

68 Wing and Atwood, 1987; Wing, 1987; Realmuto and August, 1991; Rogers et al., 1991; Moise and Petrides, 1996; Dhossche and Bouman, 1997a,b; Dhossche, 1998; Cohen et al., 1999; Zaw et al., 1999; Wing and Shah, 2000a; Thakur A, Jagadheesan K, Dutta S and Sinha VK. Incidence and phenomenology of catatonia in children and adolescents: A descriptive study. Personal communication, August 2001.

69 Hynes and Vickar, 1996.

70 Ghazziudin et al., 2002.

71 Bromocriptine (1.25 increased to 2.5 mg twice daily); lorazepam (1–2 mg thrice daily.

72 Mac Keith Conference, *Catatonia in Childhood*, London, September 2001.

73 Taieb et al., 2001.

74 Moise and Petrides, 1996.

75 Thakur A, Jagadheesan K, Dutta S and Sinha VK. Incidence and phenomenology of catatonia in children and adolescents: A descriptive study. Personal communication, August 2001.

76 Hynes and Vickar, 1996.

77 Meterissian, 1996; Sharma et al., 1996; Hasan and Buckley, 1998; Bahro et al., 1999; Robb et al., 2000; Bottlender et al., 2002.

78 The report comes from the UK National Autistic Society's tertiary referral center at the Elliott House Centre for Social and Communication Disorders in London.

79 Bush et al., 1996a.

80 Gillberg and Wing, 1999.

81 Chakrabarti and Frombonne, 2001.

82 Dhossche, 1998.

83 Realmuto and August, 1991.

84 Zaw et al., 1999.

85 Holm et al., 1993.

86 Dhossche and Bouman, 1997b.

87 Rogers et al., 1991.

88 Black et al., 1985.

89 Carr et al., 1983.

90 Powell et al., 1988.

91 Cizadlo and Wheaton, 1995.

92 Fink, 1999a.

93 Fink 1999a; American Psychiatric Association, 2001.

94 Taylor, 1999; chapters 11 and 12.

95 Fink and Klein, 1995.

96 Tinuper et al., 1992, 1994; Palmieri 1999.

97   Mac Keith Conference,*Catatonia in Childhood*, London, September 2001.

98   Segarra and Angelo, 1970; Altshuler et al., 1986; Ungvari and Rankin, 1990; Taylor, 1999.

99   Tinuper et al., 1992, 1994; Palmieri 1999.

100 Plum and Posner, 1980. For reviews of EEG findings in psychoses see Carroll and Boutros, 1995; Sengoku and Takagi, 1998.

101 Taylor, 1999.

102 Patterson, 1986.

103 Blacker, 1966.

104 Johnson and Lucey, 1987; Hermesh et al., 1989a.

105 Krüger et al., 1995, 2000a, b.

106 Bräunig et al., 1998, 1999; Krüger et al., 2000b.

107 Wing 1987; Rogers et al., 1991; Dhossche and Bouman, 1997a,b; Dhossche, 1998; Wing and Shah, 2000a,b.

108 Fink, 1999a.

109 Araneta et al., 1975; Shapiro et al., 1988; Cohen et al., 1988; Kushner, 1999.

110 Realmuto and Main, 1982.

111 Guttmacher and Cretella, 1988; Rapaport et al., 1998.

112 Baxter et al., 1987; Nordahl et al., 1989.

113 Cummings and Mendez, 1984; Lauterbach 1995.

114 Caroff et al., 1998a; Lazarus et al., 1989; Davis et al., 2000.

115 Heckl, 1987; Blum and Jankovic, 1991; Barker et al., 1998.

116 Bauer et al., 1979.

117 Bricolo, 1977.

Catatonia is measurable and common

Kahlbaum correctly states that once one recognizes the many characteristic and
conspicuous signs of catatonia, it is not possible to confuse them with other illnesses.
Secondly, I willingly add, that not only the individual characteristic signs which
Kahlbaum so masterfully identified, but the total syndrome that the patients present, is
identifiable.

Neisser, 1887[1]

Of the motor signs described by Kahlbaum, how many are useful in making
the diagnosis of the catatonia syndrome? How often is the syndrome identified? In studies of incidence, researchers used the more prominent items
of mutism, posturing, negativism, catalepsy, and stereotypy as criteria for
catatonia. More recently, rating scales with more extensive lists of signs have
been developed. In the search for a structure among the signs of catatonia,
factor analytic studies have been done. Despite this experience with catatonia
over the past few decades, its role in the DSM and ICD psychiatric classification systems remains restricted and problematic. In this chapter, we describe
this experience and suggest modifications in classification systems.

DSM classification of catatonia

After Kahlbaum's 1874 description, many reports confirmed the presence of
catatonia in patients with psychotic and mood disorders (see Chapter 1). In
a decision that strongly influenced posterity, Kraepelin incorporated catatonia as a feature of dementia praecox. He described the onset as subacute,
often beginning with a depressed mood. About 13% of his catatonic patients
achieved a cure that could last up to 10 years, a better prognosis than that
found in the other forms of dementia praecox where the recovery rate was
considerably lower.[2] His concept limiting catatonia to dementia praecox was

adopted by Bleuler, and this image has dominated psychiatric classification systems for much of the 20th Century, despite many descriptions of catatonia among patients with manic-depressive illness, toxic states, and neurologic disorders.

The American classification of psychiatric disorders DSM-II (1952) identified abnormalities in behavior as 'reactions' to stressors. Catatonia was identified as a subtype of schizophrenic reaction and was one of many disorders of psychogenic origin.[3] DSM-III (1980) and DSM-IIIR (1987) classifications recognized patients with catatonia only as a subtype of schizophrenia, catatonic type (295.2). DSM-IV (1994) continued this practice but added a category of "*Catatonic disorder due to . . . general medical condition or side-effect of a medication [293.89]*." It also included a specifier within the diagnoses of mania and depression, but without a numeric category designation.[4]

The International ICD classification system is similar to the DSM. ICD-10 includes a class of "organic catatonic disorder" (F06.1).[5] To meet the criteria, a patient must be suffering a psychiatric disorder due to brain damage or "physical illness," with stupor and/or negativism, excitement, and rapid alternation between stupor and excitement.

The limited role of catatonia in the present DSM and ICD classifications is inconsistent with the scientific literature and clinical experience. In DSM-IV, the criteria for the diagnosis of the catatonic subtype of schizophrenia [295.20], requires the patient to exhibit two of the following:

(1) Motoric immobility, as evidenced by catalepsy, (including waxy flexibility) or stupor.
(2) Excessive motor activity (that is apparently purposeless and not influenced by external stimuli).
(3) Extreme negativism (an apparently motiveless resistance to all instructions or maintenance of a rigid posture against attempts to be moved) or mutism.
(4) Peculiarities of voluntary movement as evidenced by posturing (voluntary assumption of inappropriate or bizarre postures), stereotyped movements, prominent mannerisms, or prominent grimacing.
(5) Echolalia or echopraxia.

No duration of these signs is stated, although the paragraph heading states that "*the subtypes of Schizophrenia are defined by the predominant symptomatology at the time of evaluation*."

These criteria are problematic for the clinician. The nonspecific features of immobility and excitement are sorted equally with the more specific features

Table 5.1 Recommended diagnostic criteria for catatonia

A. Immobility, mutism, or stupor of at least one hour duration, associated with at least one of the following: catalepsy, automatic obedience, or posturing, observed or elicited on two or more occasions

B. In the absence of immobility, mutism, or stupor, at least two of the following, which can be observed or elicited on two or more occasions: stereotypy, echophenomena, catalepsy, automatic obedience, posturing, negativism, ambitendency

of catalepsy, waxy flexibility, negativism, and mutism. While catalepsy and echophenomena are specific catatonic features, excessive motor activity and severe immobility are not. The excessive motor activity associated with catatonia is related to activity that is stimulus bound, i.e., influenced by external stimuli. Activities within the excitement phase may seem *purposeful* unless the patient is in a manic delirium. Also, the DSM-IV items 1, 3, and 4 include postural immobility, creating a redundancy within the criteria. Patients who are stuporous (criterion 1) are also often mute (criterion 3), another redundancy. Further, the duration criterion compromises reliability among observers, since echolalia and echopraxia come and go and the other features can be quite variable. Instead of the DSM criteria, we prefer the criteria in Table 5.1.

The dissatisfaction with the present DSM and ICD classification systems is widespread. Consideration is already underway for the development of DSM-V. The dissatisfaction was highlighted in discussions at recent meetings of the American Psychiatric Association where Professor Paul McHugh offered different perspectives, paralleling the classifications of medical disorders.[6]

An alternative classification for catatonia

It is necessary to discard the direct connection of catatonia with schizophrenia and find an alternative way to classify patients with catatonia. We propose that catatonia be defined as a separate entity with its own classification number, using the diagnostic criteria of Table 5.1. In DSM-IV, delirium is coded as 293.0, providing a model for catatonia. A similar separate category could be used for catatonia, perhaps co-opting the number now assigned to

Table 5.2 Proposed catatonia classification

29x.0 Catatonia
.1 Non-malignant catatonia (Kahlbaum syndrome) [criterion A]
.2 Delirious mania (excited catatonia) [severe mania or excitement plus criterion B]
.3 Malignant catatonia (MC/NMS) [criterion A plus fever, autonomic instability]

Modifiers
.y1 Secondary to a mood disorder
.y2 Secondary to a general medical condition or toxic state
.y3 Secondary to a brain disorder
.y4 Secondary to a psychotic disorder

---

another category. Each of the many faces of catatonia (Chapter 3) is evidence of similar pathology. For heuristic purposes, we see merit in providing subtypes for catatonia, following the classification model for other disorders. Such subtyping will encourage a closer look at symptomatology, course of illness, and more specific treatment algorithms (Table 5.2).

These subtypes also reflect differences in degrees of lethality, with the non-lethal form responding to benzodiazepines. The delirious forms are worsened by antipsychotic drugs, require higher doses of benzodiazepines (lorazepam, 10–20 mg daily), and respond best to ECT. The malignant forms require life support measures in addition to intensive ECT.

This classification recognizes the broad category of psychiatric conditions in which catatonia appears, separates the concept of catatonia from its restriction to a subtype of schizophrenia, and replaces "catatonia" as a modifier of affective states. It recognizes catatonia as reproducible and relatively stable even in diverse psychopathological states. Catatonia meets the definition of a syndrome because its characteristics are often found together, respond to treatment together, and are associated with a wide range of etiologies. Classifying catatonia as a separate entity encourages the definition of what is common among the signs, independent of a specific etiology. Using more specific criteria will reduce diagnostic false positives, i.e., labeling a patient as catatonic when he is not.

Categorizing catatonia in its own diagnostic class has consequences for treatment. Catatonic schizophrenia is usually treated with antipsychotic drugs in the same manner as patients with other types of schizophrenia (chapters 6 and 7). Other psychotropic drugs (antidepressant drugs and mood stabilizers) are rarely added, and if they are prescribed, it is timidly. ECT is rarely considered for a patient with schizophrenia. In contrast, psychiatrists who consider catatonia to be a syndrome look for the etiology and seek to treat it specifically. They prescribe sedative drugs (barbiturates and benzodiazepines), and when these fail, ECT for catatonia. The prognosis for recovery with such broad diagnostic and treatment approaches is excellent.

Placing catatonia in its own category also has implications for research. When researchers view a patient with catatonia as necessarily suffering from schizophrenia, as if catatonia is pathognomonic for the disorder, they lump schizophrenic patients into non-homogeneous samples for genetic, brain imaging, and biological marker assessments. Researchers have an optimism that these measures will provide specific markers, but the evidence for such specificity is lacking today. It is possible that the failure to find biological markers may result from the study of non-homogeneous samples of patients, including psychotic manic-depressive patients and catatonic patients in the populations sampled.

Historical basis for change in classification

The change in classification for catatonia from a subtype of a disorder to a separate entity would follow the recognition and change in other classifications in the past few decades. One example is the shift from identifying all patients with delusions as suffering from schizophrenia. During the first half of the 20th Century in the U.S., this association was strong. Epidemiology studies in the 1960s found an inflated incidence of schizophrenia in the U.S. compared to that in Europe. When the same patients were examined by U.S. and U.K. psychiatrists, U.S. psychiatrists labeled most as schizophrenic whereas U.K. psychiatrists identified many as suffering from manic-depressive illness or a personality disorder. Subsequent studies supported the U.K. judgements.[7] These observations weakened the connection between delusions and schizophrenia.

Despite these internationally recognized findings, the presence of delusions in a depressed patient required the DSM diagnosis of schizophrenia even when patients were predominantly depressed. A modest shift occurred when there developed a willingness to classify psychotic depressed patients in their own subtype following the observations that some depressed patients failed to recover despite adequate serum levels of imipramine and its metabolites. The presence of delusions was the defining marker for the poor responders.[8] The concept of a separate identifiable delusional form of depression gained credible support and a diagnostic class of major affective disorder "with psychotic features" was included in DSM-III in 1980 and in subsequent DSM versions.[9]

Another example of the classification change is in the consideration of delirium, "*a transient organic mental syndrome of acute onset, characterized by global impairment of cognitive functions, a reduced level of consciousness, attentional abnormalities, increased or decreased psychomotor activity, and a disordered sleep-wake cycle.*"[10] Delirium presents many patterns with characteristic signs and symptoms, has many causes, follows an unfavorable course when untreated or poorly treated, and another when treated properly.[11]

Catatonia is also a reversible brain disorder occurring as a feature of many psychiatric conditions. Like delirium, catatonia requires special management and treatments not typically prescribed for patients with schizophrenia. Like delirium, catatonia resolves fully when treated appropriately. Further, the prognostic implications are much more optimistic than are those associated with schizophrenia.

Using the behavioral response to treatments is another diagnostic method. Applying treatments to patients with diverse symptoms identifies the behaviors with good and bad response.[12] In a study of psychiatric patients assigned randomly to imipramine or chlorpromazine, various subtypes were identified.[13] Phobic adolescents responded and psychotic adolescents worsened with imipramine.[14] Patients with psychotic depression responded to chlorpromazine.[15] Although rejected by DSM-III and DSM-IV committees, the response to a test medicine is a valid method of classification. The response of catatonic patients to barbiturates and benzodiazepines and their worsening with antipsychotic drugs further justify their independent classification.

A helpful analogy also comes from congestive heart failure (CHF). It is recognized as a syndrome defined by the signs of fluid retention and pulmonary congestion. It has many causes including valvular heart disease, hypertension, and pericardial disease. It suggests a probable list of etiologies and prognoses. It calls for specific, and usually effective, acute treatments. Recognizing the syndrome of CHF has clinical usefulness, as does recognizing the syndrome of catatonia.

Frequency of identification

Since the introduction of psychotropic drugs and their rapid, broad, and symptomatic relief of psychiatric symptoms, detailed assessment of psychopathology has become an endangered art. Few training programs focus on it beyond describing the bare bones of the DSM classification. Catatonia was not recognized except when mutism, posturing, and rigidity dominated the condition. At one point, clinicians concluded that the syndrome had disappeared, despite systematic studies that reported it to be common (see Chapter 1).

Since 1980 American psychiatric residency programs have taught psychopathology to their students based on the DSM classification system. The students learn the criteria for the principal disorders, their definitions, and examples of each criterion. For example, auditory hallucinations are the signature criterion of schizophrenia. Hearing voices commenting about the patient's actions, echoing the patient's thoughts or voices talking to each other are the usual criteria. Classic texts of psychopathology, however, consider other characteristics, e.g., the clarity and duration of the voices. The neuropsychiatric literature also considers the time of day, prodromal and post-hallucinosis behavior, and the attributes associated with different etiologies. Paying attention to these aspects of psychopathology alters diagnostic considerations.

Patient 5.1   A 28-year-old man with a 10-year history of "schizophrenia" heard voices daily for many years. He had not worked. Antipsychotic medications allowed him to stay out of the hospital, but helped little more. The hallucinations were experienced only on awakening in the morning, ending after an hour or so. A consultant suggested the symptom might be evidence of a seizure disorder, and a trial of the anticonvulsant carbamazepine ended the hallucinosis.

Another example.

Patient 5.2   A 38-year-old married man with two children was hospitalized after a "suicide attempt." His wife found him pressing a gun to his chest. The man had a 10-year history of psychosis characterized by episodic delusions of persecution, being attacked by demons, and seeing and hearing them. During such episodes he was irritable. There was no evidence of a mood disorder, and the diagnosis of schizophrenia had been made. A consultant elicited the experience that the "demon" appeared in the distance as a small object that, as it approached, became bigger and changed to a shadowy figure standing next to the patient (Dysmegalopsia). Each episode was accompanied by anxiety, irritability, and auditory hallucinations. On the occasion of the "suicide attempt," the patient was holding the gun, waiting for the demon who recently had been seeking to "gain entry" into his body. The patient thought that he could shoot the demon, but would not harm himself. Because marriage in schizophrenic patients is infrequent, and their fertility rates are 1/10 that of the general male population, the consultant sought another explanation. Epilepsy was diagnosed and treated. The episodes of post-ictal psychosis ceased.

While the frequency with which catatonia was identified decreased during the 20th Century, particularly in the U.S. where almost all psychotic patients were diagnosed as schizophrenic during the DSM-II era (1952–80), the numbers of catatonic patients appears to have actually remained steady.[16] In 1919, Kraepelin diagnosed almost 20% of his 500 long-term hospitalized dementia praecox patients as catatonic.[17]

May (1922) surveyed the percentages of schizophrenic patients who were diagnosed as suffering from the catatonic subtype in different psychiatric institutions in the U.S. The range was wide, with 7.6% in New York and 23.2% in Massachusetts, averaging 12.1% nationally.

Comparing the diagnoses of patients within the same Finnish hospital, Achte (1961) reported 37% of 100 acutely admitted patients in the 1930s to have been diagnosed as catatonic compared with 11% in the 1950s. Another study found the incidence of catatonia to be 38% in the 1950s compared to 25% in the 1960s (Hogarty and Gross, 1966). The frequency of diagnoses of catatonia in the Iowa Psychopathic Hospital in the 1920s and the 1960s were reported as 14% and 8%.[18]

More recently, Carpenter et al. (1976) described the variation in the proportion of schizophrenic patients diagnosed as the catatonic subtype in samples from different parts of the world. The percentages averaged 8.2% (54 of 658 patients), with the highest as 21.8% in India and the lowest as 3.0% to 3.8% in U.K., Taiwan, and Denmark.

In a population survey in a single New York State county, Guggenheim and Babigian (1974a,b) found little change in the prevalence of catatonia over an 18-year period (1948–66) and concluded the population of catatonic

Table 5.3 Prevalence of catatonia in hospitalized psychiatric patients

Authors	Years surveyed	Sample size	Percent catatonic
Kraepelin	1920	500	20
May	1922	Several thousand	7.6 in NY
			23.1 in MA
			12.1 All USA
Achte	1930	100	37
Achte	1950	100	11
Hogarty and Gross	1950s	140	38
	1960s	166	25
Guggenheim and Babigian	1948–66	Countywide	16
Morrison	1920s, 1960s	500	14, 8
Carpenter et al.	1976	Worldwide	8.2 (India 21.8)
Velek and Murphy	1890–1970	Six 100-patient cohorts	10–20
Abrams and Taylor	1976	250 acutely hospitalized patients (13.5% catatonic). Of these, 120 manic	20
Pataki et al.	1985–90	43	7
Rosebush et al.	1990	140	9
Ungvari et al.	1994	212	8
Bush et al.	1996	215	9
Bräunig et al.	1998	61	31
Bush et al.	1999	249 ER patients	7.2
Healy	2000	112 (Wales)	14
		114 (India)	15
Lee et al.	2000	160	15

ER: emergency room; NY: New York; MA: Massachusetts

patients of their county to be steady at 1 per 1000 inhabitants. About 10% of all schizophrenic patients and 16% of all chronically hospitalized schizophrenic patients were of the catatonic type, similar to Kraepelin's original figure (Table 5.3).

In another study, the prevalence of catatonia was determined in cohorts of 100 schizophrenic patients each in the decades 1890, 1900, 1920, 1940, 1960, and 1970.[19] About 16% of the cohort on admission in 1890 (rediagnosed by these authors as schizophrenic) were catatonic (9% "withdrawn," 7% "excited"). In 1970, about 10% were catatonic on admission, with 9% "withdrawn" and only 1% "excited." Between 1900 and the 1960s, however, the diagnosis of catatonia increased to a peak of 20% of the cohort from 1940 to 1960. Most of the patients were of the "withdrawn" type. The disappearance of excited types in 1970 was due to their being classified as "manic" since there was no classification of catatonia in excited patients (American Psychiatric Association, 1952).

Catatonia was also identified prospectively among acutely hospitalized patients. Abrams and Taylor identified catatonic symptoms in 13.5% to 20% of patients who met their research criteria for mania. In their overall sample of 250 acutely hospitalized patients, 13.5% met criteria for catatonia (Abrams and Taylor, 1976). In a prospective study of patients with one or more catatonic symptoms, the same authors found that 62% were manic, 16% had neurologic disorders, 9% were depressed, and 7% met their research criteria for schizophrenia (Abrams and Taylor, 1977).

In a retrospective review of the records of patients diagnosed with schizophrenia, catatonic type (295.20) between 1985 and 1990, seven of 20 (35%) patients met criteria for manic depressive illness, with six of the patients meeting criteria for current mania (Pataki et al., 1992). A prospective study followed, and the criteria of two or more signs of catatonia readily identified 15 of 215 consecutive adult admissions (7%). Almost all the catatonic patients met DSM criteria for diagnoses other than schizophrenia (Bush et al., 1996a).

Using a check-list for catatonic symptoms in a survey of patients admitted to a Canadian university psychiatric facility, Rosebush et al. (1990) diagnosed catatonia in 9% (12 of 140) of patients. Less than 17% of the catatonic patients met the criteria for schizophrenia. And 8% (18 of 212) of admissions to a Hong Kong university hospital met criteria for catatonia (Ungvari et al., 1994a,b).

Studying the consecutive admissions of patients with the diagnosis of manic-depressive illness (manic or mixed type), confirmed by the structured clinical interview for DSM-IIIR, Bräunig et al. (1998, 2000) reported 19 of 61 (31%) patients had signs of catatonia. The patients with catatonia had more mixed episodes, more severe manic symptoms, more severe psychopathology, longer periods of hospitalization, and a more severe course than did the patients without catatonia.

Surveying the frequency of the diagnosis of catatonic schizophrenia before 1960 ("pre-neuroleptic era") as 30% to 38%, Höfler and Bräunig (1995) reported a decreased frequency to 10% in the subsequent period ('neuroleptic era'). They ascribed the difference to changes in diagnostic criteria, improved diagnosis of patients with structural brain lesions, and improvement in the rehabilitation and acute treatments of psychiatric patients.

The relevance of diagnostic criteria for studies of the frequency of catatonia is further analyzed by Bräunig et al. (1995b). They contrasted the criteria of Kahlbaum (1874), Bleuler (1911), Kraepelin (1913), Kleist (1943) and Leonhard (1957), ICD-10 (Dilling et al., 1991), and the symptomatic approaches of Morrison (1973), Gelenberg (1976), Abrams and Taylor (1976), Taylor and Abrams (1977), and Taylor (1990). They concluded that catatonic signs are non-specific, occurring in both patients with endogenous psychoses and with brain disorders. The reports by early authors of higher frequency of diagnoses of catatonic schizophrenia is due, in part, to the use of more signs of catatonia than defined by DSM and ICD criteria.

The role of changed diagnostic criteria is affirmed in another report.[20] Population samples from three different Austrian institutions were pooled and assessed by DSM and by Leonhard's diagnostic criteria for catatonic schizophrenia. The rates of diagnosis of catatonia among 174 consecutively admitted patients were 10.3% by DSM and 25.3% by Leonhard's criteria. The Leonhard system recognizes more behaviors (it includes about 49 features) as catatonic than do most North American psychiatrists. Many Leonhard features are traditional (e.g., grimacing, mumbling, automatic responses) but others are not generally considered catatonic (e.g., embarrassed smiles, incoherence, distractibility). The authors also report a decrease in frequency of diagnoses from 35% to 25% when they compare their samples with those of Leonhard's cohorts (1938–68, 1969–86).[21]

Healy used a catatonia rating scale to report the frequency of catatonia in two independent samples of hospitalized patients in Wales and India. He reported 16 of 112 (14%) in-patients in Wales and 17 of 114 (15%) in-patients in India met catatonia criteria.[22]

Thus, recent assessments that use standardized rating instruments in diverse academic medical centers find 6–15% of adult in-patients to meet criteria for catatonia. Using the broader criteria of European authors yields even higher frequencies.

Considering these various estimates and surveys among acute psychiatric inpatients, what is a likely annual figure for the prevalence of catatonia? Among a randomly selected one-third of non-Federal U.S. hospitals

($n = 6022$) for the year October 1996 to September 1997, there were 254,979 patients discharged with an ICD-9-CM major psychiatric diagnosis.[23] Of 160,135 patients who were classified with a mood disorder (296.xx), 42,581 were considered bipolar (296.4x, 296.5x, 296.60). Additionally, 68,298 patients were classified as schizophrenic (295.xx, but with no listing for catatonic subtype), and 17,816 as schizoaffective (295.70), a designation usually given to psychotic patients in manic or mixed manic states who have become chronically ill. Of other conditions often associated with catatonia, 5982 patients were discharged as suffering from drug withdrawal states (292.0), and 2748 with extrapyramidal disorders (333.xx). NMS was not listed as a discharge diagnosis. Assuming the 10% figure suggested by most studies of the incidence of catatonia, and that 20% of manic-depressive episodes are associated with catatonia, we estimate that 11,700 depressed, 8500 bipolar, 2000 schizoaffective, 6800 schizophrenic, 600 drug-related, and at least 275 patients with a discharge diagnosis of extrapyramidal disorder had sufficient catatonic features to meet DSM-IV criteria. This total of 29,875 acute psychiatric patients with catatonia annually is sampled from one-third of the hospitals.[24] Considering re-admissions of 20% (about 6000 patients), and then multiplying by three, the number of patients discharged from U.S. hospitals is substantially larger than the estimate of 30,000 suicides in the U.S. annually.[25] Not only is catatonia not rare, it is a major mental health issue.

The prevalence of catatonia in younger patients, however, is unclear. A summary of the published reports between 1977 and 1997 calculated that about 0.6% of adolescent acute in-patients exhibited catatonia, but these authors did not use systematic assessments.[26] In a forthcoming report, investigators using a catatonia rating scale found 18% of patients attending a child psychiatric out-patient clinic to have two or more signs of catatonia.[27]

Associated psychopathology

Excitement, impulsivity, and combativeness are nonspecific signs of catatonia in various rating scales. Their inclusion, however, likely reflects the lingering impression that catatonic excitement differs, in some unspecified ways, from catatonia in a manic patient. In an in-patient survey of the prevalence of catatonia, 7% of the patients exhibited two or more signs, with almost all patients exhibiting bradykinesia rather than excitement.[28] The surveyors assumed that any excited patients were heavily sedated in the emergency room before admission, masking the presentation. In another survey, to be published, of 249 patients over a two-month period in a psychiatric emergency room, 18 (7.2%) exhibited two or more signs of catatonia. Four patients (1.6%) were excited, eight (3.2%) retarded, three (1.2%) with fluctuating excitement and retardation, and three (1.2%) with neither excitement nor retardation.[29] In assessing specific signs of catatonia among the excited and the retarded patients, impulsivity, mannerisms, combativeness, and verbigeration were more frequently identified among excited patients, while mutism, staring, and rigidity were more frequent among retarded patients. Agitation, scored on a separate agitation rating scale, was present in 23% of the patients. Those rated as agitated had a fourfold increase in the incidence of catatonia. Using three or more signs as the criterion for catatonia, the prevalence was 11/249 (4.4%), and using four or more signs it was 7/249 (2.8%).[30]

The onset of catatonia and the relation to pre-morbid behavior has also been studied. At a 1932 catatonia symposium, two-thirds of patients (samples ranged from 20 to 154 cases) were reported to be irritable, seclusive, or stubborn before catatonia appeared, while one-third were normal.[31] These authors identified the catatonia syndrome by immobility and mutism, ignoring other features.

Abrams and Taylor, examining 55 catatonic patients, reported most patients to have from three to five features, among which mutism, stereotypy, and posturing were the most frequent (Abrams and Taylor, 1976). They did not test for patterns of symptoms and reported no differences among diagnostic groups. But inspection of the identified features in their manic-depressive and schizophrenic samples suggests that the schizophrenic patients exhibited posturing, stereotypy, and mutism, with 75% also showing stupor. These signs are included in the classic catatonic syndrome associated with dementia praecox. Their manic-depressive patients showed these features less often, but also exhibited echophenomena and automatic obedience.

The differences in findings among studies reflect different procedures or different populations. Hearst et al. (1971) and Benegal et al. (1993) studied patients who had been diagnosed as suffering from catatonic schizophrenia. Bush et al. (1996a) examined all patients admitted to an academic in-patient psychiatric unit. They used a formal rating scale and identified the patients with catatonia as those exhibiting two or more signs. Peralta et al. (1997)

looked at consecutive admissions who had a "cyclic alternating course" meeting criteria for manic and depressive episodes, co-occurring with catatonia and stupor. They sought to use Kahlbaum's definition of the syndrome. Abrams and Taylor (1977) took all consecutive admissions and assessed each for catatonic features. Interestingly, Peralta et al. (1997) initially identified 96 of 567 consecutive patients as catatonic (16.9%) whereas Abrams and Taylor (1977) identified 55 catatonic patients from about 350 consecutive admissions (15.7%). Both figures are strikingly similar to Kraepelin's, and despite Peralta et al.'s more restrictive criteria, confirm the finding by Abrams and Taylor that a patient having any one feature usually means that the patient will have several features, thus meeting criteria for the syndrome.

Stupor, mutism, and immobility were also the more common catatonic features in two other studies. The sample sizes were 20 and 45 patients.[32]

In developing a rating scale, Bush et al. (1996a) found mutism, withdrawal, posturing, negativism, and stupor to be the most common signs among acutely ill inpatients, and also among those examined in a hospital for chronic psychiatric patients.[33] A second study of catatonia in a chronically hospitalized sample found automatic obedience and posturing and catalepsy in more than 70% of the patients, with mutism and rigidity in 60%.[34] In a patient sample from India (Benegal et al., 1993), stupor, posturing, and negativism were the most frequent signs.

Factor analytic studies

Factor analytic studies have sought patterns among the signs of catatonia. In an early study of 55 catatonic patients, two factors were described.[35] One factor consisted of stupor, mutism, and negativism, corresponding to the classic picture of catatonia; the second consisted of automatic obedience, mutism, stereotypy, and catalepsy. The first factor was unrelated to diagnosis, gender, age-of-onset of illness, family history, or treatment response. The second factor was more often associated with mania.

Berrios (1996a) assessed the factor structure among the signs in Kahlbaum's 26 patients. A *neurological* factor of duration of illness, seizures, and hallucinations accounted for 29% of the variance, and a *psychotic depression* factor of hallucinations, delusions, and verbigeration accounted for 22% of the variance. He also found a robust correlation between age and waxy flexibility, with younger patients having a greater likelihood of displaying this sign. These factors differ from those presented by Abrams et al. (1979), described in the paragraph above.

In another study, four factors were abstracted from examinations of the motor, mood, and behavioral features of 34 catatonic patients.[36] One factor was similar to that described by Abrams et al. (1979) and a second factor added mania to these items. A third factor suggested compulsivity rather than catatonia, while the fourth was that of an unspecific mixed picture of signs.

Another factor analytic study concluded that the presence of three or more of 14 diagnostic signs was sufficient to confidently delineate the syndrome.[37] The study group consisted of 187 psychotic in-patients derived from 392 consecutive psychiatric admissions. Catatonia features were assessed using the Modified Rogers Scale identifying 14 catatonic signs that they deemed of diagnostic value.[38] Of 187 patients, 32 (17%) were included in the catatonia group after cluster analysis. Eleven of the 14 diagnostic signs discriminated among the groups, and any three signs were sufficient to include a patient in the catatonia group.

In a study of the incidence of catatonia in a cross-sectional assessment of a randomly selected cohort of 225 patients with chronic schizophrenia, 27.6% met the DSM-IV criteria.[39] The catatonic subjects had more negative symptoms, akinesia, and more severe illness globally than the non-catatonic counterparts. In a factor analysis, immobility-mutism, impulsivity, mannerism-stereotypy, and passive obedience were the identified factors. The authors conclude that while catatonia constitutes a distinct symptom cluster in schizophrenia, they failed to validate a separate catatonia subtype of schizophrenia.

The factor analyses suggest that different signs of catatonia cluster together (Table 5.4). Do these analyses offer a heuristic subtyping of catatonia? We see the following three clusters as derived from these factor studies.

The patterns of catatonic features that emerge reinforce clinical experience. The pattern in stupor fits the classic Kahlbaum syndrome. Those in delusional/delirious mania are easily recognizable but fluctuate in intensity as psychotic features and the patient's excitement wax and wane. The absence of observed catatonic features, even for hours, does not mean that the patient is no longer in catatonia. In contrast, the features observed in acute manic patients typically require the examiner to hunt for them. Their presence

Table 5.4 Catatonia symptom clusters

Acute mania	Delirious mania	Stupor
Echophenomena	Psychosis with excitement	Catalepsy
Ambitendency		Posturing
New accents in speech	Posturing	
Automatic obedience	Catalepsy	Mutism
(Verbigeration)	Waxy flexibility	Negativism
(Posturing)	Verbigeration	
(Mannerisms)	Automatic obedience	

( ): observed less commonly.

has the same diagnostic and treatment implications as other patterns of catatonia.

Rating scales

Interest in psychopharmacology and the need to systematically assess outcome encouraged the development of behavior rating scales to identify and measure the individual symptoms and signs that make up syndromes of interest. The first rating scales were used to evaluate mood and thought disorders. Some, like the Hamilton Depression Rating Scale and the Brief Psychiatric Rating Scale, are in wide use in research studies four decades after their introduction. Interest in motor disorders came later, with rating scales for Parkinson disorder,[40] tardive dyskinesia,[41] akathisia,[42] and retardation.[43] A detailed discussion of the merits and limitations of rating scales for motor disorders is supplied by Sachdev (1995). Rating scales for catatonia are a more recent development, although lists of motor signs to identify catatonia are reported as early as 1924.[44] An example of a recently developed rating scale is presented in Appendix I.

The variety of motor disorders that are definable, like the variety of delusional thoughts, is large.[45] Almost all scales begin with the signs reported by Kahlbaum. Each research group tailored their list of items to define catatonia as they understood the syndrome.[46] Seventeen motor signs are recognized in Kahlbaum's descriptions of his patients. From 21 to 40 signs are included in the rating scales by other authors.[47]

Three of the rating scales published between 1996 and 2000 report good inter-rater reliability with each instrument and across instruments. For example, four raters, using the Bochum-German rating scale, examined 71 catatonic subjects, reported pair-wise correlations of 0.96 to 0.97.[48] The University of Frankfurt scale inter-rater reliability for all individual items is also about 0.9.[49] The Stony Brook scale pair-wise inter-rater reliability was 0.9.[50]

Rating scales remind us of the catatonic features that need to be looked for. They are also used to monitor changes during treatment, allow comparison studies of prevalence, and to define subtypes. The characteristics of the retarded and excited types and the overlap of MC and NMS are promising applications. Rating scales are also educational tools used to teach students how to examine for and recognize the syndrome.

ENDNOTES

1 *Mit Recht aber sagt Kahlbaum, dass in allen Stadien dieser Krankheitsform (sc. der Katatonie) die charakteristischen Symptome so auffallende sind, dass eine Verwechselung mit anderen Krankheitsformen nicht wohl möglich ist, wenn man die Krankheitsform der Katatonie als solche überhaupt einmal anerkennt und kennen gelernt hat. Und ich möchte diesem Satze noch einen zweiten, freilich zunächt völlig subjectiven hinzufügen, dass nämlich nicht nur die einzelnen Symptome, welche Kahlbaum mit Meisterschaft gekennzeichnet, so charakteristisch sind, sondern auch das Totalgepräge, welche die Kranken darbieten.* Neisser, 1887: 84–85.

2 Kraepelin, 1976.

3 Coded as 000.x23, and 300.2. American Psychiatric Association, 1952.

4 American Psychiatric Association, 1994.

5 Ahuja, 2000b.

6 McHugh and Slavney, 1998.

7 Cooper et al., 1972.

8 Glassman et al., 1975; Kantor and Glassman, 1977; Avery and Lubrano, 1979; Kroessler, 1985.

9 Coded in the fifth digit as "4".

10 Lipowski, 1990.

11 Delirium is coded as 293.0 in DSM.

12 Fink and Kahn, 1961.

13 Klein and Fink, 1962a,b; Fink et al., 1964.

14 Klein, 1964, 1968; Pollack et al, 1965.

15 Fink et al., 1965.

16 Rogers, 1991, 1992.

17 Kraepelin, 1919.

18 Morrison et al., 1973; Morrison 1973.

19 Velek M and Murphy HB. The changing profile of catatonia: 1890–1970. Personal communication, 1979.

20 Stompe et al., 2002.

21 Leonhard, 1995.

22 Healy D. Incidence of catatonia in India and Wales, using the Stony Brook catatonia rating scale. Personal communication, May 12, 2000.

23 HCIA, 1998. The records of in-patient discharges from one-third of the non-Federal U.S. hospitals for the period October 1996 to September 1997 are coded by ICD-9-CM criteria. For comparison, the same records report 73,557 patient discharges for appendectomy, 72,539 for CAT-scan of the head, 16,439 for MRI of the head, and 84,728 for spinal tap. The numbers discharged with senile-presenile dementia [290.x] is 12,600 and for alcoholic psychoses [291.0] is 21,167.

24 HCIA, 1998.

25 American Association of Suicidology, 1999/1998.

26 Cohen et al., 1999.

27 Thakur A, Jagadheesan K, Dutta S and Sinha VK. Incidence and phenomenology of catatonia in children and adolescents: A descriptive study. Personal communication, August 2001.

28 Bush et al., 1996a

29 Bush G, Petrides G, Kaplan R, Fitou A, Balkunas M, Lerman M and Francis A. Excited and retarded catatonia. Personal communication, 1999.

30 Bush et al., personal communication, see endnote 26.

31 Hinsie, 1932a,b.

32 Hearst et al., 1971; Peralta et al., 1997.

33 Bush et al., 1996a, 1997.

34 Malur C. and Francis A. Prevalence and features of catatonia in a chronic psychiatric population. *Schiz Res.* (Submitted.)

35 Abrams et al., 1979.

36 Northoff et al., 1999b.

37 Peralta and Cuesta, 2001a,b.

38 Lund et al., 1991.

39 Ungvari et al., 2001b.

40 Webster rating scale for parkinsonism. (Webster, 1968).

41 Abnormal involuntary movement scale (AIMS). (Guy, 1976).

42 Akathisia rating scale. (Braude et al., 1983; Barnes, 1989).

43 Depressive retardation rating scale. (Widlocher, 1983).

44 Guiraud, 1924; Steck, 1926; Bonner and Kent, 1936.

45 Rogers, 1991. *Note 17, Chapter 1.*

46 Taylor and Abrams, 1977; Gelenberg, 1976; Lohr and Wisniewski, 1987; Rogers 1991, 1992, (modified by Lund et al., 1991 and McKenna et al., 1991); Rosebush et al., 1990; Bush et al., 1996a,b; Melo M. Catatonia: Symptoms, diagnostic criteria and concepts. Personal communication, May 27, 1998. Northoff et al., 1999b; Bräunig et al., 2000.

47 The number of items in different rating scales are: Bräunig et al., 2000 (21); Bush et al., 1996a (23); Lohr and Wisniewski, 1987 (27); Lund et al., 1991 (36); Northoff et al., 1999b (40).

48 Bräunig et al., 1998, 2000.

49 Northoff et al., 1999b.

50 Bush et al., 1996a.

6

Past treatments for catatonia

Knowledge is not a fixed thing but a stage in human development, with a past and a future.

Neil Postman, 1992

Reading the description of the treatments available to Kahlbaum in 1874, we can see how great our options are today.[1] Patients were ill for months to years, recovering after an unusual emotional or traumatic experience, a febrile episode, or most often, inexplicably. In pages titled "*Therapy*," Kahlbaum apologizes for his meager experience:

... only later was I to concentrate on the more practical subjects of prognosis and therapy, and the latter only at a late stage, since the proposal of a new disease form calls for abandoning old forms of treatment and performing multidimensional and precise experimental research to devise the correct therapy.

He offers hospital care:

In respect to the details of treatment, I must emphasize that there is no specific drug, and that as in other mental diseases, the preliminary experiences are on the whole rather negative.

Tonics are useful:

In some cases which were cured, the use of iron and quinine, combined with a diet and with a regulation of daily routine of the patient (when necessary implemented against his will) appear to have contributed greatly to the favorable outcome.

He opposes blood-letting, laxatives, withdrawal of fluids in dieting, and taking "the waters at spas":

... it is self-evident that the drugs and methods which are based on opposite viewpoints – debilitating treatments – which were formerly widely accepted and extensively applied in all psychoses, are absolutely contraindicated in catatonia.

He confirms:

... the total ineffectiveness, at any stage, of those superior medicaments of the old school – stibium tartrate in small doses and blistering drugs applied to the skull and head (stibium tartrate ointment, croton oil).

And he finds belladonna, zinc oxide, potassium bromide, and opium ineffective. He was attracted by innovative suggestions:

On the other hand, it seems we have methods of very great therapeutic importance in faradic and galvanic electricity, although for the time being the indications have not yet been worked out, and in many cases the action might be explained more on the basis of mental than of physiopathological effects.

An extensive review of catatonia in 1912 concluded that no effective treatment then existed.[2] Little progress had been made by 1921 when August Hoch described patients with catatonia in *Benign Stupors: A Study of a New Manic-Depressive Reaction Type* (Hoch, 1921). Hoch separated patients with manic-depressive illnesses, considered to have a good prognosis, from those with the malignant forms of dementia praecox and dementia paralytica. In the absence of effective treatments, doctors sought to maintain good general health, awaiting the hoped-for transition from illness to recovery that is a feature of episodic disorders. He insisted that patients be dressed daily, and that they keep themselves clean and active to avoid bedsores. Family visits were encouraged, although he recognized the hazards of delusional and angry interactions doing harm to a patient or to a visitor. Hoch found many patients to brighten when allowed to return home, and he mused:

Such experience makes one wonder whether perhaps these alone of all our insane patients would not recover more quickly at home than in hospitals, provided nursing care could be given them.

Fever therapy

A dramatic change in the therapeutics of psychiatric disorders followed the 1918 report by Wagner-Jauregg that malaria fever therapy relieved dementia paralytica (neurosyphilis). He had been studying the effects of fevers on psychiatric illnesses for two decades. The availability of a fever inducing agent (malaria) and a treatment (quinine) made it possible for him to give malaria by injection of blood from malaria patients. He did so in nine patients, reporting that three had obtained dramatic relief after six weeks of treatment; three had some improvement; and three showed little benefit. He assessed the induced fevers as the therapeutic agent.[3] The interpretation that psychiatric patients could be helped by calling on the individual's defenses in response to a physical illness justified the development of the somatic treatments of sleep therapy (Klaesi in 1922), insulin coma therapy (Sakel in 1933), chemical convulsive therapy (Meduna in 1934), lobotomy (Moniz in 1935), and electroconvulsive therapy (Cerletti in 1938).

Was fever therapy applied in catatonia? A review of the published clinical material of 314 patients in whom fever was induced, and a survey of the opinions of 301 practitioners on the benefits of infectious diseases and induced fevers in psychiatric disorders, makes no specific mention of its use in catatonia.[4] We infer its possible merits from the descriptions of fever therapy in patients with mood disorders. Among 242 "*cases demonstrating definite affective impairment*," 104 (43%) achieved notable benefit when they suffered an intercurrent infectious disorder. Of 72 "*cases suggestively featuring impaired affective involvement*," 68 (94%) achieved notable benefit. Patients who responded to fevers were those with a disturbed mood but otherwise intact affect (i.e., they were not emotionally blunted), were under age 40, and had an episodic illness of acute onset that was less than two years in duration. Febrile episodes of unusual intensity or duration, accompanied by general medical illnesses, were the most effective.

The following report describes the recovery from catatonia following an intercurrent infection.[5]

Patient 6.1   A 20-year-old man developed fluctuating brief phases of exaltation and severe depression over 18 months. "In the former there was an unusual voracious appetite, with restlessness and a very pronounced tendency to use profane language. In the latter there was a succeeding state of stupor, motor immobility, with a catatonic attitude. Resistiveness with a tendency to carry out orders diametrically opposite to the meaning of the requested ones was striking. For example, when the patient was told to flex his head, he extended it; to stretch out a limb, he flexed it; to lean forwards, he leaned backwards; to open his mouth, he closed it tightly with the teeth held firmly together, etc. During the catatonic state the patient contracted lobar pneumonia. The latter ran a typical course. When the temperature was at its height a subsidence of the mental symptoms was in evidence. The inhibitory phenomena, the antagonistic behavior to external stimuli, and the immobility were gradually decreasing. There was no stupor and no depression.

This patient made a complete recovery during the high fever of pneumonia. At the time of the report, the patient was in his seventh month of recovery without recurrence of catatonia.

An attending neurologist at the New York Neurological Institute described remissions of psychoses occurring with fever.[6]

Remissions were observed in manic stupors and depressed states, also in catatonia. Off-hand I would state that the remission was more lasting in the depressed cases and only temporary in the schizophrenic.

A superintendent of the Hudson River State Hospital in Poughkeepsie, New York testified:

A twenty-year-old man was admitted to hospital in an acute catatonic "reaction" (March 1934). He was impulsive and assaultive, reacted to auditory hallucinations, thought he was hypnotized and that he was poisoned by radium, and had cataleptic symptoms. Six months after admission he developed pulmonary tuberculosis, with pleurisy. At the same time his psychiatric disorder began to improve. Later he was able to give a good account of his illness. He was paroled from hospital (May 1936) in a greatly improved state.[7]

Another testimonial by a physician at Traverse City Hospital in Michigan:

I have noticed instances of relation of psychoses associated with fever...We recently had a case, one of Katatonic Dementia Praecox, who was quite active and markedly suicidal, striking her head against walls, etc. As a result of the latter she developed an extensive abscess of the scalp resulting in a fever of 106 °F. which persisted for about six to eight hours. Following the subsidence of this fever she did appear to improve considerably and has remained improved since then, a matter of perhaps two or three months. She appears to be in more or less mental conflict with some delusional ideas, but is no longer active and suicidal as she previously had been. I believe that most of such phenomena have been observed in Manic-Depressive Psychoses. In this group the remissions have appeared to be fairly permanent, in schizophrenic disorders only partially permanent or improved, and I have noticed no improvement whatever in epileptics.[8]

Similar experiences are described for patients treated by induced fevers. A woman with recurrent depression developed mutism, withdrawal, and rigidity (*Patient 2.6*). Venous thrombosis and pulmonary embolus led to a week of high fever. When the fever resolved, so did her catatonia. A year later, depression and catatonia with mutism, withdrawal, negativism, posturing, rigidity, and explosive speech recurred. These did not respond to pharmacotherapy, and after two months of illness she accepted ECT which relieved the syndrome.

Barbiturates

Morphine, hyoscyamus, hyoscine (scopolamine), chloral hydrate, and sodium bromide were among many sedatives used to treat catatonic patients. The discovery of barbiturates in 1903, with their ability to induce sleep, was a boon to therapy. Credit is given to the Swiss psychiatrist Jakob Klaesi for the development of continuous sleep therapy (Dauernarkose).[9] Patients were asleep most of the day, awakened periodically to eat, wash, and toilet. Treatments were given for many weeks, and although some patients recovered, a high death rate impeded its use.

The relief of catatonia with barbiturates was reported by W. J. Bleckwenn of Madison, Wisconsin in 1930.[10] The intravenous administration of a 5% solution of amobarbital sodium, in doses of 0.5 to 1.0 Gm, resulted in deep sleep of 2 to 8 hours duration. He reported dramatic, though transient, effects in three catatonic patients.

Patient 6.2   A.G., aged 35, weighing 66 pounds, with catatonic dementia praecox, had been fed by tube for over two years. She had received at least ten anesthesias with carbon dioxide and oxygen about one year before coming to the hospital, after each of which she talked normally for from five to fifteen minutes and then sank back into catatonia.

"She was given 0.48 Gm of sodium amobarbital, and she slept for four hours. She answered questions for two hours; she told me that she had missed her own physician while she was in Europe for six months (a fact); she was perfectly oriented as to time, place and person; she recalled the anesthesia with carbon dioxide and oxygen a year previously; she had perfect memory and insight. She refused, however, to take food and was fed by tube. She slept all night. She awakened at 6 a.m. and said she was going to die. She was fed by tube and showed a similar response on the next day. This patient was unable to relax completely because of muscular contractures."

A second patient reported by Dr. Bleckwenn also showed the dramatic, although transient, benefit of amobarbital.

Patient 6.3 T.W., aged 33, had catatonic dementia praecox. The onset occurred with delusions and hallucinations one year before, following a pregnancy. She became disturbed and attempted to run away from home; later, she was stubborn and resistive and refused food. She lost weight from 130 to 80 pounds in six months. For four months, she had been in cataleptic stupor and had been fed by tube.

0.48 Gm amobarbital sodium was administered intravenously. The patient slept for four hours, and was drowsy for 3.5 hours; then she asked for a glass of water and took a glass of milk. She asked the score of a football game that was being played on that afternoon; she asked also for her baby and wanted to talk to her. She was fully relaxed and went to sleep for four hours. When awake, she was negativistic, but not cataleptic. She was given daily doses (of amobarbital). She argued against venipuncture. She was fed by tube when asleep, but took considerable nourishment while awake.

Although the benefits of amobarbital were extended by daily administrations in this patient, the effects were transient. Bleckwenn reported a third patient.

Patient 6.4 J.L., aged 20, a university student, had catatonic excitement, which had had a sudden onset with confusion and mutism and refusal of food; after three weeks he went into a state of marked excitement with active hallucinations and bizarre gesticulations and grimacing. He set fire to his bed and yelled "fire."

He was given 0.6 Gm amobarbital sodium. Just before he went to sleep he said that he realized he was having a terrible time and hoped to recover to enter school in February. When he awakened, he behaved in a normal way, and discussed current topics, his illness, school, and his future plans. This lucid interval lasted for almost two hours. After a short sleep, he returned to an excited state. At the time of writing, he had made similar responses after further treatment, and was less hyperactive.

These examples were so compelling that they encouraged the use of sodium amobarbital to treat catatonia, in both the retarded and excited forms. Its use was of particular interest to psychoanalysts who saw barbiturates as an opportunity to reach unconscious material of interest in the analysis. Mutism, negativism, and stereotypy were interpreted as signs that the patient's unconscious thoughts intruded into their present behavior.

McCall and colleagues in 1992 assessed the effects of amobarbital in long-term psychiatric patients with catatonic mutism.[11] Half the patients were relieved after repeated dosing, allowing further treatment to be focused on the associated psychiatric or general medical disorder.

Benzodiazepines

Barbiturate use was associated with neurotoxic complications, drug dependence, and death by overdose. The development of chlordiazepoxide in 1958, and diazepam, lorazepam, midazolam, and zolpidem soon thereafter, provided alternatives with higher safety margins. These agents soon became the preferred treatment for catatonia.[12]

An experimental study of lorazepam for the relief of catatonia and the reversal by the intravenous injection of the benzodiazepine antagonist Ro 15-1788 (flumazenil) is instructive.[13]

Patient 6.5 A 42-year-old housewife was hospitalized for depression, nihilistic ideas, motor retardation, insomnia, weight loss, and thoughts of worthlessness. She had seven previous depressive episodes in a 10-year period. On admission, a prescription for maprotiline was discontinued.

A day later, she was mute and stuporous. General medical, neurologic, and laboratory examinations found no abnormalities. She was given 2.5 mg lorazepam orally. Fifty-minutes later, all her symptoms were reversed. She was improved and asked for discharge.

With her informed consent, she was given a bolus of 0.7 mg flumazenil, and almost immediately complained of dizziness, nausea, anxiety, and fears concerning accidents of family members. These fears condensed to certainty. Within two minutes, she was again mute and stuporous, and remained in this state for almost two hours.

That night she slept well but on awakening she was mute and stuporous. Oral lorazepam (1.5 mg) was again administered and about 60 minutes later she was given 0.3 mg flumazenil. The effects of each drug were identical to those observed the day before.

Lorazepam (1.25 mg four times daily) was prescribed and her symptoms remitted. Dosage of lorazepam was gradually reduced and carbamazepine added for long-term prophylactic management. In follow-up she was doing well with lorazepam (2 mg) and carbamazepine (400 mg) daily.

The efficacy of benzodiazepines in treating catatonia in patients with acute illnesses are almost always favorable. In one study of chronically ill, however, lorazepam failed to relieve the syndrome.[14] These patients had a mean age of 44 years and an onset of their illness at ages of 18 to 23 years. The most frequent catatonic signs were stereotypy, posturing, mannerisms, perseveration, withdrawal, grimacing, staring, and negativism. These signs did not change with treatment, but the dosages were limited to less than 6 mg daily, well below the 12–20 mg recommended today. In another report, patients with chronic forms of catatonia did respond to higher doses of lorazepam.[15] Patients with long-term catatonic conditions are likely to be successfully treated with convulsive therapy.[16]

The efficacy of lorazepam in treating MC/NMS is highlighted in the report of four patients by Fricchione et al. (1983). Each patient was hospitalized because of a general medical illness and then developed an excited delirium that was treated with haloperidol or trifluoperazine. MC/NMS developed. Withdrawal of the antipsychotic medicine, supportive measures, and intravenous lorazepam relieved the syndrome. The authors compare the benefits of lorazepam to those described for barbiturates a half-century earlier. One of their patients is reported.

Patient 6.6 A 43-year-old man with a history of rheumatic fever was hospitalized for elective aortic and mitral valve replacements. The operations were performed successfully but nine days post-operatively he became anxious, negativistic, mute, fearful, intrusive, grandiose, and sexually inappropriate. He described auditory hallucinations. He had numerous previous hospitalizations for depression that were treated successfully with ECT.

Haloperidol was prescribed with dosing of 10 mg intramuscularly and 20–40 mg intravenously. The next morning he was pale, diaphoretic and mute, with cogwheel rigidity, tongue protrusion, posturing, waxy flexibility, and opisthotonus. His temperature rose to 100.4 °F with leucocytosis, and blood pressures to 175/90 mm Hg. He became tachypneic and tachycardic. Intravenous diphenhydramine was not beneficial.

Several hours later, intravenous lorazepam elicited an immediate opening of his eyes, conversation with ease, and he was able to walk. The abnormal motor and autonomic signs disappeared within two hours. The next day, the behavioral examination showed no pathology. He was maintained on oral lorazepam 2 mg every 12 hours and discharged six days after recovery.

Insulin coma therapy

Insulin coma therapy (ICT) was introduced in 1933 for patients with dementia praecox.[17] As the first somatic treatment developed after fever and sleep therapies, sweeping claims were made for its benefits – that it relieved 50–80% of patients when they were given many daily comas. At first, 10 daily inductions was considered an adequate course, but the numbers of comas progressively increased until a course of 50 comas became the standard for care by the late 1940s. Despite such heroic efforts, success rates were low, affecting 5–30% of treated patients. The risk of prolonged coma, persistent seizures, and mortality varied widely, with death reported in 2–30% of treated patients.[18] From its beginning, doubts were raised as to the efficacy and safety of insulin induced coma.[19] The absence of more effective treatments for the severely psychotic ill encouraged the leading psychiatric hospitals to make ICT available.[20] The indications for ICT were the presence of paranoia, delusions, grandiosity, and excitement; catatonia is not featured in the published reports.

One study that compared the effects of coma induced by barbiturates with that produced by insulin found the outcomes were reported as not different.[21]

The introduction of chlorpromazine provided an alternative that was quickly tested.[22] In a study of schizophrenic patients referred for ICT, patients were assigned randomly to either insulin coma (for 50 comas over 12 weeks) or to chlorpromazine (to 2 Gm daily, with a median dose of 800 mg daily for 12 weeks).[23] Sixty patients were admitted to the study. Of 30 patients receiving ICT, 5 (17%) were considered as recovered and 15 (50%) as improved; of the chlorpromazine patients, 6 (20%) were evaluated as recovered and 17 (57%) as improved. The results for ICT were comparable to earlier reports. Of 317 patients discharged from the same hospital in 1950, 48 (15%) were treated with ICT. At discharge, 7 (14%) were considered recovered and 9 (19%) as improved. This compared to 107 referred for ECT of whom 42 (39%) were considered recovered and 29 (27%) as improved.[24]

As chlorpromazine relieved psychosis as rapidly (if not more so), with greater safety and at less cost than did insulin coma, ICT was quickly abandoned and gradually the special insulin coma facilities were converted to other uses.

Convulsive therapy

An effective advance in treating catatonia was made by Laszlo Meduna when he suggested that induced seizures would benefit patients with dementia praecox. It was fortuitous that the first patient that he treated was suffering from the catatonic form of the illness. He first elicited seizures with intramuscular injections of camphor-in-oil, but soon intravenous pentylenetetrazol was adopted as a safer induction agent.[25]

Meduna came to the idea from his examinations of autopsied brain tissues at the Hungarian Neurological Institute in Budapest.[26] In patients who died with a history of epilepsy, he found an overabundance of glia cells, while in those who died with a history of dementia praecox, he observed a scarcity of these cells. Following the logic that one disease could be used to ameliorate the defects caused by another – an idea that grew from the treatment of dementia paralytica by malarial fevers – Meduna sought ways to safely induce epileptic fits.

On January 24, 1934, a 30-year old Budapest laborer was injected with camphor-in-oil. He had been hospitalized for four years suffering from what was considered dementia praecox, catatonic type. He had been mute and stuporous much of the time, requiring full nursing care. After a wait of 45 minutes, the patient seized and survived.

Without a guideline as to how often seizures should be induced, Meduna adopted the schedule of malarial fever treatment of neurosyphilis. He injected camphor at three-to-four-day intervals. Two days after the fifth seizure, the patient awakened, looked about him, asked where he was, got out of bed, and requested breakfast. He did not believe that he had been in hospital for four years, and knew nothing of the intervening history. Later that day, he relapsed to stupor again.

With each of the next three seizures, he remained alert for increasingly longer periods. After the eighth injection, catatonia was fully relieved, and he returned to his home and to work. Five years later, when Meduna left Europe for America, the patient was well and working.

In quick order, Meduna treated five additional patients with dementia praecox, and each recovered. Such an experience was remarkable since the disease was considered relentlessly progressive and hopeless, and no prior treatment had been considered successful.

Camphor injections were painful, however, and the seizure developed after an agonizing and frightening delay of more than 30 minutes. An injection of pentylenetetrazol (Metrazol) induced a fit quickly, but its use was associated with missed and incomplete seizures, panic, delayed (tardive) seizures, and fractures. Ways were sought to reduce its risks.

Italian investigators developed the technique of using electric currents to replace the chemical induction.[27] A 39-year old man was admitted to the University Hospital in Rome suffering from his second manic, psychotic, and excited episode. A seizure was induced on April 11, 1938 using electric currents applied to the head. The seizure was just as effective as those induced by Metrazol, and its ease of use quickly established ECT as the mainstay of modern convulsive therapy.

The efficacy of ECT to relieve catatonia in its malignant manifestations in depression, mania, psychosis, and neurotoxic states is remarkable and the literature is extensive.[28] Examples are scattered throughout this book.

Other treatments of catatonia

Following their introduction in 1954, antipsychotic drugs quickly became the established treatment for schizophrenia. In the widespread belief that the catatonic type of schizophrenia is no different from other forms of schizophrenia, antipsychotic drugs have been widely used to treat it. Many patients so treated develop acute toxic reactions, especially those in whom the high potency antipsychotic drugs like haloperidol have been used. Examples are dotted throughout this book, and the literature citations are extensive. Indeed, our experience confirms the risks of administering antipsychotic drugs, including the newer atypical antipsychotic drugs, in precipitating MC/NMS, leading us to dissuade such use.

Nevertheless, some reporters describe the use of antipsychotic drugs in MC/NMS without reinstating the syndrome. The drugs are usually part of a mixture of prescriptions, including benzodiazepines. A well-documented report relates that a patient with persistent mutism, akinesis, and negativism of many years standing responded to risperidone at 6 mg/day. When this dosage was reduced, catatonia returned, and was again relieved by reinstating the dosage of risperidone.[29] An adolescent with catatonia responded slowly, over many months, to treatment with olanzapine, lorazepam, and valproic acid.[30] This experience is balanced by the many reports of the development of MC/NMS with risperidone and other atypical antipsychotic medicines.[31]

Carbamazepine, amantadine, valproic acid, biperidine, and alcohol are among treatments that have been anecdotally reported to be helpful in relieving catatonia. Carbamazepine helped resolve MC/NMS that developed in a patient treated with sulpiride.[32] It also resolved the condition in two days in two patients in whom it was administered by nasogastric tube. The psychosis of each patient was then treated with haloperidol, and both patients were discharged in stable condition within a few weeks.[33] In two patients with MC/NMS, carbamazepine treatment resulted in quick recovery, but its withdrawal resulted in relapse.[34] A report in 2001 finds carbamazepine as effective as benzodiazepines for nine patients with DSM-IV diagnosed catatonia.[35] Each patient was challenged with a 2 mg intramuscular injection of lorazepam and the response assessed at 1, 2, 24 and 48 hours allowing the patients to be classified as 'responders', 'partial responders', and 'non-responders'. Six of the nine patients had a good response to the lorazepam challenge within two hours. All patients were then treated with carbamazepine (600–1200 mg daily for 10 days). Four had a complete resolution of their catatonia within six days of treatment; one had a partial response, and four did not show improvement. The authors note that in two patients the psychiatric symptoms also resolved and in one patient, evidence of a present or pre-existing psychiatric disorder could not be found.[36]

On the other hand, catatonia has accompanied treatment with carbamazepine[37] and with its withdrawal.[38]

A similar experience is described for amantadine. It relieves catatonia.[39] Yet, its sudden withdrawal is associated with the precipitation of catatonia.[40]

A recent letter cites valproic acid as relieving a male patient with excited catatonic schizophrenia who had multiple hospitalizations.[41] The patient was treated with high dose monotherapy (4 Gm daily) and responded with a 30% reduction in catatonic symptoms. The addition of lorazepam reduced the catatonic symptoms by 90%.

Intravenous biperidine effectively relieved catatonia in 10 of 11 patients.[42] Dosing was 5 mg every 30 minutes up to 15 mg.

In the 1930s, Russian authors reported that they had relieved catatonic stupor with ethyl alcohol.[43] They administered 40% brandy in 15 ml doses every 3–6 minutes (150–400 ml in 1 to 2 hours) orally. When oral dosage was not feasible, a 20% watery solution of alcohol was administered intravenously in amounts varying from 100 ml to 500 ml introduced in 20 to 60 minutes. Stupor was reported to resolve in each of seven patients.

In a report in 1877, inhalations of amyl nitrite relieved a persistent cataleptic condition with delusions in a 26-year-old clerk. The relief after the first inhalation was for a few hours, but after repeated administration the psychiatric illness improved.[44]

A patient in catatonic stupor received transient relief from transcranial magnetic stimulation. The patient had not responded to haloperidol but showed a slow improvement when rTMS (rapid Transcranial Magnetic Stimulation) was applied over the right prefrontal area.[45] The authors conclude that the patient exhibited an "ECT-like effect" although in summarizing the experience they state: "*She performed daily activities and smiled occasionally, although she remained mute for another month while taking haloperidol (3 mg daily) before full remission of psychosis.*" Persistent mutism is not like the benefits commonly reported for such patients with adequate management with lorazepam or ECT. These usually relieve mutism within a few hours or a few treatments.

ENDNOTES

1 Kahlbaum, 1874, 1973.

2 Urstein, 1912: 641.

3 Wagner-Jauregg received the Nobel Prize for Medicine in 1928.

4 Terry, 1939.

5 Terry, 1939: 49. The patient is reported by Friedlander, 1901.

6 Dr. Lewis J. Doshay, cited in Terry, 1939: 66.

7 Dr. Ralph P. Folsom, cited in Terry, 1939: 67.

8 Dr. Melvin K. Knight, cited in Terry, 1939: 71.

9 Klaesi, 1945.

10 Bleckwenn, 1930; A videotape of his patients is available at the National Library of Medicine, Washington, D.C.

11 McCall, 1992; McCall et al., 1992.

12 Gelenberg, 1976; Fricchione et al., 1983; McEvoy and Lohr, 1983; Wetzel, et al., 1988; Menza and Harris, 1989; Rosebush et al., 1990; Delisle, 1991; McDonald and Liskow, 1992; Marneros and Jäger, 1993; Ungvari et al., 1994a,b, 2001a; Gaind et al., 1994; Mastain et al., 1995; Thomas et al., 1997; Koek and Mervis, 1999; Hirose and Asaby, 2002.

13 Wetzel et al., 1987.

14 Ungvari et al., 1999.

15 Gaind et al., 1994.

16 Meduna, 1937, 1985.

17 Sakel, 1935, 1938; Braunmühl, 1938.

18 Rinkel and Himwich, 1959; Rinkel, 1966.

19 Bourne, 1953.

20 Dr. John Nash (Nobel laureate in Economics in 1994) and Paul Robeson (actor and singer) were treated with insulin coma therapy. See Duberman, 1988; Nasar, 1998.

21 Ackner, et al., 1957.

22 Boardman et al., 1956;

23 Fink et al., 1958.

24 Rachlin et al., 1956.

25 Meduna, 1937. Pentylenetetrazol is commercially known as Metrazol and Cardiozol.

26 Meduna, 1985; Fink, 1984, 1999a, 2000a,b.

27 Cerletti, 1950, 1956; Bini, 1995.

28 Arnold and Stepan, 1952; Tolsma, 1967; Häfner and Kasper, 1982; Geretsegger and Rochowanski, 1987; Weller and Kornhuber, 1992b; Bush et al., 1996b; Davis et al., 1991; Fink, 1997b, 1999a; Mann et al., 1986, 1990; Philbrick and Rummans, 1994; Rohland et al., 1993; Troller and Sachdev, 1999.

29 Cook et al., 1996.

30 DelBello et al., 2000.

31 Meterissian, 1996; Sharma et al., 1996; Hasan and Buckley, 1998; Robb et al., 2000; Sing et al., 2002; Bottlender et al., 2002.

32 Peet and Collier, 1990.

33 Rankel and Rankel, 1988.

34 Thomas et al., 1998.

35 Kritzinger and Jordaan, 2001.

36 A suggestive example of a primary catatonia?

37 O'Griofa and Voris, 1991; Nisijima et al., 1998.

38 Keepers, 1990.

39 Gelenberg and Mandel, 1977; McCarron et al., 1982; Sakkas et al., 1991; Weller and Kornhuber, 1992a; Kornhuber and Weller, 1993; Northoff et al., 1997, 1999c.

40 Simpson and Davis, 1984; Brown et al., 1986; Hermesh et al., 1989b; Coulter and Corrigan, 1990; Dalkin and Lee, 1990; Keepers, 1990; Thomas et al., 1998; Terao, 1999.

41 Krüger and Bräunig, 2001.

42 Franz et al., 1994.

43 Kantrovich and Constantinovich, 1937.

44 Kiernan, 1877.

45 Grisaru et al., 1998.

7

Management of catatonia today

Your image of catatonia will not be accepted. The treatments that you recommend cannot be patented; neither ECT nor lorazepam can lead to commercial exploitation or have industrial advocates.

Robert Michels, M.D.[1]

The failure to recognize catatonia in a timely fashion allows depressed, manic, and psychotic patients to remain ill for want of proper diagnosis and treatment. Clinicians offer their patients many medications and combinations, hoping that the next regimen will be effective, despite the experience that when the first choice of a drug treatment fails, additional therapy trials are unlikely to improve outcomes. Such tactics prolong illness and risk severe consequences.

Treatment failure can also occur when officially sanctioned treatment guidelines are at variance with clinical experience. For example, the American Psychiatric Association (APA) treatment guidelines for schizophrenia do not mention the catatonic subtype. This omission leads to the failure to comment on the need to avoid antipsychotic drugs, the benefits of the initial use of benzodiazepines, and the efficacy of ECT in these patients.[2] In contrast, the APA guidelines for the treatment of depression and "bipolar" mood disorder recognize that catatonia may occur within depression and recommend that if "*relief* [from catatonia] *is not immediately obtained by administrating barbiturates or benzodiazepines, the urgent provision of ECT should be considered.*"[3]

We are fortunate in our present skills to treat catatonia and in our ability to recognize its many variants. Once recognized, catatonia can be effectively and rapidly relieved. Our treatment algorithms apply to patients whose illness is so severe as to be life-threatening, or whose illness is so prolonged that chronicity and early death are likely. While many different treatments have been tried to treat patients with the many varieties of catatonia, modern treatment is almost wholly based on anticonvulsant drugs and on convulsive therapy. Amobarbital was the first effective treatment, and soon other barbiturates were found to be effective. These medications were replaced by the benzodiazepines and these medicines are the mainstay of the treatment of catatonia.[4] When these treatments fail, ECT is called into play.[5] The benefits of these treatments are well established and in this chapter we describe our protocols and rationale for the treatment of different forms of catatonia.

Acute treatment

Catatonic patients, especially those with syndromes of acute onset, need protection and care, usually best done in a hospital. In a population survey, over a seven-year period, catatonic patients were three times more likely to die than age-matched individuals in the general population.[6] The death rate for persons of lower socioeconomic means was three times greater than for persons of upper socioeconomic means. This finding is likely to still be true, as ECT is more likely to be used at academic than at public hospitals.[7] For example, the State of Illinois does not permit ECT in its state hospitals, and only one state hospital in Texas has a facility for ECT.

Catatonia responds well to treatment, regardless of the underlying cause. Neither the number nor the pattern of catatonic features predicts the response to treatment. A patient with many catatonic signs is just as likely to improve as is a patient with only two or three signs.

The duration of catatonia also does not affect the outcome. Patients with acute illness and those with prolonged illness have benefited from proper treatment. Mute and immobile patients recover as well as patients who speak and move about. Associated history or examination features, however, predict the response of the present episode (the catatonia and comorbidity) Table 7.1.[8]

We recognize treatment algorithms for four principal varieties of catatonia, that of retarded catatonia, excited catatonia and delirious mania, malignant catatonia and the neuroleptic malignant and toxic serotonin syndromes.

Table 7.1 Features suggesting good outcome in a catatonic patient

Previous episode with recovery
Present (or past) diagnosis of mania or depression
Hyperactivity, rapid and pressured speech, and lability of mood
Rapidity of episode onset (days or weeks from wellness to full illness)
Good social functioning prior to the episode

Retarded catatonia (Kahlbaum syndrome)

The retarded or stuporous form of catatonia is most easily recognized. Patients are in a prolonged stupor or rigid posture. Self-care is compromised and they become dehydrated and lose weight. Skin care is poor, and if they are bed-ridden, bedsores develop. If allowed to remain in a posture for extended periods, contractures develop. Stasis of the blood leads to thrombosis, pulmonary embolism, and death.[9] Such states are common in the reports of patients in the 19th and first-half of the 20th centuries. Some families, immobilized by fear or shame, tolerate patients in prolonged stupor. The following vignette illustrates the difficulties of a family faced with a psychiatrically ill member.

Patient 7.1   A 19-year-old son spent increasing time standing in his parents' living room, speaking only when addressed, and responding in whispers of few words. He said he was "thinking." He ate and drank only when encouraged, but by the end of a week he was losing weight. He could be led to his room at night but his parents were not sure that he slept. After three weeks, they brought him to the hospital.

He was in cataleptic stupor, showing automatic obedience. ECT was recommended, but was refused. Lorazepam relieved some features, but it was not given above 8 mg daily (then considered an adequate dose).

ECT was finally accepted and, after one treatment, the catatonic features were so relieved that the parents took their son home and refused further treatment. He relapsed, was re-hospitalized a week later, received a full course of ECT, and catatonia resolved. His pre-morbid emotional blandness and interpersonal aloofness became prominent. He admitted to hearing voices when catatonic, but said they were now gone. His parents refused further treatment and he was lost to follow-up.

Comment: Although ECT ameliorated this patient's catatonia and the psychosis, he was left in a defect state. By present day practice standards, this patient would have received higher doses of lorazepam or a longer course of ECT that might have more fully relieved both the catatonia and the psychosis. We realize that outcomes are often won or lost during discussions with distraught relatives in consulting rooms. This patient's parents, knowledgeable about medicine, nevertheless could not be persuaded or educated to the proper continued care of their son.

The difficulties in convincing family members of the efficacy and safety of ECT are worsened by state legislative restrictions placed on the use of ECT, by public antipathy expressed by vocal anti-psychiatry groups, and by the ignorance of its practice and its benefits by health professionals and the public media.[10] To assist the education of patients and their families and to enhance the consent process, videotapes, pamphlets, and books are available.[11]

Before the present treatments were available, patients remained in stupor or excitement for weeks, months, and even years.[12] Today, there is little excuse for a patient to remain in a catatonic state longer than a day or so once he has come to the attention of a knowledgeable physician.

The severely retarded and often stuporous catatonic patient requires careful nursing care for hydration, nutrition, mobilization, and skin care. Patients should be clothed daily and urged to take part in group activities. Family visits are encouraged, and despite a poverty of response by the patient, family members, friends, and professional staff should attempt normal conversation and communication. When catatonic patients recover, they often remark about events during their "stupor." They relate details of conversations and thank staff members who spoke with them, despite their inability to reply. Patients say "I knew what was happening, I just couldn't get myself to say anything ... I couldn't move."

To avoid precipitating a neurotoxic reaction, treatment with antipsychotic drugs is discontinued. Many authors believe that atypical antipsychotic drugs are safer than their typical counterparts because the atypical agents are thought not to induce NMS. They suggest that these medicines may be safely continued. But NMS is reported for each atypical antipsychotic medicine that has been in the market long enough to gain extensive exposure.[13]

For re-hydration of a patient in reasonably good cardiovascular health, 500–1000 ml of intravenous fluids and electrolytes can be infused quickly, once or twice daily through a central venous line or peripheral "hep-lock." When patients will not eat, parenteral lorazepam (1–2 mg), given 30–60 minutes before meals often facilitates the patient taking fluid and food to maintain homeostasis and avoid the more intrusive methods of intragastric or intravenous lines, or on occasion, a gastrostomy.[14] Soon after injection, patients often eat and drink with nursing assistance. They may then, within an hour or two, return to the stuporous state. This tactic can be repeated several times each day until the catatonia is resolved.

If a specific cause is identified, its treatment takes priority (e.g., nonconvulsive status epilepticus). If no specific cause is considered likely, the stuporous patient is best treated with barbiturates or benzodiazepines and because these medicines are not always effective, the patients are simultaneously evaluated for ECT. Most experience has been described for lorazepam and diazepam, although it is probable that other benzodiazepines with similar pharmacologic properties would be useful. In one double-blind cross-over study of 21 patients with catatonia treated with either oxazepam or lorazepam, both agents achieved an initial effective response. The response to lorazepam was more sustained, however, possibly as a result of its longer pharmacokinetic duration of action.[15]

Lorazepam is initially prescribed at 3–4 mg a day. If well tolerated, and catatonia does not resolve in two days, the dosage may be doubled, and increased progressively to 8–16 mg a day. If, after a few days, catatonia does not show signs of resolving, or does so transiently with each dosing, ECT becomes a prime consideration.[16] Patients with chronic illness and persistent catatonic features are also less likely to respond to benzodiazepines, making ECT the principal treatment in such patients.[17]

A form of retarded catatonia accompanied by fever and severe autonomic instability is often malignant in outcome. The treatment is discussed subsequently.

Excited patients with catatonia

Excited patients with catatonia, those with delirious mania (almost all of whom exhibit catatonic features), and those with a febrile catatonic state are on a continuum of severity. They are clinically similar being overactive, verbose, euphoric, grandiose, and irritable. They disrupt in-patient ward routines, interrupt or leave meetings, break into conversations, make peremptory demands, and seek to leave the treatment unit. They need protection from harming themselves and others. Despite efforts to redirect their attention and limit their activity to their bedroom or to a quiet room, they are often unmanageable, and placing them in physical restraints or in an isolation room becomes necessary.

There are many etiologies for such excited states. When a specific cause is entertained, as in an anticholinergic-induced delirium or an alcohol toxicity syndrome, the treatment of these conditions takes precedence. If no such cause is a consideration, treatment with sedatives is the first option, but the doses need to be large. It is not unusual for the patient to need large doses repeated at frequent intervals. A common protocol is 1–2 mg lorazepam (5 mg diazepam) every 20–30 minutes, up to 10 mg lorazepam (40 mg diazepam) within a few hours. (The amobarbital equivalent is 0.5–1 Gm intravenously every few hours.) In extreme instances, general anesthesia has been required (*Patient 7.2*).

High potency antipsychotic drugs, especially haloperidol, are commonly used to reduce excited and aggressive behavior, but in these patients such use risks the development of MC/NMS. More than half the reports of patients with MC/NMS occur with haloperidol and most of the remainder are associated with other high-potency antipsychotic agents.[18] A toxic reaction is particularly likely in patients who are dehydrated, are given repeated doses of antipsychotic drugs in a short period, or who are also receiving high doses of lithium. The report of the neurotoxicity of the combination of haloperidol and lithium was first interpreted as an idiosyncratic neurotoxic syndrome.[19] In the original report, however, the dosages of both drugs were high and the patients were acutely ill. Admonitions about the use of the combination followed but further experience with the combination failed to support the initial fears. Many patients have received the combination safely. Subsequent experience with MC/NMS syndromes allows the original report to be re-examined, and it is likely that these patients had a haloperidol-induced MC/NMS rather than an independent idiosyncratic reaction to the combination.[20] The manic patients who are febrile or who have had a prior episode of catatonia are even more susceptible to develop MC/NMS with haloperidol and other high potency antipsychotic drugs.

We favor the benzodiazepines and barbiturates to sedate excited patients. These are effective and their risks are small when patients are well monitored.

The drugs are not associated with MC/NMS and the likelihood of respiratory depression is minimal even when given intravenously and in high doses. Cardiac arrhythmia is extremely rare and reduced excitement and sleep occurs long before respiratory depression (i.e., the sedation threshold is much lower than the threshold for respiratory depression). Intravenous administration also permits careful dosing.

Delirious mania is diagnosed in patients with the sudden onset of a confusional, dream-like state, excitement and overactivity, flights of ideas, and fluctuating periods of mutism and depression.[21] Between 15 and 25% of acutely hospitalized manic patients are so excited and disoriented as to meet criteria for manic delirium.[22] There are no DSM or ICD criteria or classifications for this condition, although it is mentioned in APA practice guidelines. Fever, autonomic instability, mutism, negativism, posturing, rigidity, and echophenomena make it difficult to distinguish these patients from those with MC. Delirious mania is a life-threatening condition that warrants rapid escalation of parenteral benzodiazepines. If these are not quickly effective, or the patient's temperature rises, or dehydration cannot be effectively treated, daily or twice daily ECT for three to four days may be required to achieve a rapid result.[23]

Although antipsychotic drugs are widely used, such use should be avoided in catatonic patients.[24] In patients in acute manic states, some authors recommend rapid dosing with valproic acid or lithium.[25] Such a prescription is problematic when the patient is febrile, dehydrated, or catatonic. One recommended regimen is to give a single afternoon dose of valproic acid (20–30 mg/kg of body weight) on the first day of treatment. The same, or double the dose, is given on the second day and daily thereafter. Such dosing is expected to establish effective serum levels and interrupt excitement.[26] If a patient has catatonic features, however, valproic acid loading is ill-advised as it may trigger the more malignant forms of catatonia. A similar loading-dose of 600–900 mg of lithium carbonate (depending on the patient's body weight) may also be effective for simple mania with excitement. Supplementary benzodiazepine dosing may be needed. If excitement is not controlled by these loading-dose tactics, or the tactics cannot be used because of the patient's poor general health, or the presence of catatonic features, then benzodiazepines or barbiturates are useful.

Malignant catatonia/neuroleptic malignant syndrome

MC is a life-threatening condition with the characteristics of catatonia, and associated fever and autonomic instability. It warrants intensive treatment. We consider NMS to be a variant of MC precipitated by antipsychotic drugs (Chapter 3). The immediate need in management is the discontinuation of antipsychotic medicines, protection of the patient when excited and delirious, control of temperature and hydration, and intensive nursing care (Table 7.2).

Table 7.2 Management steps for MC/NMS

Goal	Measures to take
Reverse hyperthermia	Aspirin or acetaminophen suppositories; place patient under cooling blankets or give alcohol bath; gastric lavage with ice water
Reverse dehydration	Intravenous normal or half normal saline. Ringer's lactate is avoided as it may increase acidosis. Glucose loads may precipitate a Wernicke's encephalopathy in a chronic alcoholic or other persons with chronically low thiamine levels
Maintain stable blood pressure and cardiac rhythm	Blood pressure and pulse rate are monitored. Hyperkalemia from muscle breakdown is prevented or resolved. Hypertension is controlled with labetolol or esmolol; and hypotension by increasing blood volume, and giving vasopressors
Ensure adequate oxygenation	Continuously monitor oxygen saturation. Maintain airway artificially if rigidity blocks air exchange. Use 100% oxygen if oximetry shows blood saturation less than 95%
Avoid complications of immobility: thrombosis, embolism, aspiration pneumonia, bed sores	Critical care nursing, moving of limbs, changing of position, skin care
Avoid renal failure	Frequent monitoring of serum creatinine phosphokinase (as an indicator of muscle necrosis), creatine, and urea nitrogen. Check urine for myoglobinuria to monitor renal function. Dialysis may be required if the syndrome is not promptly and fully resolved

ECT is effective in malignant catatonia. It needs to be administered early and intensively in febrile patients to contain the illness. When treatments are deferred, mortality increases sharply. The grace period for effective ECT is within the first five days of hospital care.[27]

The recognition of NMS as a defined toxic response to antipsychotic medicines in 1980 elicited two different treatment approaches. One strategy is based on the idea that NMS results from dopaminergic dysfunction with elements of malignant hyperthermia.[28] The second strategy considers NMS to be an MC variant.[29] Two treatment algorithms have been developed (Table 7.3).

Benzodiazepine-ECT approach

Benzodiazepines are a common initial treatment for patients with catatonia. A literature review of catatonia treatments summarizes "*the response rate as 70%, with lorazepam demonstrating the highest frequency of use and a 79% complete response rate.*"[30] Benzodiazepines are also effective in patients with NMS. In a chart review, rigidity and fever resolved within two days with benzodiazepines, and the other signs within three days, without adverse effects (Koch et al., 2000). Another chart review found 16 NMS patients who had received lorazepam within 24 hours of the onset of the illness (Francis et al., 2000). Fever and rigidity abated within 48 hours, while secondary features were relieved within 64 hours. An adolescent patient with NMS was successfully treated with lorazepam.[31]

ECT relieves NMS.[32] In a 1991 survey of the published experience, 29 patients with NMS were treated with ECT (Davis et al., 1991). Three patients had died – a death rate of 10.3%. In each of these patients, however, antipsychotic drugs had been maintained throughout the course of treatment and ECT had been delayed. The authors concluded that if pharmacologic dopamine-muscle relaxation therapy is not effective within "*a few days, a delayed response is unlikely, and ECT becomes an important consideration.*"

In another literature review, 23 of 27 patients with NMS responded to ECT (85%) within two days and most symptoms were relieved by three days (Mann et al., 1990). A 1999 survey of 54 clinical reports found 63% of the patients completely recovered and an additional 28% partially recovered with ECT (overall 91%) (Troller and Sachdev, 1999). The recovery from NMS with four ECT within six days is also described.[33]

Table 7.3 Comparison of the dopamine-muscle relaxant and benzodiazepine/ECT approaches in the treatment of MC/NMS

Dopamine-muscle relaxant approach	Benzodiazepine/ECT approach
Advantages	*Advantages*
• Better studied	• Benzodiazepines are easier to use and are safer than the alternative drugs
• When dantrolene works its effect is almost immediate and, if so, hyperthermia also improves	• If ECT is given, treatment of the primary condition (e.g., mood disorder) in most patients need not be interrupted
	• Treatments can be continued into the maintenance period to prevent relapse
	• Mortality rate may be lower if ECT used as the initial treatment, particularly within 5 days of the onset of the illness
Disadvantages	*Disadvantages*
• Treatment of the primary condition must be interrupted	• ECT requires specialized equipment and trained personnel to administer ECT
• Risky use if patient extremely psychotic or has severe liver dysfunction	• Signed consent needed[a]
• Dosing of each drug or combination more difficult	• Effects on cognition in this patient group is unknown
• 5–15% of patients relapse if drugs stopped, and dantrolene cannot be continued long because of liver toxicity	

[a] In some states (e.g., Michigan) written consent is needed to prescribe psychotropic drugs. Illogically, the Michigan rules permit a family practitioner to prescribe a psychotropic medication without signed consent but do not allow a psychiatrist to do so. Prescribing valproic acid for migraine does not require signed consent but prescribing it for bipolar disorder does.
ECT: electroconvulsive therapy.

Hawkins et al. (1995) reviewed the somatic treatment of catatonia and concluded that: "*Electroconvulsive therapy was also efficacious (85%) and was more likely to provide a positive outcome in cases of malignant catatonia.*"

Dopaminergic-muscle relaxant approach

This treatment approach considers NMS as an idiosyncratic response to the dopamine blockade accompanying antipsychotic drugs, both the typical and the atypical varieties, and dopamine-depleting drugs such as tetrabenazine and alpha-methyltyrosine. The sudden withdrawal of levodopa, carbidopa, and amantadine, dopamine agonists, also elicits the syndrome. The notion that NMS specifically derives from acute dopamine blockade led to the strategy using:

(1) the presynaptic dopamine agonist amantadine (100 mg given 2–4 times daily);

(2) the post-synaptic dopamine receptor agonist bromocriptine (5–45 mg daily is the usual dose, with a starting dose of 2.5 mg orally 2–3 times daily);

(3) the muscle relaxant dantrolene sodium (100–300 mg daily in divided doses, starting with an IV dose 1–2.5 mg/kg of body weight). When acidosis, rigidity, and fever resolve, then dantrolene 1.0 mg/kg is given every six hours for 48 hours. If improvement continues, the dose is reduced to 1.0 mg/kg every 12 hours and then 1 mg/kg daily for eight days of treatment. These measures are usually effective within 48 hours. If a benefit is not apparent within 48 hours, an alternate treatment is warranted. (Dantrolene, however, is hepatotoxic in high doses and should be avoided in patients with liver disease.)

Amantadine also lowers body temperature and may not increase psychotic symptoms as do other dopaminergic drugs.[34] Such drugs are used in combination, but looking at the sequence of events in clinical reports, dantrolene is prescribed first. After two or three days, if the effects are disappointing, bromocriptine or amantadine is added. If results are still not fully satisfactory, the remaining drug is added.

The treatment is not easy. Bromocriptine in high doses exacerbates psychosis, lowers blood pressure, and elicits vomiting with the opportunity for aspiration pneumonia. High doses of dantrolene are associated with liver damage. A satisfactory response may be slow, requiring several days to weeks.

The claim of the merit of this treatment algorithm is based on uncontrolled clinical trials. In almost all reported patients, the antipsychotic drug was discontinued, and this alone may have been the therapeutic factor.

For *amantadine*, 19 patients received amantadine alone and 63% improved. One death was reported and six patients worsened when amantadine was discontinued.[35]

Bromocriptine was used alone in 50 patients and a beneficial effect was observed in 94% (88% when used in combination). The mortality of NMS was reduced by 50%, and 10 patients became worse when bromocriptine was stopped.[36] In a Japanese survey of 33 patients receiving bromocriptine alone, 82% did well (Yamawaki et al., 1990).

Dantrolene benefited 41 of 50 patients with NMS. Half the patients showed muscle relaxation within a few hours, and the estimated mortality rate was reduced by half. In the Japanese survey cited above, 56% had "moderate" or better improvement with dantrolene. One patient died.

The literature finds some patients to respond quickly and dramatically to dantrolene and perhaps dantrolene plus bromocriptine, while the majority shows modest to good recovery in two to eight days. About 15% relapse when the medications are discontinued; 5–10% die.

A scattering of clinical reports describe patients with MC/NMS responding to levodopa, dopamine hydrochloride, calcium channel blockers, corticosteroids, and atypical antipsychotic medicines. The responses are usually reported as delayed or partial. In view of the efficacy of benzodiazepines and ECT, their use is best limited to research centers rather than in clinical practice. The use of anticholinergic medicines (as if the patient had a malignant form of Parkinsonism) is also not recommended, as these medications block sweating, hinder fever reduction, and may induce a febrile delirium.

Useful treatment techniques in malignant catatonia/neuroleptic malignant syndrome

Two aspects of the benzodiazepine and ECT treatment algorithm for MC/NMS warrant special attention. First, the intravenous benzodiazepine challenge test sets the criteria for continued benzodiazepine treatment. Second, to maximize an effective course of ECT, monitoring of seizures by EEG is essential.

Benzodiazepine challenge and treatment

In a patient with a new onset rigidity, mutism, posturing, and stupor, regardless of the associated psychopathology, intravenous sedatives typically resolve the syndrome rapidly. Intravenous amobarbital was the favored treatment, usually administered in a solution of 50 mg/ml at a rate of 1 ml in 40–60 seconds until symptoms resolved or the patient fell asleep. After 3–7 ml was administered, about half of the patients answered questions and responded to commands. Nowadays, lorazepam is favored, and is adminis-tered intravenously in 1 mg/ml concentration, with up to 2 mg administered in five minutes. (Diazepam is administered in higher concentrations, usually 2.5 mg/ml with dosages up to 10 mg.)

In the challenge test, a syringe with 2 mg of lorazepam is prepared and a "butterfly" or similar intravenous setup established. The patient is examined for signs of catatonia; 1 mg lorazepam is injected. The patient is observed for signs of catatonia and questioned. If, after five minutes, there has been no change, the second dose is given, the patient again observed and questioned. Favorable responses usually occur within 10 minutes, although patients are observed for longer periods. The degree of change is recorded. A standardized catatonia rating scale is useful as a guide to a complete examination (see Bush et al., 1996a). The score values are not prognostic, however, for patients with few signs and those with many signs have the same response to treatment with medications or ECT.

In those who have a positive response to intravenous dosing, continued treatment with lorazepam relieves catatonia in 90% of patients.[37] Larger dosages must be administered than are ordinarily prescribed. The dosing schedule varies with the severity of catatonia and the presence of fever and vegetative signs. For stuporous patients, dosing starts at 3 mg daily, increasing daily to 6 mg, 9 mg, and 12 mg as tolerated. For excited patients, dosing may be escalated more rapidly. For patients with fever, hypertension, tachycardia, and tachypnea, intravenous dosing of 1 mg lorazepam, up to 6 mg, every two hours may be prescribed. Further dosing depends on response, and fail-ure to respond within two days warrants ECT scheduled on a daily basis.[37] Equivalent single doses of diazepam are 5 mg, up to 60 mg daily, although higher doses have been used.[38] To maximize the effects, the longer-acting benzodiazepines are preferred. A successful acute treatment course will take from 4–10 days.

When a benzodiazepine challenge fails to relieve the symptoms, some au-thors continue with high doses of benzodiazepines with an eventual good result.[39] A failed benzodiazepine challenge and a failed clinical trial of ben-zodiazepines warrants treatment with ECT. If the benzodiazepine challenge does not elicit measurable relief, preparation for ECT should begin imme-diately as a failed challenge suggests a prolonged and often failed clinical trial. To wait until the treatment is considered failed to obtain the necessary consents, laboratory assessments, and examinations for ECT will needlessly prolong the patient's illness. In discussions with family members, from whom consent is usually required, the treatment plan needs to be explicit: a benzodiazepine challenge test, benzodiazepine treatment for several days, and if no response or an inadequate response after 20 mg of lorazepam or its equivalent, the administration of ECT.

Electroconvulsive therapy

For patients in catatonic stupor, manic excitement, or delirious mania, seizures are induced daily until the syndrome abates substantially. Thereafter, ECT is given at a customary frequency. We prefer bitemporal electrode placement with brief-pulse currents. The experience with bifrontal electrode placement is still too new to be assured of its efficacy, but we anticipate that it will be associated with good clinical outcomes. The inefficacy of unilateral electrode placements, even at high multiples of the measured seizure threshold, for patients with depression argues that this method of ECT has little justification in treating catatonia.[40]

Our present knowledge encourages us to treat our catatonic and manic patients with initial energies estimated at half the patient's age.[41] (Thus, a 60-year-old patient would be started at 30% of the ECT device's maximum energy output, a 40-year-old patient would be started at 20% of the maximum, and so on. These guidelines are for US devices, calibrated to deliver 100 mC at the maximum settings. Appropriate adjustments are to be made for devices set at double energy (200 mC)).

Seizure thresholds may be high after benzodiazepine treatment and the first seizures may not be considered adequate. To be sure that each treatment has a benefit, the EEG characteristics of each seizure are monitored. If a high seizure threshold interferes with efficacy, the benzodiazepine antagonist flumazenil (0.5 mg IV) may be given in the ECT induction process. In more than 13 years of direct treatment of catatonia by these means, we have rarely failed to relieve catatonia. (Our *patients 7.2* and *7.3* are examples.) In two patients, seizure thresholds were extraordinarily high and despite maximum energies of modern brief-pulse devices, bilateral electrode placement, double stimulations, and augmentations with hyperventilation and intravenous caffeine, we were unable to achieve effective seizures. Were we faced with such an instance again, we would consider etomidate anesthesia, sinusoidal ECT device (these deliver higher energies) or augment the seizure with pentylenetetrazol (Metrazol). Our willingness to use higher energies and pentylenetetrazol is encouraged by the experience that when benzodi-azepines in our customary doses failed and ECT was interrupted, barbiturate anesthesia was successful (*Patient 7.1*).

ECT not only relieves catatonia, but may also affect the underlying psy-chopathology. Most catatonic episodes occur in patients with a manic-depressive disorder. When catatonia is relieved with the first few seizures, continuing ECT will usually resolve the mood disorder and psychosis.[42] When catatonia is relieved by benzodiazepines, further treatment of the as-sociated psychopathology follows standard treatment algorithms.

When catatonia is dramatically relieved by ECT, often within two or three treatments, family members and practitioners ask that the ECT course be discontinued. But discontinuation risks quick relapse, and as a rule of thumb, at least six ECT should be administered in the first course.

Questions are often raised as to the safety of ECT in patients with general medical illnesses that are co-morbid with or the cause of catatonia. With modern procedures in experienced hands, ECT is remarkably safe even in the medically compromised, the elderly, and in all trimesters of pregnancy.[43] The principal risk for teratogenicity with medications in pregnant patients occurs during the first trimester.[44] In decades past, such patients could be protected in hospital settings without medication. In the present demands for ultra-short hospitalization, ECT is an effective and safe alternative to reduce severe depression, excitement, or catatonia. In pregnant patients during the second and third trimesters, ECT is safe and it is a preferred treatment when a rapid benefit is needed or when medications are not tolerated or fail.[45] Although medical illnesses may limit the use of benzodiazepines, dantrolene, or dopamine agonists, we find no contraindication to the use of ECT, making it the preferred treatment for catatonia, of any severity, in the widest range of patients, and with virtually any comorbidity.[46]

Toxic serotonin syndrome

TSS has many features of MC/NMS with the addition of diarrhea, nausea, vomiting, tremulousness, shivering, myoclonus, and sweating. No specific treatment is established. It is reasonable to discontinue the ongoing medica-tions and assure essential homeostatic care. Parallel to the use of dopamine agonists and dantrolene for NMS, some authors offer the serotonin antag-onist cyproheptadine (4–24 mg daily).[47] Others consider benzodiazepines, dantrolene, propranolol, and ketanserin.[48]

In *Patient 3.6*, we described a patient hospitalized with the signs of NMS – rigidity, stupor, posturing, and fever, accompanied by nausea and diarrhea. Medications were discontinued and lorazepam prescribed. Examination of a detailed treatment record found no mention of antipsychotic drugs. Two weeks before the episode, a second SSRI (selective serotonin reuptake inhibitor) had been added to one prescribed for a depressive condition. Despite the withdrawal of all medications, catatonia persisted. In the absence of the use of antipsychotic drugs, we made the diagnosis of TSS. She was successfully treated with ECT.[49] The similarities of the signs of TSS to NMS suggest that TSS is another type of catatonia, arguing for the treatment for catatonia in its resolution.[50]

Treatment failure

Despite the frequent success of our present treatments, it is useful to review the failures. In some instances, catatonia was recognized late and the patients were referred to our attention after many weeks of unsuccessful treatments. Such delay occurs because the treatment of patients with catatonia is complex. First, multiple medication trials drag on for months and under such circumstances the course of ECT needed to effectively reduce catatonia is many times the number needed to relieve syndromes of onset of several days or even weeks. Second, ECT requires special consent, delaying treatment further. For example, a consultant while lecturing at a Long Island New York State Office of Mental Health facility was asked to see a woman with a "bizarre" behavior, said to be unresponsive to all medications and a treatment failure with ECT.[51] On examination, he found her to exhibit mania with catatonia. When given antipsychotic drugs, she developed fever and rigidity. ECT had been tried at a schedule of once every 7–12 days, since ECT was only available at that facility once weekly. The schedule was inadequate for a useful benefit. Lorazepam had been given to 6 mg daily, the maximum allowed by the rules at the facility. Sadly, neither the psychiatrists at the hospital nor the officers at the state central office were aware of the deficits in their treatment program.

In our experience, each catatonic patient with a poor outcome had been initially diagnosed as suffering from a neurologic illness of unknown etiology, had undergone extensive neurologic assessment, and had been treated intensively with anticonvulsant medicines. This treatment made it almost impossible to achieve effective seizures with ECT, and is the probable explanation for the failure of ECT. An example of a difficult, though successful, treatment course occurred in *Patient 3.5*, admitted in a manic delirium during an exacerbation of lupus erythematosus. The course of another difficult patient is described.

Patient 7.2   A 23-year-old woman became stuporous. Extensive neurologic, EEG, and general medical testing failed to define an etiology. She developed bed-sores and pneumonia. Four weeks into her illness, a consultant administered a test dose of intravenous lorazepam and within a few minutes she opened her eyes and then moved her limbs and eyes on command. With repeated higher doses of lorazepam, periods of alertness and responsiveness were longer, but rigidity, mutism, and lack of motility persisted. ECT was recommended and consent obtained from the patient's mother and fiancé in the sixth week of her hospital course.

Seizures were induced on successive days with a rapid improvement in vigilance and responsiveness. After the fourth ECT, she recognized her family, hesitantly answered questions, turned her body on command, and took oral feedings. An EEG was done on the day after her fourth treatment; it showed high voltage slow waves in bursts with spike activity. A neurologist erroneously interpreted the record as evidence of status epilepticus and ECT was interrupted. Her stupor recurred despite high doses of anticonvulsants. After an additional two weeks of care, she was anesthetized in barbiturate coma for one week. Recovery was slow and six weeks after anesthesia treatment, she was ambulatory and verbal. One year later she was married and working.

Comment: The EEG did not exhibit epileptic activity before ECT. Treatment with anticonvulsants was unsuccessful. Improvement began within a week of ECT but was erroneously interrupted by the neurologist's misinterpretation of an interseizure EEG done the morning after a treatment. The neurologist had not been aware that the inter-treatment EEG records during a course of ECT show progressive slowing of frequencies, with increases in amplitudes and in rhythmicity that simulate records found in patients with seizure disorders.[52] These physiologic changes are short-lived, and abate rapidly. Within a few weeks of the last ECT, the slow EEG frequencies have disappeared to be replaced by high amplitude and very well modulated alpha (8–12 Hz) frequencies. To the unsophisticated neurologist, the EEG records during a course of ECT are easily mistaken for status epilepticus, especially if the record is "read" in the absence of concurring behavioral observations.

Barbiturate anesthesia was successful in this patient. While many episodes of catatonia resolve spontaneously, and others require sedation only, a few conditions are so severe that they require the more intensive effects of ECT. Anesthesia appears to be another more intensive treatment for catatonia.

Two other patients with catatonia did not recover with ECT and were transferred to nursing homes for their continued care. In both, adequate seizures could not be induced. In hindsight, double stimulation or the use of older high-energy devices may have elicited adequate treatments.

Patient 7.3 A 38-year-old mother of two children was admitted to the hospital in a depressed state. She had been sleepless and had lost weight in the prior weeks. She was slow in speech and echoed the examiner's phrases. At times, she was mute, staring beyond the examiner. Her extremities were rigid, and she stood in the same position for many minutes. Retarded depression with catatonia was diagnosed. Lorazepam in high doses was administered for five days; when she did not improve, ECT was recommended.

During the pre-ECT general medical examination, a temperature of 100.3 °F was recorded and a putative diagnosis of encephalitis was made by the consulting neurologist. She was transferred to the care of the neurologist for further assessment. EEG, MRI, CSF, and neurologic examinations were negative. Her temperature became normal. The stupor persisted, however. Pneumonia developed, fever returned, and antibiotics were prescribed. The fever resolved but the stupor worsened. She required intubation. After this cascade of unfortunate events, psychiatric consultation was again requested. The stupor was interpreted as a depressive stupor and ECT again recommended.

Consent for ECT was obtained from her husband and mother. When bitemporal ECT was attempted, adequate seizures could not be elicited on two successive days. The anticonvulsants and sedatives were withdrawn without change in stupor. After 10 days, ECT was again attempted. Seizures were inadequate despite many maneuvers to enhance seizure activity. After 10 attempts, ECT was abandoned. At that time, the patient was afebrile, in stupor, requiring continuing nursing care. She was transferred to a nursing home.

Comment: The patient's treatment was interrupted by the assessment that fever in the presence of catatonia represented an example of encephalitis. During the neurologic work-up, taking more than a week, the patient was treated with antibiotics and anticonvulsants. The diagnosis of encephalitis was not confirmed. Many similar examples of erroneous diagnoses of encephalitis in patients in manic delirium with fever and catatonia dot the medical literature.[53]

Electroconvulsive therapy-induced electroencephalogram changes

At one time, any motor convulsion in ECT was considered therapeutic. But once the finding that the efficacy of seizures induced with unilateral electrode placement was sensitive to dosing, greater attention was placed on the brain seizure and its association with clinical efficacy. At first, the duration of the motor convulsion was considered a criterion.[54] But the experience that the sub-therapeutic seizures with RUL ECT were adequate in duration led to the discard of this criterion.[55]

Attention is now directed to the EEG characteristics of the seizure. We consider an adequate seizure in the ictal EEG to be characterized by a rapid build-up of amplitudes after the stimulus; high voltage bursts of slow waves (delta) that include "spikes" (they look like the spires on top of church steeples); strings of symmetric and rhythmic slow waves; followed by a period of waxing and waning of slow waves; and an abrupt (sharp) end-point to the rhythms leading to a period of relative electrical quiescence (Figure 7.1). The duration of EEG seizures between 30 and 120 seconds are considered therapeutic. Longer seizures seem not to be associated with better clinical results so the present practice is to abort longer seizures by intravenous benzodiazepines.

Patient 7.4 A 46-year-old woman became depressed and was treated with antidepressant medications for four months. She expressed suicidal and psychotic thoughts. When seen in consultation, her speech was slow with echolalia. She sat rigidly, postured, stared into space, and resisted passive movement. She was hospitalized. Treatment with high doses of lorazepam was without benefit, and consent for ECT was obtained from her husband.

Her seizure threshold was measured and found to be very high. None of the first three induced seizures were deemed adequate despite the use of double energies, flumazenil to antagonize lorazepam, and double-stimulation. She remained depressed and catatonic. The next three seizures were considered "effective". She became more verbal and expressed delusional thoughts of her husband's infidelity. Catatonia waned and then, despite maximum energies and various technical maneuvers to assure adequate seizures, she remained depressed, slow in movement, and periodically mute. She became confused and incontinent, and ECT rate was reduced. Olanzapine was prescribed. After 14 ECT, there was little change in her condition, and her husband asked that the treatments be discontinued. One month later she was discharged for long-term nursing care.

Comment: When the seizure threshold is very high, making it difficult to elicit a therapeutic seizure, the following steps are recommended. The dose of

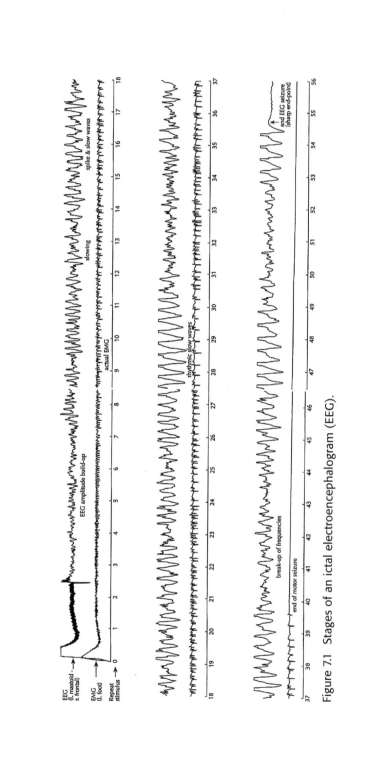

Figure 7.1 Stages of an ictal electroencephalogram (EEG).

the anesthetic is reduced. If propofol has been used, it is replaced by a barbiturate, or by etomidate or ketamine. Anticonvulsants are discontinued, and if the patient has been given benzodiazepines, flumazenil (a benzodiazepine antagonist) is given (in doses of 0.3–0.8 mg) in the anesthesia induction process. Intravenous caffeine (0.5–1.0 g; 5–10 minutes before stimulation) or theophylline (single doses of 200–400 mg the night before treatment by rectal suppository), and hyperventilation are considered useful augmentations of seizure duration, but their contribution is small. Double stimulation effectively increases the stimulus energy. When devices are delivering their maximum energy (a factor in U.S. devices), it may be warranted to resort to treatment with an older higher-energy device.

Maintenance treatment protocol

To prevent relapse, continuation treatment is necessary for most psychiatric conditions. The duration of the continuation period and the treatments used vary with the underlying disorder. In general, whatever prescription was effective during the acute illness is continued during aftercare. A single long-term outcome study assessed depressed patients with catatonic features after courses of ECT. The patients did well with continuation medications, referred to as "anti-melancholic medications" (lithium, tricyclic antidepressants, venlafaxine, buproprion).[56] The duration of continuation treatment is arbitrary, customarily stated to be for at least six months for ECT and 6–12 months for medications.[57]

In traditional ECT experience, benzodiazepines are discontinued before a course of ECT is begun. That was the accepted practice because benzodiazepines raise seizure thresholds, making it more difficult to develop an effective course of treatment. When unilateral electrode placement was widely used in ECT, the energies that were delivered were just above seizure threshold. Such seizures were clinically less effective than those with more robust energies measured against the seizure threshold. Such inefficacy was worsened in patients who had received or continued to receive benzodiazepines during ECT.[58] Practitioners eschewed benzodiazepines during ECT and indeed, they were admonished to discontinue such medicines during ECT. Now that the interaction of seizure threshold and treatment induction dosage is better understood, we are able to effectively treat most patients who are prescribed benzodiazepines, even when dosages affect seizure thresholds. Benzodiazepine antagonists (flumazenil) are administered during the drug sequence before the seizure. Also, seizure thresholds can be determined and treatments then given at 1.5 times the seizure threshold with bitemporal electrode placement. The adequacy of each treatment can be assessed by EEG criteria (Figure. 7.1).

When lorazepam or diazepam is used to treat catatonia today, and is unsuccessful, the patient is referred for ECT. Despite high benzodiazepine tissue concentrations, effective treatments (seizures) can be elicited. As patients improve, lorazepam or diazepam may again become the mainstay of treatment.[59] In difficult-to-treat patients, lorazepam in 2–6 mg daily is continued, and periodically augmented with ECT. In such instances, the energies for the seizure are adjusted upwards, and the EEG examined to assure an adequate seizure. When an adequate seizure is not seen, treatment is repeated immediately with higher energies, usually increased by 50% if possible, or flumazenil is given before the treatment.

Our patients have been sustained in the community with continuation ECT at bi-weekly, monthly, and bi-monthly intervals, with or without daily benzodiazepine dosing. We are unable to predict scientifically the optimal schedule for such treatment. Either we treat a patient within 48 hours of the first sign of recurrence, or we establish a schedule of regular treatments, and decrease the frequency as the patient maintains his well-being.

Sustaining a relapse-free maintenance phase of treatment depends on several factors cited in Table 7.4. None of these indicators have been established scientifically but they guide decisions as to the frequency of treatments or the length of continuation treatments.

The continued care of patients suffering with a manic-depressive illness depends on lithium, antipsychotic drugs, mood stabilizing anticonvulsants, and benzodiazepines. If one drug is insufficient to maintain clinical health, others are added. It is not uncommon for such patients to be sustained on combinations of two to five medicines. Indeed, polypharmacy is the standard of modern treatment for these severely ill patients, despite the evidence that this strategy is marginally effective. A course of ECT is a more reasonable option for patients who have failed the first and second combinations of medicines, or for patients who are cycling between depression

Table 7.4 Planning maintenance treatment in a catatonic patient

Less likely to relapse	More likely to relapse
Rapid dramatic response to benzodiazepine challenge	High doses of benzodiazepines needed to ameliorate catatonia
Episodic course of illness with high functioning between episodes	Catatonia associated with oneiroid state[a]
Catatonia as part of primary mood disorder	Chronic manic patient with signs of limbic sensitization[b]
ECT easily induced and ictal EEG changes meet criteria for adequate seizures	Co-morbid alcoholism, substance-induced mood disorder with catatonia, or coarse neurologic disease

[a] See Meduna (1950).
[b] See Post et al. (1984); Taylor (1999).

and mania with short intervals. For rapid cycling patients and those in mixed affective states, ECT is a better option than complex polypharmacy. Once responding to ECT, many patients who could not be well-maintained with polypharmacy, now respond to simpler prescriptions of one or two medications.

Depression and catatonia

A similar treatment regimen is adopted for a patient with a depressive mood disorder and catatonia, except that the primary continuation medication is an antidepressant. We generally prescribe a broad-spectrum non-specific or partially specific reuptake inhibitor antidepressant, such as desipramine or nortriptyline, if the patient can tolerate it. These have modest anticholinergic and quinidine-like side-effects, are well tolerated by most otherwise healthy patients. Newer agents with a broad pharmacodynamic profile may be alternatives. Our preference for broader spectrum antidepressants is their clear efficacy in the severely depressed patient, their tendency toward sedation rather than the arousal that occurs with a pure SSRI, their lesser effects on sexual function, and their lesser expense.

A recent report reminds us that the efficacy of the newer antidepressants is still poorly understood. In a comparison of sertraline and imipramine treatment in 235 men and 400 women with unipolar depression, men and post-menopausal women were better served by imipramine, while pre-menopausal women were better served by sertraline.[60]

Schizophrenia and catatonia

For patients with schizophrenia and catatonia, we prefer not to use antipsychotic drugs until all signs of catatonia are resolved. We aim to sustain the improvement of the catatonic type of schizophrenia by relying on the antipsychotic activity of ECT when it is available. When ECT and lorazepam have failed or produced a partial response, an antipsychotic medicine may be added during the continuation treatment. In open clinical trials at University Hospital at Stony Brook, New York and at the Long Island Jewish Hillside Medical Center for more than a decade, the augmentation of clozapine by ECT in clozapine-resistant patients has been safe and effective.[61] The successful use of continuation ECT without medication is described in a patient with catatonic schizophrenia (see Üçok and Üçok, 1996).

Catatonia in other conditions

When a patient exhibits a neurotoxic reaction, we do not prescribe the precipitating agent again. For patients who developed catatonia as a manifestation of their general medical illness, we usually prescribe continuation lorazepam in doses of 3–8 mg daily for six months or longer after the acute episode has been successfully treated.

Patient 7.5 A 23-year-old man had a history of persecutory ideas. He was self-isolating, without friends, and was brought to the hospital when he lost weight, refused food, and was mute and negativistic. On examination, he repeated phrases, postured in a soldier-like stance, staring into space. A diagnosis of paranoid schizophrenia with catatonic features was made and treatment begun with fluphenazine. The catatonic features were treated with lorazepam without success. Persistent psychosis and catatonia led to referral for ECT. A course of 16 bilateral ECT resolved both the psychosis and catatonia. He was cooperative, responsive, and alert and was returned home with prescriptions for fluphenazine.

After three weeks the catatonic signs returned and he was re-admitted. Treatment with lorazepam again failed but he responded to ECT. Continuation ECT every two to three weeks was able to sustain him in his home. Seeking to increase the time between treatments, lorazepam was prescribed at increasing doses. When lorazepam was given at 6–8 mg daily, the intervals became longer, and after nine months of combined treatment, it was possible to forego ECT. The antipsychotic prescription was changed to risperidone, requiring no further ECT for at least two years when his care was transferred to a community psychiatrist.[62]

Additional strategies

If the etiology of the catatonia is associated with a mood or a psychotic disorder, maintenance treatment and perhaps indefinite prophylactic treatment will be needed. Patients who cooperate in their long-term care relapse less frequently when attention is also paid to reducing the expressed emotion in their environment. Stress can induce immobility with rigidity in laboratory animals, particularly those with increased cholinergic sensitivity that results from exposure to drugs with anti-cholinergic properties. Psychotropic drugs with anticholinergic properties sometimes cannot be avoided, but reducing the negative intense, hypercritical emotional interactions in a patient's environment reduces relapse in general, and may be specifically important in reducing the risk of the relapse being catatonic. The reduction of expressed emotion in the presence of psychotic patients in remission is an established strategy for reducing relapse rates – in some studies by 50%. Characteristics of a high-expressed emotion environment include the frequent expression of hostility, making critical comments, being overly involved in the patient's daily activities and over-controlling on large issues, and often intensely expressing positive and negative emotions. Typical family and crisis oriented therapies that rely on "getting things out in the open" are counterproductive for these patients. The education of the family and the professional staff of alternative ways to interact with the patient work best.[63]

Prophylaxis

Catatonia that is not effectively treated may persist for years. In Morrison's Iowa survey of 250 patients, about 25% remained symptomatic for longer than a year and 10% were symptomatic after 5 years (Morrison, 1973, 1974a). Kraepelin's catatonic patients had a recovery prevalence of 10–15%. Patients with symptoms lasting longer than six months were "common" and 22% had "protracted admissions," with some patients continuously hospitalized for decades. When appropriately treated, however, catatonia almost always resolves.[64]

Because catatonia can be long-lasting and episodic, tactics to prevent recurrences are needed. When catatonia results from a general medical, toxic, or neurologic condition that is resolved or well controlled, prophylaxis is usually not necessary. When catatonia results from a psychotic disorder or manic-depressive illness, it is likely to recur when the condition exacerbates. In such patients, prophylaxis is typically needed. What was effective during the continuation phase is likely to be effective when used in prophylaxis. In some patients, catatonia persists even though the initial illness process appears to have resolved or the patient appears to be chronically symptomatic. For these patients, continuation ECT is prescribed, or lorazepam for those who can be sustained with it or who refuse ECT.

In patients with mood disorder, prevention should focus on correcting behaviors that lead to electrolyte and fluid imbalance, reducing excitement, and knowing when *not* to prescribe an antipsychotic agent. *Hyponatremia* is associated with an MC/NMS picture in patients treated with antipsychotic agents. It elicits catatonia when sodium loss is corrected overly rapidly.[65] Starvation or substantial weight loss, as seen in anorexia nervosa, is associated with hypoperfusion biparietally as demonstrated by SPECT, and is a precursor to catatonia.[66]

When catatonia is expressed in a patient with a mood disorder, it reflects an increase in severity. Severe excitement in mania or the stuporous state of melancholia may disrupt frontal circuitry and elicit catatonia. The best protection is to control excitement with a benzodiazepine rather than with an antipsychotic agent, and to relieve stuporous depression with ECT.

Patients with pre-existing intrinsic frontal-basal ganglia thalamic disease, or those who are epileptic, or who are suspected of an epilepsy spectrum disorder and psychosis, should not receive drugs that lower the seizure threshold or that antagonize dopamine or GABA. Because cholinergic deficiency aggravates hyperthermia, potent anticholinergic drugs should be avoided. Some clinicians, however, have argued that acute catatonia may be a cholinergic/dopaminergic imbalance, and one report describes a catatonic patient who improved when the anticholinergic agent benztropine was administered.[67] She had discontinued taking thiothixene, thereby eliciting cholinergic sensitivity. Catatonia has also been reported to occur after withdrawal of an anticholinergic agent.[68]

Since catatonic patients may be more likely than non-catatonic patients to have a history of perinatal distress and infectious disease, such history should be sought routinely in all mood disorder and psychotic patients, and the risks of catatonia then weighed against the use of antipsychotic drugs.[69] Antipsychotic agents should be avoided in mood disorder patients with the

Table 7.5 Laboratory test risk indicators for catatonia

Study	Findings indicating increased risks
Serum electrolytes	Low sodium
Body weight	>5% loss of body weight in 3 weeks, >20% of body weight loss in 6 months
Serum iron and creatine phosphokinase	Low iron levels, elevated CPK are indicators of a degree of excitement leading to high risk
EEG	Findings *consistent* with epilepsy
MRI (functional MRI)	Lesion in frontal-basal ganglia thalamic circuits, pons, or parietal lobes
SPECT	Fronto-parietal hypoperfusion L > R

CPK: creatine phosphokinase; EEG: electroencephalogram; MRI: magnetic resonance imaging; SPECT: single photon emission computed tomography.

cited risk factors. Mood disorder patients with a family history of epilepsy or basal ganglia disease may also be at risk, but the extent is unknown.

These observations suggest some laboratory studies that may identify a patient at risk for catatonia (Table 7.5).

Preventive procedures in patients with a non-mood disorder psychosis follow similar guidelines. Dehydration and weight loss need to be corrected and antipsychotic agents avoided for patients with prominent risk factors. Epileptic patients should be treated with anticonvulsant agents but lorazepam is immediately helpful to reduce anxiety or agitation until the definitive treatment with an anticonvulsant has time to work. ECT is also useful in treating epileptic psychosis.[70]

For patients with a metabolic disorder, a likely mechanism precipitating catatonia is electrolyte imbalance. Correcting the imbalance, controlling excitement, and avoiding antipsychotic drugs should be treatment guidelines.

Table 7.6 lists risk factors for catatonia. Although no study has systematically assessed the risk factors in Tables 7.5 and 7.6 in a multivariate approach, the more immediate or severe the risk factor, the higher the risk for catatonia. Several risk factors are more ominous than one, but to what degree is unknown. Our advice is to play it safe. Although gratifyingly treatable, catatonia can be lethal. Thus, if the risk is high, assume that catatonia will occur unless you treat with agents that reduce that risk. The overall strategy

Table 7.6 Risk factors for catatonia

- Perinatal infectious disease history
- Previous catatonia
- Previous drug related extrapyramidal side-effects
- Mood disorder with substantial psychomotor retardation or excitement or psychosis
- Epilepsy and epilepsy associated conditions (e.g., migraine)
- Frontal circuitry, brainstem, pontine-cerebellar disease
- An acute behavioral syndrome associated with dehydration or hyponatremia, or substantial weight loss
- Recent exposure to medications that lower the seizure threshold, block dopamine, increase serotonin
- Acute psychotic episode associated with substantial cocaine use
- Any abnormality listed in Table 6.2
- Long-term exposure to anticholinergic drugs and recent withdrawal or reduction in their dose

---

is to avoid antipsychotic agents, use lorazepam for sedation, and consider ECT and anticonvulsant mood stabilizers as definitive treatments.

ENDNOTES

1 History of Psychiatry Section, Cornell Medical College, June 23, 2001.

2 American Psychiatric Association, 1997.

3 American Psychiatric Association, 1996.

4 Fricchione et al., 1983, 1990; Rosebush and Stewart, 1989; Rosebush and Mazurek, 1991b; Rosebush et al., 1990; White and Robins, 1991; White, 1992; Hawkins et al., 1995.

5 Arnold and Stepan, 1952; Hermle and Oepen, 1986; Geretsegger and Rochawanski, 1987; Lauter and Sauer, 1987; Mann et al., 1990; Ferro et al., 1991; Rummans and Bathingthwaite, 1991; Cape, 1994; Cizaldo and Wheaton, 1995; Hawkins et al., 1995.

6 Guggenheim and Babigian, 1974a.

7 Thompson et al., 1994; Hermann et al., 1995.

8 Morrison, 1974b; Abrams and Taylor, 1976, 1977; Abrams, Taylor, and Stolurow, 1979.

9 McCall et al., 1995; Carroll, 1996; Mashimo et al., 1995.

10 Fink 1979, 1991, 1997c, 1999a; Lebensohn 1984, 1999.

11 Fink, 1999a; American Psychiatric Association, 2001.

12 Bell, 1849; Kahlbaum, 1874; Kraepelin, 1903, 1919; Hoch, 1921; Stauder, 1934; Meduna, 1937, 1985; Laskowska, 1967.

13 Sachdev et al., 1995; Meterissian, 1996; Hasan and Buckley, 1998; Johnson and Bruxner, 1998; Karagianis et al., 1999, 2001; Caroff et al., 2000; Meltzer, 2000; Robb et al., 2000; Martényi et al., 2001; Biancosino et al., 2001.

14 *Patient 2.1.*

15 Northoff et al., 1995; Bush et al., 1996b; Zaw and Bates, 1997; Schmider et al., 1999.

16 The benzodiazepine challenge and treatment, and ECT are discussed subsequently.

17 Ungvari et al., 1999.

18 Shalev and Munitz, 1986; Hermesh et al., 1992; Wilkinson et al., 1999.

19 Cohen and Cohen, 1974.

20 Normann et al., 1998.

21 Klerman, 1981; Fink 1999b.

22 Bell, 1849; Bond, 1980; Fink, 1999a,b.

23 This form of ECT, known as *ECT en bloc*, is to be differentiated from *Multiple Monitored ECT* (MMECT). In MMECT, four to eight seizures are rapidly induced in a single anesthetic session. This form of ECT is riskful and has been discarded. Also, before the number of treatments in a course was well defined, some psychiatrists treated patients daily or twice daily for weeks to develop a severe delirium. This practice, known as "regressive ECT," is also discarded (Fink, 1979, 1999a; Abrams, 1997).

24 Keck et al., 1989, 1991; Osman and Khurasani, 1994; Blumer, 1997; Berardi et al., 1998.

25 Fava et al., 1984; Keck et al., 1993; Hirschfeld et al., 1999.

26 Jefferson et al., 1983; Goodwin and Jamison, 1990.

27 Arnold and Stepan, 1952; Geretsegger and Rochawanski, 1987; Mann et al., 1990; Weller et al., 1992; Weller and Kornhuber, 1992b; Philbrick and Rummans, 1994; Frey et al., 2001.

28 Rosenberg and Green, 1989; Caroff et al., 1998a,b; Davis et al., 2000.

29 Rosebush and Stewart, 1989; White, 1992; Fink 1996a.

30 Ungvari et al., 1994b; Hawkins et al., 1995; Koek and Mervis, 1999; Schmider et al., 1999.

31 Woodbury and Woodbury, 1992.

32 Addonizio and Susman, 1987; Mann et al., 1990; Davis et al., 1991; Sheftner and Shulman, 1992; Nisijima and Ishiguro, 1999; Troller and Sachdev, 1999.

33 Nisijima and Ishiguro, 1999.

34 Birkhimer and DeVane, 1984; Lazarus, 1986.

35 Davis et al., 2000.

36 Davis et al., 2000

37 Bush et al., 1996b; Fink, 1997a; Petrides and Fink, 2000.

38 Takeuchi, 1996.

39 Rosebush and Stewart, 1989; Rosebush and Mazurek, 1991b; Rosebush et al.,1990.

40 Fink 2001; Fink et al., 2001.

41 Petrides and Fink, 1996.

42 Abrams, 1997; Fink, 1999a.

43 Abrams, 1997; American Psychiatric Association, 1990, 2001.

44 Walker and Swartz, 1994; Miller 1994.

45 American Psychiatric Association, 1990; Abrams 1997.

46 American Psychiatric Association, 1990, 2000; Abrams, 1997; Fink, 1999a.

47 Lappin and Auchincloss, 1994; Graudins et al., 1998.

48 Keck and Arnold, 2000.

49 Fink, 1996b.

50 Caley, 1997; Richard, 1998; Birbeck and Kaplan, 1999; Carbone, 2000; Keck and Arnold, 2000.

51 Dr. Georgios Petrides, personal communication, March 2001.

52 Fink and Kahn, 1957; Abrams et al., 1972; Sackeim et al., 1996

53 Carroll et al., 1994; Caroff et al., 1998b.

54 Fink and Johnson, 1982.

55 Sackeim et al., 1987, 1993, 2000, 2001.

56 Swartz et al., 2001.

57 Fink et al., 1996.

58 Pettinati et al., 1990.

59 Petrides et al., 1997; Petrides and Fink, 2000.

60 Kornstein et al., 2000.

61 A prospective study supported by NIMH began in 2001; the principal investigator is Georgios Petrides, M.D.

62 For another example of continuation see *Patient 4.4.*

63 Falloon et al., 1982; Overshett et al., 1986; Bebbington and Kuipers, 1994a,b; DeJesus and Steiner, 1994.

64 Abrams and Taylor, 1976.

65 Tormey et al., 1987; Dierckx et al., 1991; Morinaga et al., 1991; Sechi et al., 1996; Chalela and Kattalh, 1999.

66 Nazoe et al., 1995; Delvenne et al., 1997.

67 Tandon and Greden, 1989.

68 Menza and Harris, 1989; Panzer et al., 1990; Spivak et al., 1996.

69 Wilcox, 1986.

70 Kalinowsky and Hoch, 1952; Kalinowsky et al., 1982.

8

The neurology of catatonia

Whatever the practical merits of emphasizing differences rather than the similarities between neurological and psychiatric motor disorders, this has had the effect of holding back a much needed neurological approach to the motor disorder of psychiatric illness. By far, the best way forward is accepting catatonic motor disorder, whether forming part of neurological or psychiatric disorder, as an extrapyramidal motor disorder.

Rogers, 1992: 25

Almost all the neuropathological studies so far performed have been prone to errors of subjectivity. The brain is easily duped when it studies itself.

Lohr and Wisniewski, 1987: 218

The pathophysiology of catatonia has yet to be defined. Kahlbaum, Kraepelin, and Bleuler thought that catatonia was an expression of a deficit in *will* because that interpretation suited their views in defining behavioral syndromes. The accepted notion was that the mind was comprised of three parts: *will or volition*; *emotion or feelings*; and *thinking*. Kraepelin's ideas about psychological disease were rooted in the tripartite mind concept and his cross-sectional criteria for dementia praecox included deficits in all three spheres. He described manic-depressive illness as a disturbance in feeling, sparing the other two spheres. He delineated two disorders by their course: dementia praecox beginning in the decade after puberty and deteriorating into dementia; and manic-depressive insanity beginning after age 25 years, marked by episodes and good remissions. He incorporated Kahlbaum's concept of catatonia into dementia praecox because it was "clearly" a disorder of will or volition. Kahlbaum, wedded to the mid-nineteenth century idea of unitary psychosis (i.e., all psychoses were phases of the same process that could end in dementia), characterized catatonia as a phase of illness leading to dementia. Kahlbaum's construct of catatonia fit Kraepelin's construct for

Table 8.1 The tripartite mind concept and diagnostic criteria for schizophrenia

	Emotion	Will/volition	Thinking
Kraepelin	Dullness, indifference, apathy, no sense of shame	Catatonia, stubbornness, stupor	Denial of illness, noncompliance with treatment
Bleuler	Affective flattening	Ambivalence, passivity	Autistic thinking, associational loosening, formal thought disorder
DSM	Flat or grossly inappropriate affect, residual-phase features (marked social isolation and withdrawal, blunted and inappropriate affect)	Catatonia, residual-phase features (markedly decreased initiative, interests, energy, marked impairment in personal hygiene and grooming)	Incoherence or marked loosening of associations; residual beliefs or magical thinking; digressive, vague speech; poverty of speech

dementia praecox.[1] Modern diagnostic criteria for schizophrenia still follow the footprints of the tripartite mind construct as shown in Table 8.1.

In this view, a catatonic patient could not will himself out of a posture once in it and so remained in that position. He could not resist the manipulations of the examiner because he had no will to resist.

Although the concept of the tripartite mind has failed the tests of time and scientific scrutiny, modern neuropsychiatric interpretation of catalepsy and posturing can be considered expressions of *pathological inertia* (i.e., the inability to initiate or stop movement) observed in patients with frontal lobe disease. This distinction, however, describes the same phenomena without clarifying their neurophysiologic meaning.

Our understanding of catatonia is made complex because it seems so specific – there is something wrong with the patient's ability to move normally. But catatonia results from so many etiologies that it is likely that the syndrome has a final common pathway. For what? Why do so many conditions affecting brain function induce catatonia? Why do some persons with a catatonia-producing disease process develop catatonia, while others do not? If half the catatonic patients have a mood disorder, and 15–20% of manic episodes are associated with catatonia, why are not all manic episodes associated with catatonia? How does a manic patient with catatonia differ from one without catatonia? Why do only some patients on high doses of antipsychotic drugs develop MC/NMS?

In this chapter we discuss the brain processes associated with catatonia. We have picked our data carefully, seeking those findings that may offer clinical guidance toward its prevention and treatment.

Motor system dysfunction

The pathophysiology of catatonia is linked to dysfunction in the motor system. Kleist (1960) considered catatonic features to be identical to those of basal ganglia disease. Summarizing decades of observations, he concluded that catatonia characterized by prominent "*lack of spontaneity . . . impairment of active and creative thought*" was "*observed in injuries and diseases of the frontal brain.*" Further, "*In all the other varieties of catatonia psychomotor signs due to the disorders of the brain stem are predominant.*" Periodic catatonia, which he considered to be a milder disorder with remissions, was "*localized in the striatum, particularly in the caudatum.*" Taylor (1990) made a similar case for catatonia as resulting from disruption in frontal lobe regulatory functions and brainstem arousal mechanisms.

Clinicopathological correlations implicate motor system lesions in catatonia, supporting Kleist's views. Frontal lobe and basal ganglia lesions are commonly observed.[2] But lesions in the cerebellum–pons and in the brainstem between the frontal circuitry and the cerebellum–pons have also been implicated.[3] Frontal lobe degeneration, ruptured anterior cerebral artery aneurysms, traumatic brain injury, vascular malformations, neoplasms, general paresis in the frontal lobes, and lesions in the medial aspect of the dominant supplementary motor area have been associated with catatonia.

Luria described patients with frontal lobe war injuries who developed catatonia, and other Russian neuropsychologists described dogs with experimentally ablated frontal lobes exhibiting ambitendency, catalepsy, and waxy flexibility.[4] In an experiment by Pavlov and Anokhin, dogs with ablated frontal lobes were placed in front of two bowls of food. Although hungry, the dogs could not choose which bowl of food to eat. They looked and sniffed, first at one and then the other bowl, stuck between two equally powerful stimuli. Their behavior was similar to the catatonic patient with ambitendency who cannot resist moving his hand toward the examiner's hand despite instructions to the contrary.

Basal ganglia pathology of post-encephalitic parkinsonism, bilateral lesions of the globus pallidus, and von Economo's encephalopathy are associated with catatonia. During the outbreak of von Economo's encephalitis, catatonic features were described.[5]

French psychiatrists reported catatonic features to be similar to the motor signs of parkinsonism.[6] They described autopsy findings of pathology in the basal ganglia and sub-optic area in schizophrenic patients. Similarly, theorizing about the effects of rheumatic fever causing lesions in the basal ganglia, Wilcox (1986) compared the records of 60 catatonic patients to 134 surgical controls, 189 non-catatonic schizophrenic patients, and 325 patients with mood disorder. More catatonic patients had such histories than did patients in either of the other groups.

Recently, a syndrome of "Pediatric Autoimmune Neuropsychiatric Disorder Associated with Streptococcal infection" (*PANDAS*) has been recognized.[7] Boys at ages six to seven are at particular risk for the development of acute attention deficit hyperactivity features, tics, and obsessive–compulsive disorder. It is too early in the history of these patients to know if they too are at risk for catatonia.

Neuropathological studies of catatonic schizophrenic patients, however, are inconsistent and fraught with sampling, diagnostic, and technical problems. Nevertheless, they support a role for the basal ganglia in catatonia, finding cell loss in the globus pallidus, the substantia innominata, and nucleus accumbens, and a decrease in microneuron size in the striatum. Because of the diagnostic heterogeneity of these patients, the findings likely reflect a risk factor for catatonia rather than a specific pathophysiology, e.g., structural lesions in frontal brain circuitry disrupt motor regulatory functions leading to catatonia. Catatonia resulting from a disruption in the basal ganglia-frontal lobe circuitry rather than a direct lesion in the basal ganglia is consistent with our understanding that the responsibility for the automatic execution of learned motor programs lies in the frontal lobes.[8]

In patients with catatonic schizophrenia, Joseph et al. (1991) reported more vermal and brainstem atrophy compared to examinations in other schizophrenic patients. Wilcox (1986) found mild cerebellar atrophy in 20%

of catatonic schizophrenic patients compared with 8% of those with other forms of schizophrenia, 5% of manic-depressive patients, and none in control patients. Akinetic mutism has been reported to occur in patients with bilateral thalamic infarcts.[9]

Several *neuro-metabolic studies* support the association between catatonia and motor system dysfunction. Luchins et al. (1989) and Ebert and Feistel (1992) found basal ganglia hypometabolism (right more so than left) that returned to normal with resolution of catatonia. The right temporo-parietal cortex also had low metabolism. Using functional MRI, Northoff and colleagues (1999a) found decreased motor cortex activation contralateral to a posturing limb, and reduced activation in the motor cortex of catatonic patients contralateral to a motor task, but increased activation ipsilateral to the task, a pattern opposite to that of normal controls. These and other investigators report disturbed metabolism of the basal ganglia. Atre-Vaidya (2000) reported a patient whose catatonia persisted beyond resolution of what was likely a drug induced psychosis, and who also had basal ganglia hypoperfusion on SPECT, right more so than left. As the number of patients in these reports is small and the asymmetries vary, the most parsimonious conclusion is that basal ganglia functional imbalance is associated with catatonia rather than an exclusive left or right problem.

In contrast, Satoh and colleagues (1993a,b) and Galynker et al. (1997) observed frontal lobe and posterior temporal and parietal lobe hypoperfusion on SPECT in their catatonic patients. Galynker et al. (2000) report five additional patients with motor cortex and partial temporal cortex cerebral blood flow hypoperfusion that normalized with successful treatment. Northoff and colleagues (1999e) also report orbito-frontal metabolic problems in catatonic patients. These findings are confirmed by Miozzo et al. (2001) but not by Escobar et al. (2000).

Catatonia typically resolves fully, suggesting that the motor system dysfunction is one of regulation rather than due to a structural loss of pyramidal motor neurons. Anterior frontal lobe basal ganglia circuitry is fundamental to motor regulation, suggesting a neurocognitive explanation for catatonia. Indeed, the association between frontal lobe basal ganglia dysfunction and catatonia is not surprising given the role of these circuits in attention and arousal, emotional expression, and motor regulation.[10] Dysfunction in each of these domains is the hallmark of catatonia, and all the classic catatonic features are recognized in the neurologic literature as signs of frontal lobe disease.

Catatonic features have been interpreted as neuropsychological manifestations of frontal lobe dysfunction. The patients have problems with working memory and visuospatial tasks, consistent with frontal circuitry dysregulation.[11] For example, echolalia, echopraxia, and passive resistance are seen as stimulus-bound phenomena. Stereotypy and mannerisms have been likened to motor perseveration, and catalepsy as profound pathological inertia.

Some patients with frontal lobe disease exhibit a dissociation between "knowing" and "doing," such that verbalization no longer controls active behavior. When instructed "to let you do all the work" while you manipulate his limbs, a patient with frontal lobe disease may be able to tell you what you want him to do, but once you start moving his limb, he must "help" and move with you, despite repeated instructions not to do so. The patient responds to your touch, not to your words, but has no other catatonic features. Some patients with frontal lobe defects are aware of their errors, but cannot use their knowledge to modify what they do. This is exemplified by a patient with automatic obedience. He responds to the examiner's touch, but his response is disconnected from the examiner's verbal commands and he is unable to respond to them. Milner (1982) suggested that patients with frontal lobe disease have difficulty in the use of external cues to direct responses and lack adequate self-monitoring. The patient who postures or who maintains positions for prolonged periods appears to have such an inability, suggesting a disconnection from appropriate or sufficient sensory information resulting in an inability to properly evaluate and alter motor behaviors. The patient with catatonia, like one with a frontal lobe lesion, cannot match the action with its original intention, and the action is inappropriately maintained. Patients with frontal lobe lesions experience abnormal body awareness and exhibit inattention, neglect, and denial. The patient with catalepsy or posturing is usually unaware of his odd behavior, reflecting a disconnection between the systems recognizing intent and behavior.[12]

Patients with frontal lobe lesions also have a problem responding appropriately to "go/no-go" tasks requiring them to respond to one signal, but not to a second. This limitation, and their deficits in verbalization controlling action, may be the process underlying their ambitendency. Their loss of ability to start and stop behavior may also explain their stereotypes. In each case, motor monitoring systems are disconnected from sensory input (or sensory input is impaired). Stimuli are ignored or misunderstood, with garbled or insufficient sensory input leading to inappropriate responses. Disconnected from confirmatory sensory signals, the catatonic patient cannot tell if the response is adequate and so repeats or sustains the abnormal motor behavior.

Catatonia may also be elicited from lesions in the area of the thalamus connecting the cerebellar–pons with the frontal lobe circuitry and the associated lack of tone to the frontal circuitry (the thalamic "lesion" cutting off arousal input from the reticular activating system).[13] Catatonic patients without specific neurologic lesions often have metabolic dysfunction in this system.

In an early review, Roberts (1965) compared catatonic features with the disrupted functions associated with anterior-limbic cortical structures, focusing on lesions in the anterior thalamic nucleus and the cingulate gyrus. Loss of facial expression, reduced vocalizations, inhibition of voluntary movement, posturing, catalepsy, and "confusion" were typical of lesions to these areas in laboratory animals. In describing the projections of the anterior thalamus to the anterior cingulate gyrus, prefrontal cortex and parietal lobe cortex, Roberts made the case for catatonia resulting from dysfunction in the anterior-limbic cortical system. He anticipated the metabolic findings of fronto-parietal hypometabolism in catatonic patients. The anterior cingulate gyrus and the dorsolateral prefrontal cortex have roles in self-monitoring (particularly to congruent stimuli) and implementation of controlled responses, respectively.[14] Catatonic patients have problems in both these domains.

At first glance, reports that parietal lobe metabolic problems occur in some catatonic patients seem to contradict a specificity of the pathophysiology of catatonia to the motor system. Satoh and colleagues (1993a,b) and Galynker et al. (1997, 2000) report reduced cerebral blood flow and metabolism bifrontally (particularly dorsally) and in both parietal lobes in catatonic patients compared with other psychiatric patients. In another study, nine catatonic patients exhibited parietal lobe hypoperfusion on SPECT examinations, with additional temporal and frontal involvement in eight of the nine (Malur et al., 2000). Perfusion improved with clinical recovery.

Attentional-motor and visuospatial problems compared to normals consistent with frontoparietal dysfunction were reported in 13 catatonic patients (Northoff et al., 1999e). Catatonia associated with right parietal lesions has also been reported.[15] The next patient had a left parietal lobe lesion.

Patient 8.1   A 78 year-old-man was transferred from a nursing home for being "uncooperative" and striking an aide. A brain tumor that involved his skull and the left parietal lobe had been surgically removed several years earlier leaving a large skull depression. Thereafter, he had lived in the nursing home. For several weeks he had been "praying" in the hallways, kneeling on his right knee and raising his right hand as if in prayer. At times, his left hand was also raised. When asked what he was doing, or requested to stop, he became irritable and could not explain his posture, saying that nothing was amiss.

On the day of admission, while getting on an elevator, he slowly sank to one knee, blocking the elevator door. An aide became annoyed, tried to remove him from the doorway, and was slapped for the effort.

He showed no irritability as long as his posturing was ignored. He sustained his postures for many minutes and stopped only when his attention was captured by an intense stimulus. His right arm, but not his left, showed passive resistance during examination. He would converse while posturing. The features of the Gerstmann syndrome (dysgraphia, dyscalculia, right–left disorientation, and finger agnosia) and naming problems were demonstrable.

Sedatives did not relieve his unilateral posturing. He received no further pharmacotherapy. Redirection of his attention, however, minimized and shortened posturing. When discharged to another nursing home, the personnel were educated to the safe management of his behavior.

Epileptic patients with parietal lobe foci may exhibit catatonic signs.[16] These signs are usually brief and include dystonic posturing and catalepsy. The patient described above and those described by Northoff and co-workers suggest how parietal lobe dysfunction can result in catatonia. One's awareness of body position, how body parts are related to each other, and attentiveness to body space in the three-dimensional world depend on adequate parietal lobe function. Without effective somatosensory processing the sense of "body," and its location in space is lost. Patients with parietal lobe lesions experience striking forms of psychopathology, such as nihilistic delusions and alienation (a Schneiderian first rank symptom). They neglect space and their own body parts, the latter resulting in postures like those demonstrated by *Patient 8.1*. If frontal motor systems do not receive adequate somatosensory input, they are prone to shut down, resulting in catalepsy and other catatonic features.[17] Thalamic dysfunction is associated with somatosensory dysfunction, analgesia, unresponsiveness (mutism), and catatonia.[18]

Neurochemical aberrations

Dopamine has been hypothesized as having a primary role in motor functions. It is a major neurotransmitter in frontal circuitry, particularly in the basal ganglia. This concept converges neuropharmacologic with neurometabolic and phenomenologic data suggesting that the signs of catatonia result from abnormalities mediated by a motor system neurotransmitter. The literature relating neurotransmitter aberrations to psychiatric disorder, and specifically to catatonia, is large. The brain, of course, does not work in bits and pieces, so the idea that one neurotransmitter is the basis for catatonia is oversimplified. Even though dopamine provides much of the neurochemical substrate to frontal circuits, these circuits are also modified by GABA, and by serotonergic projections from the dorsal raphe nucleus.[19]

Researchers tend to focus on a specific receptor–transmitter system. As no unified theory for the role of brain neurotransmitters in behavior exists, such focusing encourages transmitter-specific notions. For example, increased GABA-A or decreased GABA-B as the basis for catatonia is one such idea. Such overly specific ideas generate substantial skepticism leading some writers to facetiously equate modern ideas of the neurochemistry of psychiatric illness to the beliefs of psychoanalysis.[20]

Other views of the role of neurotransmitters in catatonia are seen in reports that endogenous opiates modify dopaminergic and cholinergic neurons in critical areas of the forebrain. The complexity of neurotransmitter interactions using NMS as a model to suggest that in addition to dopamine, sympatho-adrenal hyperactivity is critical in the development of MC/NMS.[21]

In examining autopsied brains from three patients with fatal hyperthermia, severe brain choline acetyltransferase deficiency was reported, suggesting that a dopamine imbalance in hypothalamic syndromes, including NMS, is aggravated by cholinergic deficits.[22] A universal biochemical explanation of NMS and catatonia has also been formulated.[23] A partial review of dopaminergic drugs and catatonia, suggesting that cocaine use is a risk factor for catatonia, has been published.[24]

The presumed primary role of dopamine in the pathophysiology of catatonia rests on the following findings.

- Antipsychotic drugs that block dopamine (particularly those that affect the D_2 receptors) elicit the MC/NMS syndrome in humans. Their identification as antipsychotic agents is based on the ability to induce catalepsy in laboratory animals. D_2 receptor blockade in the nigrostriatal system also results in parkinsonian features that mimic some catatonic signs.
- Dopamine depleting drugs (e.g., methyltyrosine, tetrabenazine) and dopamine antagonists (e.g., oxiperomide, speroxatrine) are associated with catalepsy.
- The sudden withdrawal of dopaminergic enhancing drugs (e.g., l-dopa) has been implicated in the MC/NMS syndrome.
- Patients with MC/NMS have been treated successfully with dopamine enhancing drugs (e.g., bromocriptine, dantrolene, amantadine). They are also successfully treated with ECT. Seizures increase brain levels of dopamine and relieve parkinsonism.

In contrast, investigators who find increased plasma levels of the dopamine metabolite homovanillic acid in catatonic patients suggest that catatonic states may be associated with increased, not decreased, dopamine activity. These reports, however, are limited to periodic catatonia, and likely reflect the mood and arousal states of these patients rather than their catatonic features.

Some authors argue that periodic catatonia is a distinct, familial disease.[25] Stöber and colleagues (2000c) reported a genetic linkage study of 12 pedigrees with 135 relatives of patients with periodic catatonia. Using 356 markers, they report a linkage on chromosome 15 and a possible linkage on chromosome 22 with an autosomal dominant pattern of transmission. Previously these investigators reported a life-time morbidity risk of 27% for periodic catatonia in first-degree relatives. Such linkage analyses are notoriously fickle, however, and the strength of this reported linkage is modest, suggesting that replication will be difficult. A greater concern, however, is the diagnosis. The authors use the Leonhard system that gives added weight to psychotic features than to mood symptoms. Many of their patients meet the criteria for manic-depressive psychosis or schizo-affective unipolar or bipolar disorder by U.S. psychiatrists, and their patients respond to treatments for manic-depressive illness.

The neurotransmitter GABA has been implicated in catatonia. Lorazepam, a strong GABA-A agonist, is an accepted treatment for catatonia. One report describes the therapeutic reversal of lorazepam in a catatonic patient with the GABA-A antagonist flumazenil.[26] Zolpidem, a non-benzodiazepine GABA-A agonist relieves catatonia.[27] Carbamazepine and barbiturates relieve catatonia, and these agents have GABA agonistic properties. And, ECT enhances GABA-ergic systems.[28]

On the other hand, GABA-B agonists (e.g., baclofen, muscinol, valproic acid) induce catatonia. These pharmacologic observations are enhanced by studies that find reduced density of GABA-A receptors in the sensory-motor cortices of catatonic patients. These patients also have reduced cerebral blood flow to these brain areas.[29] We conclude that too much GABA-B or too little GABA-A activity contributes to the expression of catatonia. From clinical reports of patients receiving or withdrawing from drugs affecting GABA-ergic systems, the more precipitous the neurochemical change, the more likely the development of a catatonia.

GABA-ergic neurons are prominent in the thalamus, basal ganglia, prefrontal cortex circuits, the brainstem, and the pons and cerebellum – the structural brain systems implicated in catatonia. GABA's role in movement disorders is recognized in Parkinson and cerebellar-pontine diseases. Increased GABA-ergic activity in the thalamus inhibits prefrontal dopamine activity.[30] In addition, morphine increases GABA turnover in the basal ganglia resulting in immobility and other catatonic features.[31] The involvement of GABA in Parkinson disease is reported.[32] The role of GABA in another movement disorder, that of catatonia, has face validity.

Epilepsy model

A seizure-like process has also been considered in the pathophysiology of catatonia. This suggestion is based on observations that post-ictal immobility is hardly distinguishable from catalepsy, and the stereotypes, dystonias, and more complex psychosensory and psychomotor features of seizures are similar to the signs of catatonia. Also, catatonia is prominent in patients with non-convulsive, petit mal, and partial complex status epilepticus with the prevalence of epilepsy being high in samples of catatonic patients. Finally, catatonia is relieved by anticonvulsant drugs and by ECT, and both agents raise the seizure threshold.[33]

After a spontaneous tonic-clonic seizure in epileptic patients and induced seizures in laboratory animals, post-ictal torpor includes catalepsy, analgesia, and full immobility, often flaccid, but sometimes rigid, among the prominent features. This post-ictal phenomenon suggests that catatonia may arise from deep brain seizure-like (excitatory) discharges. Thalamic GABA-ergic dysfunction has been linked to seizures and petit mal status, and the thalamus is also central to frontal basal ganglia functioning, thus making it a leading candidate as the source of these deep brain discharges. Thalamic dysfunction has been implicated in the genesis of synchronized oscillations that lead to generalized seizures, and thalamic GABA-A receptor blockade induces them. Thalamic GABA-B receptor blockade moderates this activity. A similar GABA-ergic pattern is implicated in the development of some catatonias, and thalamic lesions can directly result in catatonia.[34]

The thalamus has also been implicated in the pathophysiology of schizophrenia and is central to the speech and language problems in schizophrenic patients following the model of subcortical aphasia after stroke. A developmental model of schizophrenia is considered useful.[35] Thalamic morphologic abnormalities have been observed in schizophrenic patients and thalamic volume correlated with age of onset of first psychosis.[36] The thalamic dual role in frontal circuitry and perceptual integration makes it a model for schizophrenia, explaining both positive and negative symptoms.[37]

The thalamus is an integrator of perception, a link between the anterior and posterior aspects of the central motor system. It is also a key feedback and tone-providing unit in frontal circuits. These aspects fit nicely with the hypotheses of catatonia: frontal circuit dysfunction; a disconnection between motor regulatory systems and perception; and GABA and dopamine dysregulation.

Epileptic patients, particularly those with partial complex seizures, exhibit transient catatonic behavior. Frontal lobe seizures are accompanied by stereotypes, catalepsy with arm or facial posturing, verbigerated speech or mutism, or forced speech similar to catalepsy and negativism. Temporal lobe seizures are associated with stereotypes, catalepsy, and mannerisms that are often complex. Parietal lobe seizures elicit stereotypes and posturing.[38]

The expression of catatonia in non-convulsive status and in petit mal and partial complex status is considered in Chapter 4. Non-convulsive status epilepticus is a particularly good model for catatonia, as it is a rapidly developing altered state with motor dysregulation (catatonia) that resolves with anticonvulsant therapy. The most consistent causal finding in children and adolescents who present with catatonia is epilepsy, after patients with mood disorder and schizophrenia. A striking example, however, is a report of an adolescent girl who had recurrent menstrual epileptoid psychoses during which she also had catatonic features. Her seizures and catatonia were eliminated with phenytoin.[39]

About 10–15% of adult patients with catatonia not due to a mood disorder have epilepsy. In a review of 29 acutely ill patients with catatonia, Primavera et al. (1994) identified four patients with seizure disorder, and stressed the need for EEG evaluation in patients with catatonia. That catatonia can evolve from a seizure disorder does not imply that all catatonia is of epileptic origin. The epilepsy model suggests, however, that excitatory foci in strategic brain areas involved in motor regulation can be expressed as catatonia when increasing numbers of neurons are recruited to fire synchronously until the brain seizure produces the outward convulsion. In catatonia, the excitatory focus does not spread but is strategically located so that the diverse manifestations of catatonia develop.

Synthesis and clinical implications

Present views about the pathophysiology of catatonia are convergent. The brain systems implicated in catatonia are illustrated in Figure 8.1. Catatonia is associated with frontal circuitry dysfunction. Disconnection from perceptual-integrating brain systems because of thalamic or parietal lobe lesions and limbic interference (as occurs in intense mood states) have been identified. The driving forces of this system are the neurotransmitters dopamine and GABA. When seizures induce catatonia, they derive from foci in the frontal circuitry and anterior limbic system.[40]

Table 8.2 displays the mechanisms that may disrupt the brain systems shown in Figure 8.1, resulting in a catatonia.

Our model for catatonia has practical clinical implications. The suggestions for steps to prevent catatonia are clinically useful. Patients who develop

Table 8.2 Pathophysiologic pathways to catatonia

Ablating lesion in critical area of the motor system (anterior cingulate, dorsolateral prefrontal cortex, supplementary motor cortex, basal ganglia, thalamus)

Excitatory lesion in or around the thalamus

Neurochemical imbalance in the anterior motor circuitry (drugs or disease that results in reduced dopamine activity, increased GABA-B activity, or reduced GABA-A activity)

Ablating or excitatory (rare) lesion in the parietal lobe(s) (disconnecting the motor system from perceptual integration so attention to body parts and their position in space and to each other is compromised)

Metabolic disorders that cause frontal circuitry neurochemical imbalance or that disrupt parietal lobe sensory processing via hyponatremia, reduced benzodiazepine receptors, or both

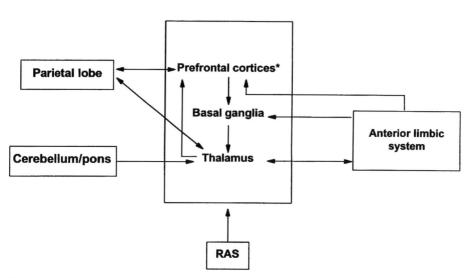

*Motor, supplementary motor area, and anterior cingulate areas

Figure 8.1 Brain systems implicated in catatonia.

catatonia fall into four broad groups: mood disorder patients; those who are psychotic and likely to get an antipsychotic agent; those with neurologic disease; and patients with metabolic disorder. The therapeutic implications of these considerations are discussed in Chapter 7.

ENDNOTES

1 Durant, 1961; Heinroth and Schmorak, 1975.

2 Joseph, 1999.

3 Joseph et al., 1991.

4 Luria, 1973: 89, 187–225.

5 Bond, 1920; Kirby and Davis, 1921; Cheyette and Cummings, 1995.

6 Dide, Guiraud and LaFage, 1921

7 Gjedd et al., 2000.

8 Alexander et al., 1986; Taylor, 1999: chapter 1.

9 Senser et al., 1993.

10 Wilcox, 1986; Roberts, 1965.

11 Northoff, 2000; Boker et al., 2000.

12 MacDonald et al., 2000.

13 Scheibel, 1997.

14 MacDonald et al., 2000.

15 Saver et al., 1993; Fukutake et al., 1993.

16 Ho et al., 1994.

17 Critchley, 1953; Kolb and Whishaw, 1996 (pp. 305–3330); Jasper, et al., 1995; Goldberg, 1992; Fuster; 1997; Miller and Cummings, 1999.

18 Roberts, 1965; Scheibel, 1997.

19 Kasture et al., 1996.

20 An example of such an imaginary association of psychodynamic constructs and neurochemistry would read:

Psychodynamic-neurochemistry equivalencies

Intrapsychic structure	Underlying transmitter	Action
Id	Dopamine	Driving force; activates frontal systems; basis for hedonistic reward system
Ego	Serotonin	Modifies dopamine; limits activity to socially acceptable limits; prevents violence, suicide
Super-Ego	Noradrenaline	Generates anxiety whenever dopamine and serotonin systems clash; encourages reward-sustaining behavior

21 Charney et al., 2000; Guerrera, 1999.

22 Kish et al., 1990,

23 Carroll, 2000.

24 Kosten and Kleber, 1988.

25 Gjessing, 1974; Stöber et al., 2000a,b,c.

26 Wetzel et al., 1987.

27 Thomas et al., 1997; Zaw and Bates, 1997.

28 Petrides et al., 1997; Carroll, 1999.

29 Northoff et al., 1999a.

30 Churchill et al., 1996a,b; Munoz et al., 1998; Kardos, 1999.

31 Wenzel and Kuschinsky, 1990.

32 Hauber, 1998; Jellinger, 1999.

33 Taylor, 1999.

34 Bowyer et al., 1996; Neuman et al., 1996; Charpier et al., 1999; Castro-Alamancos 1999; Velasco et al., 2000; Blumenfeld and McCormick, 2000.

35 Weinberger, 1987.

36 Pakkenberg, 1992; Staal et al., 1998.

37 Crosson and Hughes 1987; Andreasen et al., 1994; Pantelis et al., 1992; Weinberger et al., 1994.

38 Taylor, 1999.

39 Kramer, 1977.

40 Taylor 1990, 1999.

9

Back to the future

von Baer made the rueful remark that all new and truly important ideas must pass through three stages: first dismissed as nonsense, then rejected as against religion, and finally acknowledged as true, with the proviso from initial opponents that they knew it all along.

Gould, 2001

We define and describe catatonia from a clinician's perspective. We detail how to identify it reliably, to seek its causes, and to best treat it, regardless of the severity or the variations in its presentation. If it seems that most of the patients with catatonia that we discuss had miraculous relief and resolution of the underlying disease process, it is not a misperception, nor a misleading selection of clinical vignettes. The majority of patients with catatonia we have treated get "all better." "All better" is a phrase rarely used in discussions of patients with behavior syndromes. But, if quickly identified and properly treated, "all better" is the frequent response for catatonia. We have presented 51 patient vignettes. Of these, 15 were treated with barbiturates or benzodiazepines, nine successfully; 23 with ECT, 20 successfully; and seven successfully with lithium or anticonvulsants. With that favorable experience in mind, what do we know about this remarkable condition that supports our ability to treat it so well, and what does its study teach us?

Catatonia is a stable syndrome

We know that catatonia is a psychopathological syndrome similar to delirium and delusions. Delirium results from altered arousal and is a feature of many disorders. Delusions result from disordered thinking and are also features of many conditions. Catatonia is a parallel disorder of the motor system. Like the characteristic signs and symptoms that define delirium and delusion, characteristic signs delineate catatonia. It is a reversible syndrome that follows a defined course when untreated, and another course when properly treated. It occurs in many illnesses including mood disorders, general medical conditions, toxic and psychotic states, and neurologic pathology.

We know that the features of catatonia can be systematically and reliably assessed. We define the features and show that they can be clearly identified. The clinical ambiguities that remain are a duration requirement for the diagnosis of each feature, and whether mutism and immobility alone suffice for the diagnosis to be made. We have taken the persistence of signs for one hour as a reasonable standard, unless the feature is transient by definition (e.g. echolalia) and then, two or more expressions of it suffice. We argue that the DSM classification system overvalues mutism and immobility and that other specific features of catatonia must be also present to make the diagnosis. Otherwise, other conditions (e.g., parkinsonism, elective mutism) can be mistaken for catatonia.

False positive diagnoses (when catatonia is not present) are as clinically damaging as are false negatives (missing the diagnosis). False negative diagnoses hurt patients directly by depriving them of effective treatment. False positive diagnoses erode the clinician's ability to treat patients with the condition. If a mute patient is mistakenly diagnosed as catatonic and the administered treatment gives no relief, the disappointed clinician will be less likely to pursue catatonia in his next mute patient.

We know that catatonia is stable and reproducible. A landmark epidemiological countywide study in New York State found the diagnosis to be stable over several decades.[1] Recent factor analytic studies report similar patterns of psychopathology: stupor, mutism, and negativism make up the classic catatonia syndrome, and automatic obedience and stimulus bound behaviors, stereotypy, and catalepsy make up the syndrome that is more prevalent in manic patients.[2] Careful attention to a patient's motor behavior should identify all patients with catatonia.

Catatonia is common

We know that catatonia is frequently seen in acute care settings, with 5–10% of acutely hospitalized psychiatric patients exhibiting catatonia as defined by modern diagnostic criteria (Table 5.3). Estimating the numbers of patients likely to exhibit catatonia from hospital discharge records, we find the number much greater than the number of suicides annually. Of all that we know about catatonia, this fact is the most surprising to clinicians who do not routinely look for catatonic features, or who assume (incorrectly) that all catatonic patients are mute and immobile. The figures for the prevalence of catatonia are remarkably consistent for the last half century.

Catatonia has many faces

Catatonia has many forms. We recognize a stuporous, retarded form of the illness that is labeled catatonia, catatonic stupor, or the Kahlbaum syndrome. An excited form that represents mania with catatonia is described. A malignant (lethal) form of catatonia occurs with an acute onset, fever, and severe disturbances in body physiology. The outcome is fatal when not adequately treated. A delirious dream-like state is a feature of an excited form of catatonia and is known as delirious mania or oneiroid state. The mixed affective state during which the patient rapidly shifts between mania and depression is likely a form of delirious mania. Whether the treatment algorithms that are effective for delirious mania also benefit patients with rapid cycling manic disorders requires systematic study. Some catatonic states occur in patients with epilepsy, non-convulsive status epilepticus, and basal brain disease (e.g., akinetic mutism).

These diverse conditions are joined in the commonality of their presenting motor signs and in their response to treatment. Sedative anticonvulsant medicines and ECT are effective for each catatonic variant.

Neuroleptic malignant syndrome is malignant catatonia

Although none of these clinical presentations of catatonia is "new", recent data find NMS to be a form of malignant catatonia triggered by exposure to dopamine blocking drugs. The focus on "neuroleptic" in the neuroleptic malignant syndrome is a misnomer. Many drugs induce the syndrome.[3] NMS is also triggered by the sudden withdrawal of dopaminergic agents, a pharmacologically-induced sudden imbalance in GABA-A versus GABA-B brain neurohumors, and the sudden increase in brain serotonin. The signs and symptoms of NMS and MC and their laboratory profiles are indistinguishable.[4] The interpretation of NMS as malignant catatonia is the most important advance in the diagnosis and management of catatonia since the 1970s when the relationship between catatonia and manic-depressive illness was re-established. We recommend the treatment for NMS from this perspective.

Catatonia is not usually associated with schizophrenia

The connection between catatonia and schizophrenia established in modern classification schemes needs to be broken. Many pathophysiologies elicit the catatonia syndrome (Chapter 4). Manic-depressive illness is the most likely etiology, followed by general medical and neurologic diseases. About 10% of patients with catatonia meet criteria for schizophrenia, making it more likely that a patient with catatonia is suffering from a disorder other than schizophrenia. This fact is a paradigm shift for many clinicians and a challenge to the drafters of the next versions of the DSM and ICD classification systems. The recognition of catatonia in its many forms is essential, however, if we are to reshape our understanding of psychopathology. Treatment considerations and how the choices expand when the false link between catatonia and schizophrenia is broken are described in Table 9.1.

Table 9.1 Treatment most likely to be considered based on the etiology[a] of catatonia

Mood disorder[b]	Neurologic disease	General medical disease	Schizophrenia
Antidepressants	Anticonvulsants	Correct metabolic imbalance	Antipsychotics
Anticonvulsants	Traumatic brain injury and stroke protocols	Cardiovascular protocols	Antiparkinson protocols
Lithium	Neurosurgery	Better medication management	Augmentation
Benzodiazepines ECT	Benzodiazepines	Correct endocrine imbalance	Last resort; antipsychotic augmentation

[a] *Treatments for neurologic and general medical disease reflect the most common causes within those categories. For specifics, see Chapter 4.*
[b] *The risk for NMS in a catatonic patient with a mood disorder is substantial when an antipsychotic is given, and we avoid these agents in these patients, using them only as a last resort.*

Table 9.2 Acute management of a patient with catatonia

Hospitalization
Benzodiazepine challenge
Benzodiazepine treatment trial
Maintain fluid and electrolyte balance
Avoid antipsychotic agents
Avoid prolonged immobility
Identify and correct an underlying neurologic or general medical cause
If substantial improvement fails to occur by four days, give ECT

To accurately reflect what we know about catatonia, psychiatric nosologies will serve psychiatric patients best by listing catatonia as an independent movement disorder (as delirium is listed as an independent cognitive disorder). Subtypes are best defined as non-malignant catatonia (Kahlbaum syndrome), delirious mania, and malignant catatonia, with modifiers as secondary to a mood disorder, a general medical condition or toxic state, to a brain disorder, or to a psychotic disorder. Such designation would recognize the many syndromes in which catatonia is an identifiable feature and encourage better treatments.

Catatonia is a good-prognosis condition

The management of catatonia is well defined. Acute treatment strategies, however, must recognize that catatonia can evolve to a life-threatening stage. The guidelines for the acute management of catatonia, discussed in Chapter 7, are summarized in Table 9.2. Although we lack double-blind controlled studies of the response to treatments of patients with catatonia, the published clinical reports and our own experience indicate that when properly treated, almost all episodes of catatonia fully resolve. Recovery from the cause of the catatonia depends on the pathophysiology. The most likely cause of failure in relieving the syndrome is prolonged inadequate treatment.

For the patient in the full-blown syndrome, the steps listed in Table 9.2 need to be carefully followed to avoid prolonged morbidity or death. If the patient has catatonic features, but they do not over-shadow the causative condition, the catatonic features can be ignored and the patient treated for the causative condition as long as antipsychotic drugs are avoided. For excited manic patients, a mood stabilizer loading strategy, or a mood stabilizer and a benzodiazepine for temporary sedation, or ECT are the safest effective approaches. For severely depressed patients, ECT is the treatment of choice and should not be delayed for a drug trial.

Patients with catatonia need continuation treatment after the syndrome and the causes are successfully resolved. Continuation (maintenance) treatment is typically an extension of the acute treatment strategy, so the acute treatment choices need to be considered with their long-term efficacy and availability in mind. Because catatonia is most commonly associated with a mood disorder, a frequently recurrent condition, lifetime prophylactic treatment is often necessary. When a benzodiazepine, ECT, or their combination is the acute treatment, it is also the continuation treatment.

Catatonia is a syndrome of motor dysregulation

Although the pathophysiology of catatonia is unclear, we recognize risk factors and the involved brain processes. Catatonia is a motor dysregulation syndrome. Patients have trouble starting and stopping movement. They have severe inertia, exemplified in catalepsy, mutism, posturing, and stereotypes. They have trouble monitoring their motor behavior to keep it appropriate. They respond motorically, despite understanding the instructions to the contrary. Automatic obedience, ambitendency, and echophenomena are examples.

Such catatonic features are associated with lesions throughout the central motor system, although frontal circuitry disease is the most common. When a specific motor system lesion cannot be identified, we see thalamic and parietal lobe lesions as interfering with visuo-spatial processing and perceptual motor coordination, leaving the motor system with insufficient or confusing afferent inputs to allow an appropriate response. Hyponatremia and starvation encourage the expression of catatonia. When a specific neurologic or general medical cause for catatonia has not been determined, bilateral parietal lobe and frontal circuitry hypometabolism has been observed (Chapter 8). We see that brain levels of dopamine, GABA, and serotonin play important roles in motor regulation, and drugs that alter these neurotransmitters are often the basis for catatonia.

Future studies

What can the study of catatonia teach us?

For the *clinical neuroscientist*, catatonia is a natural laboratory of motor regulatory functioning. It is a behavior state with a rapid onset that is quickly terminated by specific interventions that have common properties. Assuming family or guardian consent, the opportunity for brain imaging, metabolic assessment, neuroendocrine, EEG, and evoked potential studies under both sick and recovered conditions are readily done. Given the many precipitants of catatonia, many clinical investigations are justified. Comparisons within subjects during and after catatonia, with other patient groups, and with normal subjects could be accomplished.

To answer what questions?

What are the brain systems that decide when to start and stop movement and then carry out the plans? What brain systems monitor movement so that we know we are doing what we planned to do? How does sensory feedback modulate voluntary movement and what brain systems integrate this feedback with movement to self-correct it? Which brain processes are dysfunctional in catatonia? Do the many etiologies of catatonia affect different or the same brain systems that subserve voluntary movement?

A rostral to caudal neural network that controls motivated behavior has been proposed.[5] The network includes the cerebral cortex, medial pre-optic area, anterior hypothalamus, descending paraventricular, ventromedial and premammillary nuclei, the mammillary body, substantia nigra, and the ventral tegmental area. The striate inhibits the network while the pallidum disinhibits it. The rostral segment of the network controls eating, drinking, reproductive, and defensive behaviors. The caudal segment of the network controls exploratory or foraging behavior with locomotor and orienting components. This segment serves behaviors required for obtaining goal-directed objects. The prefrontal cortex, particularly the supplementary motor area (SMA), has a major role in planning and preparing for these voluntary movements. Functional MRI testing finds the caudal subdivision of the SMA involved in the execution of externally cued movement, especially when the cues are unpredicted.[6] Frontal EEG changes have been correlated with "when to move" decisions,[7] and with different demands on attention to move and its execution.[8] These procedures have been applied to patients with catatonia only as diagnostic aids. The parts of the network that are dysfunctional in catatonia are unknown. Patients with catatonia are excellent subjects to test this hypothesis.

Dopamine and other neurotransmitters have different effects within this neural network.[9] Catatonia can be induced by rapidly altering neurotransmitter relationships, but systematic study with multiple procedures, looking for predicted convergences, have not been done. Because catatonia is so prevalent among patients with manic-depressive illness, it would be useful to consider the neurophysiologic aspects of mood disorder that disrupt this motor network. Are changes in attention or arousal or the intensity of the mood state central to the disruption?

Catatonic patients respond inappropriately to conflicting stimuli. Ambitendency is an example. Some patients seem unaware that their motor behavior is inappropriate. The ability to self-monitor responses to conflicting stimuli may be a function of the anterior cingulate gyrus, one of the prefrontal cortical circuits likely associated with catatonia.[10]

Without sensory input, the motor system is unguided. Patients with thalamic and parietal lobe lesions exhibit neglect and posturing. Bilateral frontal and parietal lobe hypometabolism is described in psychiatric patients with catatonia. Visuo-spatial function is central to adequate motor function, and inhibition of muscle groups is partly dependent upon reciprocal sensory information from opposing muscle groups.[11] One report found catatonic patients to have impaired visuo-spatial and attentional function on neuropsychological testing.[12] These investigators also report decreased density of GABA-A receptors in the sensorimotor cortex[13] and abnormal movement-related cortical potentials in frontoparietal areas.[14] During voluntary tasks, anterior and posterior parts of the ventrolateral nucleus of the thalamus participate at different points in preparation, initiation, and performance.[15] The thalamus is part of frontal circuits involved in action. It provides feedback to the prefrontal cortex and tone to the circuitry. It links these circuits with the cerebellum, which is also involved in attentional and visuo-spatial aspects of voluntary movement.[16] The thalamus is also involved in sensory integration. Thalamic dysfunction could explain all the features of catatonia, including the generalized analgesia in patients with the full-blown syndrome. Visual and somatosensory evoked potential studies in catatonic patients might further delineate the relationship between catatonic features and sensorimotor integration.

Kraepelin and Bleuler described different subtypes of schizophrenia, and their subtyping is accepted in DSM and ICD classifications. The genetic researcher, when he assesses the genetic bases for schizophrenia, can either treat all types of schizophrenia as having a common etiology, or he can study the subtypes separately. Separating catatonic patients from the other subtypes will examine more homogeneous samples than when all the subtypes are studied as one disorder. Recent genetic studies of patients with periodic catatonia report identifiable loci of common abnormalities based on criteria of the Wernicke–Kleist–Leonhard classification system. They identify susceptibility loci in chromosomes 15q15 and 22q13 for periodic catatonia.[17] It is reasonable, based on the many differences between catatonic psychotic patients and those that are not catatonic, to study the subtypes of schizophrenia separately.

For the *clinical researcher*, catatonia is an opportunity to examine psychopathology with measures of neuroendocrinology, electrophysiology, and experimental therapeutics. The defined treatments of catatonia are benzodiazepines, anticonvulsants, and ECT. What do these agents have in common? Benzodiazepines and anticonvulsants are strong GABA-ergic agents, and an imbalance between GABA-A and GABA-B has been suggested as a factor in the development of catatonia. These treatments raise the seizure threshold and are so effectively anticonvulsant as to be able to interrupt an ongoing status epilepticus. Is subclinical epilepsy a model for catatonia?

EEG recordings assess the impact of treatments on brain function. A dominant paradigm in quantitative EEG has been the intimate association between changes in EEG with changes in behavior.[18] This paradigm developed with the measurement of EEG changes with different psychoactive drugs. By measuring changes in EEG frequencies, amplitudes, and rhythmicity, it was possible to differentiate the cerebral effects of psychoactive drug classes – antipsychotic, antidepressant, mood stabilizing, psychostimulant, and deliriant. Digital computer methods of analysis allowed the successful prediction of the clinical activity of putative psychoactive compounds. The quantitative EEG changes induced by ECT and by benzodiazepines, the agents most useful in treating catatonia today, are well defined and distinguishable. Repeated measures allow the tracking of the interaction of treatment effects with the changes in behavior. The EEG allows the clinician to more accurately specify the presence of an epileptic disorder, the severity of delirium, and the depth of stupor. Failure of the EEG to change with treatment points our attention to reconsider the choice of treatment and the dosing. Can EEG recordings be used to monitor the treatment of patients with catatonia?

The brain imaging methods of MRI, CAT, PET, SPECT, and functional MRI are widely studied in psychiatric research. The resolution of the images of brain nuclear structures is still modest, but improving rapidly. The physiologic measures are still gross, only allowing statements about cerebral blood flow over large regions of the brain, usually the major lobes. The quantitative EEG, although equally limited in resolution, allows moment-to-moment and repeated correlations with behavior, chemistry, and physiology. It is safe, continuous, quantifiable, easily recorded, and as easily quantified on-line, in real-time, while subjects are performing specified tasks. What are the EEG characteristics of catatonia, how do these change with treatment, and what are their correlations with the severity and various expressions of the syndrome?

The relation of the neuroendocrine system to behavior is another aspect for clinical research. In seeking what is common to the treatments of catatonia, we look mainly to their effects on neurohumors. In exploring the mechanism of action of ECT, however, attention has been directed to neuroendocrine regulation. ECT profoundly affects the neuroendocrine system.[19] It elicits the immediate release and alters the continuing relationships of the hypothalamic and pituitary hormones. The most effective forms of ECT have the greatest direct effects on neuroendocrine release. When the changes in neuroendocrine levels are not forthcoming, the benefits of ECT are modest and poorly sustained. While few examples of neuroendocrine testing in patients with catatonia are recorded, the examples find the abnormalities to recover when the syndrome lifts (Chapter 4). Gjessing and his followers sought to define the role of thyroid function in their patients with periodic catatonia and reported interesting correlations. Our techniques of measurement and the range of endocrine measures have broadened. What neuroendocrine abnormalities are associated with catatonia, and how do they change with recovery and relapse? How do they change with treatment? Do schizophrenic patients with catatonia have the same or different neuroendocrine profiles than those in manic-depressive illness or under toxic conditions?

In addition to these suggestions for the neuroscientist and the clinician researcher, we call attention to the legislated restrictions on the use of ECT in the treatment of psychiatric patients.[20] The catatonic patient is served poorly by these limitations and consideration should be given to making all treatments of proven merit available in the care of our patients.

ENDNOTES

1 Guggenheim and Babigian, 1974a,b. Table 5.2 lists prevalence studies.
2 Chapter 1, endnotes 23–26; Chapter 5.
3 Table 3.2.
4 Table 3.3.
5 Swanson, 2000.
6 Thickbroom et al., 2000.
7 Kukleta and Lamarche, 2000.
8 Feige et al., 2000.
9 Yamaguchi et al., 1998.
10 Botvinick et al., 1999.
11 Botvinick et al., 1999; Leis et al., 2000.
12 Northoff et al., 1999d.
13 Northoff et al., 1999e.
14 Northoff et al., 2000.
15 Raeva et al., 1999.
16 Taylor, 1999.
17 Stöber et al., 2001.
18 Fink 1968, 1969, 1985.
19 Fink 1979, 1991, 1999a, 2000a,b.
20 Bach-Y-Rita and De Ranieri, 1992.

Appendices

I. Rating scale for catatonia

From Bush et al., 1996a.
- Use the presence or absence of items 1–14 for screening purposes.
- Use the 0–3 scale for items 1–23 to rate severity.

1. Excitement

Extreme hyperactivity, constant motor unrest which is apparently non-purposeful. Not to be attributed to akathisia or goal-directed agitation.

0 = Absent
1 = Excessive motion, intermittent.
2 = Constant motion, hyperkinetic without rest periods.
3 = Severe excitement, frenzied motor activity.

2. Immobility/Stupor

Extreme hypoactivity, immobility. Minimally responsive to stimuli.

0 = Absent
1 = Sits abnormally still, may interact briefly.
2 = Virtually no interaction with external world.
3 = Stuporous, not responsive to painful stimuli.

3. Mutism

Verbally unresponsive or minimally responsive.

0 = Absent
1 = Verbally unresponsive to most questions; incomprehensible whisper.
2 = Speaks less than 20 words/5 minutes.
3 = No speech.

4. Staring

Fixed gaze, little or no visual scanning of environment, decreased blinking.

0 = Absent

1 = Poor eye contact. Gazes less than 20 seconds between shifting of attention; decreased blinking

2 = Gaze held longer than 20 seconds; occasionally shifts attention.

3 = Fixed gaze, non-reactive.

5. Posturing/Catalepsy

Maintains posture(s), including mundane (e.g., sitting or standing for long periods without reacting).

0 = Absent

1 = Less than one minute.

2 = Greater than one minute, less than 15 minutes.

3 = Bizarre posture, or mundane maintained more than 15 min.

6. Grimacing

Maintenance of odd facial expressions.

0 = Absent

1 = Less than 10 sec.

2 = Less than 1 min.

3 = Bizarre expression(s) or maintained more than 1 min.

7. Echopraxia/Echolalia

Mimicking of examiner's movements/ speech.

0 = Absent

1 = Occasional.

2 = Frequent.

3 = Continuous.

8. Stereotypy

Repetitive, non-goal-directed motor activity (e.g. finger-play; repeatedly touching, patting or rubbing self). (Abnormality is not inherent in the act but in its frequency.)

0 = Absent
1 = Occasional.
2 = Frequent.
3 = Continuous.

9. Mannerisms

Odd, purposeful movements (hopping or walking tiptoe, saluting passers-by, exaggerated caricatures of mundane movements). (Abnormality is inherent in the act itself.)
0 = Absent
1 = Occasional.
2 = Frequent.
3 = Continuous.

10. Verbigeration

Repetition of phrases or sentences.
0 = Absent
1 = Occasional.
2 = Frequent, difficult to interrupt.
3 = Continuous.

11. Rigidity

Maintenance of a rigid position despite efforts to be moved (Exclude if cogwheeling or tremor are present.)
0 = Absent
1 = Mild resistance.
2 = Moderate.
3 = Severe, cannot be repostured.

12. Negativism

Apparently motiveless resistance to instructions or to attempts to move/ examine patient. Contrary behavior, does the opposite of the instruction.
0 = Absent
1 = Mild resistance and/or occasionally contrary.
2 = Moderate resistance and/or frequently contrary.
3 = Severe resistance and/or continually contrary.

13. Waxy Flexibility

During reposturing of patient, patient offers initial resistance before allowing himself to be repositioned (similar to that of a bending a warm candle).

0 = Absent.

3 = Present.

14. Withdrawal

Refusal to eat, drink and/or make eye contact.

0 = Absent.

1 = Minimal oral intake for less than one day.

2 = Minimal oral intake for more than one day.

3 = No oral intake for one day or more.

15. Impulsivity

Patient suddenly engages in inappropriate behavior (e.g. runs down hallway, starts screaming, or takes off clothes) without provocation. Afterwards, cannot explain.

0 = Absent

1 = Occasional

2 = Frequent

3 = Constant or not redirectable

16. Automatic Obedience

Exaggerated cooperation with examiner's request, or repeated movements that are requested once.

0 = Absent

1 = Occasional

2 = Frequent

3 = Continuous

17. Passive obedience (mitgehen)

Raising arm in response to light pressure of finger, despite instructions to the contrary.

0 = Absent

3 = Present

18. Negativism (Gegenhalten)

Resistance to passive movement that is proportional to strength of the stimulus; response seems automatic rather than willful.

0 = Absent

3 = Present

19. Ambitendency

Patient appears "stuck" in indecisive, hesitant motor movements.

0 = Absent

3 = Present

20. Grasp Reflex

Strike open palm of patient with two extended fingers of examiner's hand. Automatic closure of patient's hand.

0 = Absent

3 = Present

21. Perseveration

Repeatedly returns to same topic or persists with same movements.

0 = Absent

3 = Present

22. Combativeness

Usually in an undirected manner, without explanation.

0 = Absent

1 = Occasionally strikes out, low potential for injury

2 = Strikes out frequently, moderate potential for injury

3 = Danger to others

23. Autonomic Abnormality

Circle: Temperature

Blood Pressure

Pulse rate

Respiratory rate

Inappropriate sweating.

0 = Absent
1 = Abnormality of one parameter [exclude pre-existing hypertension]
2 = Abnormality of 2 parameters
3 = Abnormality of 3 or greater parameters

II. Examination for catatonia

From Bush et al., 1996a.

- The method described here is used to complete Catatonia Rating Scales.
- Ratings are made based on the observed behaviors during the examination, with the exception of completing the items for 'withdrawal' and 'autonomic abnormality', which may be based upon either observed behavior and/or chart documentation.
- Rate items only if well defined. If uncertain, rate the item as '0'.

Procedure:	Examines:
1. Observe patient while trying to engage in a conversation.	Activity level, abnormal movements, abnormal speech
2. Examiner scratches head in exaggerated manner.	Echopraxia
3. Examine arm for cogwheeling. Attempt to reposition, instructing patient to "keep your arm loose". Move arm with alternating lighter and heavier force.	Rigidity, Negativism, Waxy Flexibility
4. Ask patient to extend arm. Place one finger beneath hand and try to raise slowly after stating, "DO NOT let me raise your arm".	Passive obedience
5. Extend hand stating, "DO NOT shake my hand".	Ambitendence
6. Reach into your pocket and state, "Stick out your tongue, I want to stick a pin in it."	Automatic Obedience
7. Examine for the grasp reflex.	Grasp Reflex
8. Examine the patient's chart for oral intake, vital signs, and unusual incidents.	
9. Observe the patient indirectly for a brief period each day.	

References

The publisher has used its best endeavors to ensure that the URLs for external websites referred to in this book are correct and active at the time of going to press. However, the publisher has no responsibility for the websites and can make no guarantee that a site will remain live or that the content is or will remain appropriate.

Abrams R (1997). *Electroconvulsive Therapy*. 3rd edn. New York: Oxford University Press.

Abrams R, Fink M, Dornbush R, Feldstein S, Volavka J & Roubicek J (1972). Unilateral and bilateral ECT: Effects on depression, memory and the electroencephalogram. *Arch Gen Psychiatry* **27**: 88–94.

Abrams R & Taylor MA (1976). Catatonia, a prospective clinical study. *Arch Gen Psychiatry* **33**: 579–581.

Abrams R & Taylor MA (1997). Catatonia: Prediction of response to somatic treatments. *Am J Psychiatry* **134**: 78–80.

Abrams R, Taylor MA & Stolurow KAC (1979). Catatonia and mania: Patterns of cerebral dysfunction. *Biol Psychiatry* **14**: 111–117.

Achte KA (1961). *Der Verlauf der Schizophrenien und der Schizophrenormen Psychosen*. Copenhagen: Munksgaard.

Ackner B, Harris A & Olham AJ (1957). Insulin treatment of schizophrenia: control study. *Lancet* **2**: 607–611.

Addonizio G & Susman VL (1987). ECT as a treatment alternative for patients with symptoms of neuroleptic malignant syndrome. *J Clin Psychiatry* **48**: 102–105.

Addonizio G, Susman VL & Roth SD (1987). Neuroleptic malignant syndrome: review and analysis of 115 cases. *Biological Psychiatry* **22**: 1004–1020.

Adland ML (1947). Review, case studies, therapy, and interpretation of acute exhaustive psychoses. *Psychiatr Quart* **21**: 39–69.

Ahuja N (2000a). Organic catatonia: A review. *Indian J Psychiatry* **42**: 327–346.

Ahuja N (2000b). Organic catatonia. (Letter). *J Am Acad Child Adolesc Psychiatry* 1464.

Ahuja N (2000c). Founders of psychiatry: Karl Ludwig Kahlbaum (1828–1899). *Delhi Psychiatr Soc Bull* **3**: 28–35.

Ahuja N & Nehru R (1990). Neuroleptic malignant syndrome: a subtype of lethal catatonia? (Letter.) *Acta Psychiatr Scand* **82**: 398.

Akhtar S & Ahmad H (1993). Ciprofloxin-induced catatonia. *J Clin Psychiatry* **54**: 115–116.

Alexander GE, DeLong MR & Strick PL (1986). Parallel organization of functionally segregated circuits linking basal ganglia and cortex. *Ann Rev Neuroscience* **9**: 357–381.

Allen JR, Pfefferbaum B, Hammond D & Speed L (2000). A disturbed child's use of a public event: Cotard's syndrome in a ten-year old. *Psychiatry* **63**: 208–213.

Altschuler LL, Cummings JL & Mills MJ (1986). Mutism: review, differential diagnosis, and report of 22 cases. *Am J Psychiatry* **143**: 1409–1414.

American Association of Suicidology. *1999 Official Final Statistics.* In: JL McIntosh: *Supplemental Suicide Statistics 1998.* www.suicidology.org

American Psychiatric Association (1952). *Diagnostic and Statistical Manual: Mental Disorders.* Washington D.C.: American Psychiatric Association.

American Psychiatric Association (1980). *Diagnostic and Statistical Manual of Mental Disorders.* 3rd edn. Washington, D.C.: American Psychiatric Association.

American Psychiatric Association (1987). Task force on laboratory tests in psychiatry. The dexamethasone suppression test: an overview of its current status in psychiatry. *Am J Psychiatry* **144**: 1253–1262.

American Psychiatric Association (1994). *Diagnostic and Statistical Manual of Mental Disorders.* 4th edn. Washington, D.C.: American Psychiatric Association.

American Psychiatric Association (1996). *Practice Guidelines.* Washington D.C.: American Psychiatric Association.

American Psychiatric Association (1997). *Practice Guideline for the Treatment of Patients with Schizophrenia.* Washington D.C.: American Psychiatric Association.

American Psychiatric Association (1990). *Electroconvulsive Therapy: Treatment, Training and Privileging.* Washington D.C.: American Psychiatric Association.

American Psychiatric Association (2001). *Electroconvulsive Therapy: Treatment, Training and Privileging.* 2nd edn. Washington D.C.: American Psychiatric Association.

Andreasen NC, Arndt S, Swayze IIV, Cizadlo T, Flaum M, O'Leary D, Erhardt JC & Yu WTC (1994). Thalamic abnormalities in schizophrenia visualized through magnetic resonance imaging averaging. *Science* **266**: 294–298.

Anfinson TJ & Cruse J (1996). SIADH associated with catatonia. Its resolution with ECT. *Psychosomatics* **36**: 212.

Araneta E, Magen J, Musci MN, Singer P & Vann CR (1975). Gilles de la Tourette's syndrome symptom onset at age 35. *Child Psychiatry Hum Dev* **5**: 224–230.

Arnold OH (1949). Untersuchungen zur Frage der akuten tödlichen Katatonien. *Wien Z Nervenheilk Grenzgeb* **2**(4): 386–401.

Arnold OH & Stepan H (1952). Untersuchungen zur Frage der akuten tödliche Katatonie. *Wr Z Nervenheilkunde* **4**: 235–287.

Arnone D, Hansen L & Davies G (2002). Pulmonary embolism and severe depression. (Letter.) *Am J Psychiatry* **159**: 873–874.

Aronson MJ & Thompson SV (1950). Complications of acute catatonic excitement. A report of two cases. *Am J Psychiatry* **107**: 216–220.

Aschaffenburg G (1898). Die Katatoniefrage. *Allg Z Psychiatrie* **54**: 1004–1026.

Assion HJ, Heinemann F & Laux G (1998). Neuroleptic malignant syndrome under treatment with antidepressants? A critical review. *Eur Arch Psychiatry Clin Neurosci* **248**: 231–239.

Atre-Vaidya N (2000). Significance of abnormal brain perfusion in catatonia. A case report. *Neuropsychiatry Neuropsychol Behav Neurol* **13**: 136 139.

Avery D & Lubrano A (1979). Depression treated with imipramine and ECT: the deCarolis study reconsidered. *Am J Psychiatry* **136**: 559–562.

Bach-Y-Rita G & De Ranieri A (1992). Medicolegal complications of postpartum catatonia. *West J Med* **156**: 417–419.

Bahro M, Kaempf C & Strnad J (1999). Catatonia under medication with risperidone in a 61-year-old patient. *Acta Psychiatr Scand* **99**: 223–226.

Baldessarini RJ (1970). Frequency of diagnosis of schizophrenia vesus affective disorder from 1944 to 1968. *Am J Psychiatry* **127**: 759–763.

Barker RA, Revesz T, Thom M, Marsden CD & Brown P (1998). Review of 23 patients affected by the stiff man syndrome: clinical subdivision into stiff trunk (man) syndromes, stiff limb syndrome, and progressive encephalomyelitis with rigidity. *J Neurol Neurosurg Psychiatry* **65**: 633–640.

Barnes MP, Saunders M, Walls TJ, Saunders I & Kirk CA (1986). The syndrome of Karl Ludwig Kahlbaum. *J Neurol Neurosurg Psychiatry* **49**: 991–996.

Barnes TR (1989). A rating scale for drug-induced akathisia. *Br J Psychiatry* **154**: 672–676.

Bates WJ & Smeltzer DJ (1982). Electroconvulsive treatment of psychotic self-injurious behaviour in a patient with severe mental retardation. *Am J Psychiatry* **39**: 1355–1356.

Bauer G, Gerstenbrand F & Rumpl E (1979). Varieties of the locked-in syndrome. *J Neurol* **221**: 77–91.

Baxter LR, Phelps ME, Mazziotta JC, Guze BH, Schwartz JM & Selin CE (1987). Local cerebral glucose metabolic rates in obsessive compulsive disorder. *Arch Gen Psychiatry* **44**: 211–218.

Bear DM (1986). Behavioural changes in temporal lobe epilepsy: conflict, confusion, challenge. In MR Trimble & TG Bolwig (Eds). *Aspects of Epilepsy and Psychiatry*, vol. 3, pp. 19–30. New York: John Wiley & Sons.

Bebbington P & Kuipers L (1994a). The clinical utility of expressed emotion in schizophrenia. *Acta Psychiatr Scand* **89** (Suppl. 302): 46–53.

Bebbington P & Kuipers L (1994b). The predictive utility of expressed emotion in schizophrenia. An aggregate analysis. *Psychol Med* **24**: 707–718.

Beckmann H, Franzek E & Stöber G (1996). Genetic heterogeneity in catatonic schizophrenia: a family study. *Am J Med Gen (Neuropsychiatric Gen)* **67**: 289–300.

Behr A (1891). *Die Frage der "Katatonie" oder des Irreseins mit Spannung*. Thesis. Dorpat University, 1891. Riga: WF Häcker.

Bell LV (1849). On a form of disease resembling some advanced stages of mania and fever. *Am J Insanity* **6**: 97–127.

Benegal V, Hingorani S & Khanna S (1993). Idiopathic catatonia: validity of the concept. *Psychopathology* **26**: 41–46.

Benegal V, Hingorani S, Khanna S & Channabasavanna SM (1992). Is stupor by itself a catatonic symptom. *Psychopathology* **25**: 229–231.

Ben-Shachar D, Levine E, Spanier I, Zuk R & Youdim MB (1993). Iron modulates neuroleptic-induced effects related to the dopamine system. *Isr J Med Sci* **29**: 587–592.

Berardi D, Amore M, Keck Jr PE, Troia M & Dell'Atti M (1998). Clinical and pharmacologic risk factors for neuroleptic malignant syndrome: a case-control study. *Biol Psychiatry* **44**: 748–754.

Berger H (1929). On the electroencephalogram of man. *Arch Psychiat Nervenkr* **87**: 527–570.

Berman E & Wolpert EA (1987). Intractable manic-depressive psychosis with rapid cycling in an 18-year-old woman successfully treated with electroconvulsive therapy. *J Nerv Ment Dis* **175**: 236–239.

Berrios GE (1981). Stupor: A conceptual history. *Psychological Medicine* **11**: 677–686.

Berrios GE (1996a). *The History of Mental Symptoms. Descriptive Psychopathology Since the Nineteenth Century*. Cambridge: Cambridge University Press.

Berrios GE (1996b). Die Gruppirung der psychischen Krankheiten. Part III. *Hist Psychiatry* **7**: 167–181.

Berrios GE & Porter R (1995). *A History of Clinical Psychiatry*. London: Athlone Press.

Biancosino B, Zanchi P, Agostini M & Grassi L (2001). Suspected neuroleptic catatonia induced by clozapine. (Letter) *Can J Psychiatry* **46**: 458.

Billig O & Freeman WT (1943). Fatal catatonia. *Am J Psychiatry* **100**: 633–638.

Bini L (1995). Professor Bini's notes on the first electro-shock experiment. *Convulsive Ther.* **11**: 260–261.

Birbeck GL & Kaplan PW (1999). Serotonin syndrome: A frequently missed diagnosis? Let the neurologist beware. *Neurologist* **5**: 279–285.

Birkhimer LJ & DeVane CL (1984). The neuroleptic malignant syndrome: Presentation and treatment. *Drug Intellig Clin Pharm* **18**: 462–465.

Black DWG, Wilcox JA & Stewart M (1985). The use of ECT in children: Case report. *J Clin Psychiatry* **46**: 98–99.

Blacker KH (1966). Obsessive–compulsive phenomena and catatonic states – A continuum. A five-year case study of a chronic catatonic patient. *Psychiatry* **29**: 185–194.

Bleckwenn WJ (1930). The production of sleep and rest in psychotic cases. *Arch Neurol Psychiatry* **24**: 365–372.

Bleuler E (1924). *Textbook of Psychiatry*. New York: Macmillan.

Bleuler E (1950). *Dementia Praecox or the Group of Schizophrenias*, p. 211. J Zinkin (trans). York: International University Press.

Bleuler E (1988). *Dementia praecox oder Gruppe der Schizophrenien*. Tübingen: Nachbruck. Edition Dikord. (1st edn 1911, Leipzig: Deutke.)

Blum P & Jankovic J (1991). Stiff-person syndrome: an autoimmune disease. *Movement Disorders* **6**: 12–20.

Blumenfeld H & McCormick DA (2000). Corticothalamic inputs control the pattern of activity generated in thalamocortical networks. *J Neurosci* **20**: 5153–5162.

Blumer D (1997). Catatonia and neuroleptics: Psychobiologic significance of remote and recent findings. *Comprehens Psychiatry* **38**: 193–201.

Boardman RH, Lomas J & Markowe M (1956). Insulin and chlorpromazine in schizophrenia; a comparative study in previously untreated cases. *Lancet* **2**: 487–494.

Boker H, Northoff G, Lenz C, von Schmeling C, Eppel A, Hartling F, Will H, Lempa G, Meier M & Hell D (2000). The reconstruction of speechlessness: An investigation of subjective experience of catatonic patients by means of modified Landfield Categories. *Psychiatrische Praxis* **27**: 389–396.

Bolwig TG (1986). Classification of psychiatric disturbances in epilepsy. In MR Trimble & TG Bolwig (Eds). *Aspects of Epilepsy and Psychiatry*, vol. 1, pp. 1–8. New York: John Wiley & Sons.

Bond ED (1920). Epidemic encephalitis and katatonic symptoms. *Am J Insanity* **76**: 261–264.

Bond TC (1980). Recognition of acute delirious mania. *Arch Gen Psychiatry* **37**: 553–554.

Bonner CA & Kent GH (1936). Overlapping symptoms in a catatonic excitement and manic excitement. *Am J Psychiatry* **92**: 1311–1322.

Bottlender R, Jaeger M, Hofschuster E, Dobmeier P & Moeller H-J (2002). Neuroleptic malignant syndrome due to atypical neuroleptics: Three episodes in one patient. *Pharmacopsychiatry* **35**: 119–121.

Botvinick M, Nystrom LE, Fissell K, Carter CS & Cohen JD (1999). Conflict monitoring versus selection-for-action in anterior cingulate cortex. *Nature* **402**: 179–181.

Bourne H (1953). Insulin myth. *Lancet* **2**: 964–968.

Bowyer JF, Clausing P, Schmued L, Davies DL, Binienda Z, Newport GD, Scallet AC & Slikker W (1996). Parenterally administered 3-nitropropionic acid and amphetamine can combine to produce damage to terminals and cell bodies in the striatum. *Brain Res* **712**: 221–229.

Braude WM, Barnes TR & Gore SM (1983). Clinical characteristics of akathisia: a systematic examination of acute psychiatric inpatient admissions. *Br J Psychiatry* **143**: 139–150.

Bräunig P (1991). Zur Frage der "Katatonia alternans" und zur Differentialtypologie psychomotorischer Psychosen. *Fortschr Neurol Psychiatr* **59**: 92–96.

Bräunig P & Krüger S (1999). Images in psychiatry: Karl Ludwig Kahlbaum. *Am J Psychiatry* **156**: 989.

Bräunig P & Krüger S (2000). Karl Ludwig Kahlbaum (1828–1899) – ein Protagonist der modernen Psychiatrie. *Psychiat Praxis* **27**: 112–118.

Bräunig P, Krüger S & Hoffler J (1995a). Verstarkung katatoner Symptomatik unter Neuroleptiktherapie. [Exacerbation of catatonic symptoms in neuroleptic therapy.] *Nervenarzt* **66**: 379–382.

Bräunig P, Börner I & Krüger S (1995b). Diagnostiche Merkmale katatoner Schizophrenien. In P Bräunig (Ed.). *Differenzierung katatoner und neuroleptika-induzierter Bewegungsstörungen*, pp. 36–42. Stuttgart: Georg Thieme Verlag.

Bräunig P, Krüger S & Shugar G (1998). Prevalence and clinical significance of catatonic symptoms in mania. *Compr Psychiatry* **39**: 35–46.

Bräunig P, Krüger S & Shugar G (1999). Pravalenz und klinische Bedeutung katatoner Symptome bei Manien. [Prevalence and clinical significance of catatonic symptoms in mania.] *Fortschr Neurol Psychiatr* **67**: 306–317.

Bräunig P, Krüger S, Shugar G, Hoffler J & Borner I (2000). The catatonia rating scale I: development, reliability, and use. *Compr Psychiatry* **41**: 147–158.

Braunmühl A (1938). *Die Insulinshockbehandlung der Schizophrenie*. Berlin: Julius Springer Verlag.

Breakey WR & Kala AK (1977). Typhoid catatonia responsive to ECT. *Br Med J* **2**: 357–359.

Bricolo A (1977). The medical therapy of the apallic syndrome. In G Dall Ore, F Gerstenbrand, CH Lücking, G Peters & UH Peters. (Eds). *The Apallic Syndrome*, pp. 182–188. Berlin: Springer-Verlag.

Bright-Long LE & Fink M (1993). Reversible dementia and affective disorder: The Rip Van Winkle Syndrome. *Convulsive Ther* **9**: 209–216.

Brockington IF, Perris C, Kendell RE, Hillier VE & Wainwright S (1982a). The course and outcome of cycloid psychosis. *Psycholog Med* **12**: 97–105.

Brockington IF, Perris C & Meltzer HY (1982b). Cycloid psychosis: diagnosis and heuristic value. *J Nerv Ment Dis* **170**: 651–656.

Brown CS, Wittkowsky AK & Bryant SG (1986). Neuroleptic-induced catatonia after abrupt withdrawal of amantadine. *Pharmacotherapy* **6**: 193–195.

Bush G, Fink M., Petrides G, Dowling F & Francis A (1996a). Catatonia: I: Rating scale and standardized examination. *Acta psychiatr. Scand.* **93**: 129–136.

Bush G, Fink M, Petrides G, Dowling F & Francis A (1996b). Catatonia: II. Treatment with lorazepam and electroconvulsive therapy. *Acta psychiatr. Scand.* **93**: 137–143.

Bush G, Petrides G & Francis A (1997). Catatonia and other motor syndromes in a chronically hospitalized psychiatric population. *Schizophrenia Res* **27**: 83–92.

Cairns H (1952). Disturbances of consciousness with lesions of the brain-stem and diencephalon. *Brain* **75**: 109–146.

Cairns H, Oldfield RC, Pennybacker JB & Whittridge D (1941). Akinetic mutism with an epidermoid cyst of the third ventricle. *Brain* **64**: 273–290.

Caley CF (1997). Extrapyramidal reactions and the selective serotonin-reuptake inhibitors. *Ann Pharmacother* **31**: 1481–1489.

Cape G (1994). Neuroleptic malignant syndrome – A cautionary tale and a surprising outcome. *Br J Psychiatry* **164**: 120–122.

Carbone JR (2000). The neuroleptic malignant and serotonin syndromes. *Emerg Med Clin North Am* **18**: 317–325.

Carlson GA & Goodwin FK (1973). The stages of mania: A longitudinal analysis of the manic episode. *Arch Gen Psychiatry* **28**: 221–228.

Caroff SN (1980). The neuroleptic malignant syndrome. *J Clin Psychiatry* **41**: 79–83.

Caroff SN & Mann SC (1993). Neuroleptic malignant syndrome. *Med Clin North Am* **77**: 185–202.

Caroff SN, Mann SC & Campbell EC (2000). Atypical antipsychotics and neuroleptic malignant syndrome. *Psychiatric Annals* **30**: 314–324.

Caroff SN, Mann SC, Gliatto MF, Sullivan KA & Campbell EC (2001). Psychiatric manifestations of acute viral encephalitis. *Psychiatr Ann* **31**: 193–204.

Caroff SN, Mann SC & Keck PE (1998a). Specific treatment of the neuroleptic malignant syndrome. *Biol Psychiatry* **44**: 378–381.

Caroff SN, Mann SC, Lazarus A, Sullivan K & MacFadden W (1991). Neuroleptic malignant syndrome: diagnostic issues. *Psychiatr Ann* **21**: 130–147.

Caroff SN, Mann SC, McCarthy M, Naser J, Rynn M & Morrison M (1998b). Acute infectious encephalitis complicated by neuroleptic malignant syndrome. *J Clin Psychopharmacol* **18**: 349–351.

Carpenter WW, Bartko JJ, Carpenter CL & Strauss JS (1976). Another view of schizophrenic subtypes: A report from the international pilot study of schizophrenia. *Arch Gen Psychiatry* **33**: 508–516.

Carr V, Dorrington C, Schrader G & Wale J (1983). The use of ECT for mania in childhood bipolar disorder. *Br J Psychiatry* **143**: 411–415.

Carroll BJ, Feinberg M, Greden JF, Tarika J, Albala AA, Haskett RF, James NM, Kronfol Z, Lohr N, Steiner M, DeVigne JP & Young E (1981). A specific laboratory test for the diagnosis of melancholia: standardization, validation, and clinical utility. *Arch Gen Psychiatry* **38**: 15–22.

Carroll BT (1996). Complications of catatonia. (Letter.) *J Clin Psychiatry* **57**: 95.

Carroll BT (1999). GABA$_a$ versus GABA$_b$ hypothesis of catatonia. *Movement Dis* **14**: 702–703.

Carroll BT (2000). The universal field hypothesis of catatonia and neuroleptic malignant syndrome. *CNS Spectrums* **5**: 26–33.

Carroll BT (2001). Kahlbaum's catatonia revisited. *Psychiatry Clin Neurosci* **55**: 431–436.

Carroll BT & Boutros NN (1995). Clinical electroencephalograms in patients with catatonic disorders. *Clin Electroencephalogr* **26**: 60–64.

Carroll BT & Taylor BE (1997). The nondichotomy between lethal catatonia and neuroleptic malignant syndrome. *J Clin Psychopharmacol* **17**: 235–236.

Carroll BT, Anfinson TJ, Kennedy JC, Yendrek R, Boutros M & Bilon A (1994). Catatonic disorder due to general medical conditions. *J Neuropsychiatry Clin Neurosci* **6**: 122–133.

Carroll BT, Graham KT & Thalassinos AJ (2001). A common pathogenesis of the serotonin syndrome, catatonia, and neuroleptic malignant syndrome. *J Neuropsychiatry Clin Neurosci* **13**: 150. (Abstract.)

Castillo E, Rubin RT & Holsboer-Trachsler E (1989). Clinical differentiation between lethal catatonia and neuroleptic malignant syndrome. *Am J Psychiatry* **146**: 324–328.

Castro-Alamancos MA (1999). Neocortical synchronized oscillations induced by thalamic disinhibition in vitro. *J Neurosci* **19**: RC27.

Cerletti U (1950). Old and new information about electroshock. *Am J Psychiatry* **107**: 87–94.

Cerletti U (1956). Electroshock therapy. In F Marti-Ibanez, RR Sackler, AM Sackler & MD Sackler (Eds). *The Great Physiodynamic Therapies in Psychiatry: An Historical Reappraisal*, pp. 91–120. New York: Hoeber-Harper.

Chakrabarti S & Frombonne E (2001). Pervasive developmental disorders in preschool children. *JAMA* **285**: 3093–3099.

Chalela J & Kattah J (1999). Catatonia due to central pontine and extrapontine myelinolysis: case report. *J Neurol Neurosurg Psychiatry* **67**: 692–693.

Chandler JD (1991). Psychogenic catatonia with elevated creatine kinase and autonomic hyperativity. *Can J Psychiatry* **36**: 530–532.

Chandrasena R (1986). Catatonic schizophrenia: an international comparative study. *Can J Psychiatry* **31**: 249–252.

Chaplin R (2000). Possible causes of catatonia in autistic spectrum disorders. (Letter.) *Br J Psychiatry* **177**: 180.

Charney DS, Nestler EJ & Bunny BS (Eds) (2000). *Neurobiology of Mental Illness*. New York: Oxford University Press.

Charpier S, Leresche N, Deniau JM, Mahon S, Hughes SW & Crunelli V (1999). On the putative contribution of GABA (B) receptors to the electrical events occurring during spontaneous spike and wave discharges. *Neuropharmacology* **38**: 1699–1706.

Cheyette SR & Cummings JL (1995). Encephalitis lethargica: Lessons for contemporary neuropsychiatry. *J Neuropsychiatry Clin Neurosci* **7**: 125–134.

Chopra YM & Dandiya PC (1974). The mechanism of the potenting effect of antidepressant drugs on the protective influence of diphenhydramine in experimental catatonia. The role of histamine. *Pharmacology* **12**: 347–353.

Chopra YM & Dandiya PC (1975). The relative role of brain acetylcholine and histamine in perphenazine catatonia and the influence of antidepressants and diphenhydramine alone and in combination. *Neuropharmacology* **14**: 555–560.

Churchill L, Zahn DS, Duffy P & Kalivas PW (1996a). The mediodorsal nucleus of the thalamus in rats. II. Behavioral and neurochemical effects of GABA agonists. *Neuroscience* **70**: 103–112.

Churchill L, Zahn DS & Kalivas PW (1996b). The mediodorsal nucleus of the thalamus in rats. I. Forebrain gabergic innervation. *Neuroscience* **70**: 93–102.

Cizadlo BC & Wheaton A (1995). Case study: ECT treatment of a young girl with catatonia. *J Am Acad Child Adolesc Psychiatry* **34**: 332–335.

Cocito L & Primavera A (1996). Letter on catatonia mimicking NCSE. *Epilepsia* **37**: 592–593.

Cohen D, Cottias C & Basquin M (1997a). Cotard's syndrome in a 15-year-old girl. *Acta Psychiatr Scand* **95**: 164–165.

Cohen D, Dubos PF, Hervé M & Basquin M (1997b). Épisode catatoniques à l'adolescence: Observations cliniques. *Neuropsychiatr Enfance Adolesc* **45**: 597–604.

Cohen D, Flament M, Cubos P & Basquin M (1999). Case series: Catatonic syndrome in young people. *J Am Acad Child Adolesc Psychiatry* **38**: 1040–1046.

Cohen DJ, Bruun RD & Leckman JF (1988). *Tourette's Syndrome and Tic Disorders: Clinical Understanding and Treatment.* New York: John Wiley & Sons.

Cohen WJ & Cohen NH (1974). Lithium carbonate, haloperidol, and irreversible brain damage. *JAMA* **230**: 1283–1287.

Cook EH, Olsen K & Pliskin N (1996). Response of organic catatonia to risperidone. (Letter.) *Arch Gen Psychiatry* **53**: 82–83.

Cooper AF & Shapira K (1973). Case report: depression, catatonic stupor, and EEG changes in hyperthyroidism. *Psycholog Med* **3**: 509–515.

Cooper JE, Kendell RE & Gurland BJ (1972). *Psychiatric Diagnosis in New York and London: A Comparative Study of Mental Hospital Admissions.* Maudsley Monograph No. 20. London: Oxford University Press.

Coulter F & Corrigan FM (1990). Carbamazepine and NMS. *Br J Psychiatry* **158**: 434–435.

Cravioto H, Silberman J & Feigin I (1960). A clinical and pathologic study of akinetic mutism. *Neurology* **8**: 10–21.

Critchley M (1953). *The Parietal Lobes,* New York: Hafner Press.

Crosson B & Hughes CW (1987). Role of the thalamus in language: Is it related to schizophrenic thought disorder? *Schizophr Bull* **13**: 605–621.

Cummings JL & Mendez MF (1984). Secondary mania with focal cerebral lesions. *Am J Psychiatry* **141**: 1084–1087.

Cutajar P & Wilson D (1999). The use of ECT in intellectual disability. *J Intellect Disabil Res* **43**: 421–427.

Dalkin T & Lee AS (1990). Carbamazepine and forme fruste neuroleptic malignant syndrome. *Br J Psychiatry* **157**: 437–438.

Dalle Ore G, Gerstenbrand F, Lücking CH, Peters G & Peters UH (1977). *The Apallic Syndrome*. Berlin: Springer Verlag.

Davis JM, Caroff SN & Mann SC (2000). Treatment of neuroleptic malignant syndrome. *Psychiatr Ann* **30**: 325–331.

Davis JM, Janicak PG, Sakkas P, Gilmore C, Wang Z (1991). Electroconvulsive therapy in the treatment of the neuroleptic malignant syndrome. *Convulsive Ther.* **7**: 111–120.

Davis PA & Davis H (1939). The electroencephalograms of psychotic patients. *Am J Psychiatry* **95**: 1007–1025.

DeJesus MJ & Steiner DL (1994). An overview of family interventions and relapse in schizophrenia: meta-analysis of research findings. *Psychol Med* **24**: 565–578.

Delay J & Deniker P (1968). Drug-induced extrapyramidal syndromes. In Vinken PJ, Bruyn OW (Eds). *Handbook of Clinical Neurology*, vol. 6: *Disease of the Basal Ganglia*, pp. 248–266. New York: Elsevier.

Delay J, Pichot P & Lempérière T (1960). Un neuroleptique majeur non phenothiazine et non reserpinique, l'haloperidol, dans le traitement des psychoses. *Ann Med Psychol* **118**: 145–152.

DelBello MP, Foster KD & Strakowski SM (2000). Case report: treatment of catatonia in an adolescent male. *J Adolescent Health* **27**: 69–71.

Delisle J (1991). Catatonia unexpectedly reversed by midazolam. (Letter.) *Am J Psychiatry* **148**: 809.

Delvenne V, Goldman S, De Maertelaer V, Wikler D, Damhaut P & Lotstra F (1997). Brain glucose metabolism in anorexia nervosa and affective disorders influenced of weight loss on depressive symptomatology. *Psychiatr Res* **74**: 83–92.

Deuschle M & Lederbogen F (2001). Benzodiazepine withdrawal-induced catatonia. *Pharmacopsychiatry* **34**: 41–42.

Dhossche D (1998). Brief report: Catatonia in autistic disorders. *J Autism Devel Disorders* **28**: 329–331.

Dhossche D & Bouman NH (1997a). Catatonia in children and adolescents. (Letter.) *J Am Acad Child Adolesc Psychiatry* **36**: 870–871.

Dhossche D & Bouman NH (1997b). Catatonia in an adolescent with Prader-Willi syndrome. *Ann Clin Psychiatry* **9**: 247–253.

Dhossche D & Petrides G (1997). Negative symptoms of catatonia? (Letter.) *J Am Acad Child Adolesc Psychiatry* **36**: 302.

Dide A, Guiraud P & LaFage R (1921). Syndrome parkinsonian dans la demence precoce. *Rev Neurol* **28**: 692–694.

Dierckx RA, Saerens J, De Deyn PP, Verslegers W, Marien P & Vandevivere J (1991). Evolution of technetium-99m-HMPAO SPECT and brain mapping in a patient presenting with echolalia and palilalia. *J Nucl Med* **32**: 1619–1621.

Diethelm O (1971). *Medical Dissertations of Psychiatric Interest Printed Before 1750*. Basel: S. Karger.

Dilling H, Mombour W & Schmidt MH (Eds) (1991). *Internationale Klassifikation psychischer Störungen – ICD-10*. Bern: Huber.

Duberman MB (1988). *Paul Robeson*. New York: Alfred A. Knopf.

Dupont S, Semah F, Boon P, Saint-Hildaire J-M, Adam C, Broglin D & Baulac M (1999). Association of ipsilateral motor automatisms and contralateral dystonic posturing, a clinical feature differentiating medial from neocortical temporal lobe epilepsy. *Arch Neurol* **56**: 927–932.

Durant W (1961). *The Story of Philosophy, The Lives and Opinions of the Great Philosophers*. New York: Washington Square Press.

Earl CJC (1934). The primitive catatonic psychosis of idiocy. *Br J Med Psychol* **14**: 230–253.

Ebert D & Feistel H (1992). Left temporal hypo-perfusion in catatonic syndromes: A SPECT study. *Psychiatric Res: Neuroimag* **45**: 239–241.

Engel GL & Romano J (1944). Delirium II: Reversibility of the electroencephalogram with experimental procedures. *Arch Neurol Psychiatry* **51**: 378–392.

Engel GL & Rosenbaum M (1945). Delirium III: Electroencephalographic changes associated with acute alcoholic intoxication. *Arch Neurol Psychiatry* **53**: 44–50.

Epstein R (1991). Ganser syndrome, trance logic, and the question of malingering. *Psychiatr Ann* **21**: 238–244.

Escobar R, Rios A, Montoya ID, Lopera F, Ramos D, Carvajal C, Constain G, Gutierrez JE, Vargas S & Herrera CP (2000). Clinical and cerebral blood flow changes in catatonic patients treated with ECT. *J Psychosom Res* **49**: 423–429.

Ezrin-Waters C, Miller P & Seeman P (1976). Catalepsy induced by morphine or haloperidol: effects of apomorphine and anticholinergic drugs. *Can J Physiol Pharmacol* **54**: 516–519.

Falloon IRH, Boyd JL, McGill CW, Razani J, Moss HB & Gilderman AM (1982). Family management in the prevention of exacerbations of schizophrenia: a controlled study. *N Engl J Med* **306**: 1437–1440.

Fava GA, Molnar G, Block B, Lee JS & Perini GI (1984). The lithium loading dose method in a clinical setting. *Am J Psychiatry* **141**: 812–813.

Feige B, Aertsen A & Kristeva-Feige R (2000). Dynamic synchronization between multiple cortical motor areas and muscle activity in phasic voluntary movements. *J Neurophysiol* **84**: 2622–2629.

Fein S & McGrath MG (1990). Problems in diagnosing bipolar disorder in catatonic patients. *J Clin Psychiatry* **51**: 203–250.

Ferro FM, Janiri L, DeBonis C, Del Carmine R & Tempesta E (1991). Clinical outcome and psychoendocrinological findings in a case of lethal catatonia. *Biol Psychiatry* **30** (2):197–200.

Fink M (1958). Lateral gaze nystagmus as an index of the sedation threshold. *Electroenceph Clin Neurophysiol* **10**: 162–163.

Fink M (1968). EEG classification of psychoactive compounds in man: Review and theory of behavioral associations. In D Efron, JO Cole, J Levine & JR Wittenborn (Eds). *Psychopharmacology – A Review of Progress, 1957–1967*, pp. 497–507, 671–682, 1231–1239. Washington D.C.: U.S. Government Printing Office.

Fink M (1969). EEG and human psychopharmacology. *Ann Rev Pharmacol* **9**: 241–258.

Fink M (1979). *Convulsive Therapy: Theory and Practice*. New York: Raven Press.

Fink M (1984). Meduna and the origins of convulsive therapy. *Am J Psychiatry* **141**: 1034–1041.

Fink M (1985). Pharmaco-electroencephalography: A note on its history. *Neuropsychobiology* **12**: 173–178.

Fink M (1991). Impact of the anti-psychiatry movement on the revival of ECT in the U.S. *Psychiatr Clin North Am* **14**: 793–801.

Fink M (1992a). Catatonia and DSM-IV. *Convulsive Ther* **8**: 159–62.

Fink M (1992b). Why not ECT for catatonia? (Letter.) *Biol Psychiatry* **31**: 536–537.

Fink M (1992c). Missed neuroleptic malignant syndrome. (Letter.) *BMJ* **304**: 1246.

Fink M (1994). Catatonia in DSM-IV. *Biol Psychiatry* **36**: 431–433.

Fink M (1996a). Neuroleptic malignant syndrome. One entity or two? *Biol Psychiatry* **39**: 1–4.

Fink M (1996b). Toxic serotonin syndrome or neuroleptic malignant syndrome? Case report. *Pharmacopsychiatry* **29**: 159–161.

Fink M (1996c). Catatonia. In TA Widiger, AJ Frances, HA Pincus, R Ross, MB First & WW Davis (Eds). *DSM-IV Sourcebook*, vol. 2, pp.181–192. Washington DC: American Psychiatric Association.

Fink M (1997a). Catatonia. In M. Trimble & J Cummings (Eds). *Contemporary Behavioural Neurology*, vol. 16, pp. 289–309. Oxford: Butterworth/Heinemann.

Fink M (1997b). Lethal catatonia, neuroleptic malignant syndrome, and catatonia: A spectrum of disorders. Reply. (Letter.) *J Clin Psychopharmacol* **17**: 237.

Fink, M (1997c). Prejudice against ECT: Competition with psychological philosophies as a contribution to its stigma. *Convulsive Ther* **13**: 253–65.

Fink M (1999a). *Electroshock: Restoring the Mind*. New York: Oxford University Press.

Fink M (1999b). Delirious mania. *Bipolar Disord* **1**: 54–60.

Fink M (2000a). Electroshock revisited. *Am Sci* **88**: 162–167.

Fink M (2000b). Neuroleptic malignant syndrome best treated as catatonia. *Psychiatr Times* **17**: 28–29.

Fink M (2001). Modal ECT is effective: Response to letter by Sackeim HA. (Letter.) *JECT* **17**: 222–225.

Fink M, Abrams R, Bailine S & Jaffe R (1996). Ambulatory electroconvulsive therapy: Report of a task-force of the Association for Convulsive Therapy. *Convulsive Ther* **12**: 41–55.

Fink M, Bailine S & Petrides G (2001). Electrode placement and electroconvulsive therapy: A search for the chimera. (Letter.) *Arch Gen Psychiatry* **58**: 607–608.

Fink M, Bush G & Francis A (1993). Catatonia: A treatable disorder, occasionally recognized. *Directions in Psychiatry* **13**: 1–8.

Fink M & Francis A (1992). ECT response in catatonia. (Letter.) *Am J Psychiatry* **149**: 581–582.

Fink M & Francis AJ (1996). Treating the syndrome before complications. (Letter.) *Am J Psychiatry* **153**: 1371.

Fink M & Johnson L (1982). Monitoring the duration of electroconvulsive therapy seizures: "Cuff" and EEG methods compared. *Arch Gen Psychiatry* **39**: 1189–1191.

Fink M & Kahn RL (1957). Relation of EEG delta activity to behavioral response in electroshock: Quantitative serial studies. *Arch Neurol Psychiatry* **78**: 516–525.

Fink M & Kahn RL (1961). Behavioral patterns in convulsive therapy. *Arch Gen Psychiatry* **5**: 30–36.

Fink M, Kellner CH & Sackeim HA (1991). Intractable seizures, status epilepticus, and ECT. *JECT* **15**: 282–284.

Fink M & Klein DF (1995). An ethical dilemma in child psychiatry. *Psychiatric Bull* **19**: 650–651.

Fink M, Klein DF & Kramer JC (1965). Clinical efficacy of chlorpromazine-procyclidine combination, imipramine and placebo in depressive disorders. *Psychopharmacologia* **7**: 27–36.

Fink M, Pollack M, Klein DF, Blumberg AG, Belmont I, Karp E, Kramer JC & Willner A (1964). Comparative studies of chlorpromazine and imipramine I: Drug discrimination patterns. In PB Bradley, Flügel & PH Hoch (Eds). *Neuro-Psychopharmacology*, vol. 3, pp. 370–372. Amsterdam: Elsevier.

Fink M, Shaw R, Gross G & Coleman FS (1958). Comparative study of chlorpromazine and insulin coma in the therapy of psychosis. *JAMA* **166**: 1846–1850.

Fink M & Taylor MA (1991). Catatonia: A separate category for DSM-IV? *Integrative Psychiatry* **7**: 2–10.

Fink M & Taylor MA (2001). The many varieties of catatonia. *Eur Arch Psychiatry Clin Neurosci* **251** (Suppl. 1): 8–13.

Fisher CM (1989). 'Catatonia' due to disulfiram toxicity. *Arch Neurol* **46**: 798–804.

Ford RA (1989). The psychopathology of echophenomena. *Psychol Med* **19**: 627–635.

Francis A, Chandragiri S, Rizvi S, Koch M & Petrides G. (2000). Is lorazepam a treatment for neuroleptic malignant syndrome? *CNS Spectrums* **5**: 54–57.

Francis A, Divadeenam K, Bush G & Petrides G (1997). Consistency of symptoms in recurrent catatonia. *Comprehens Psychiatry* **38**: 56–60.

Francis A, Divadeenam K & Petrides G (1996). Advances in the treatment of catatonia with lorazepam and ECT. *Convulsive Ther* **12**: 259–261.

Franz M, Gallhofer B & Kanzow WT (1994). Treatment of catatonia with intravenous biperidine. (Letter.) *Br J Psychiatry* **164**: 847–848.

Freedman A (1991). American viewpoint on classification. *Integrative Psychiatry* **22**: 11–22.

Frey R, Schreiner D, Heiden A & Kasper S. (2001). Einsatz der Elecktrokrampftherapie in der Psychiatrie. [Use of electroconvulsive therapy in psychiatry]. *Nervenarzt* **72**: 661–676.

Fricchione GL (1985). Neuroleptic catatonia and its relationship to psychogenic catatonia. *Biol Psychiatry* **20**: 304–313.

Fricchione GL, Bush G, Fozdar M, Francis A & Fink M (1997). Recognition and treatment of the catatonic syndrome. *J Intensive Care Med* **12**: 135–147.

Fricchione GL, Cassem NH, Hooberman D & Hobson D (1983). Intravenous lorazepam in neuroleptic-induced catatonia. *J Clin Psychopharm* **3**: 338–342.

Fricchione GL, Kaufman LD, Gruber BL & Fink M (1990). Electroconvulsive therapy and cyclophosphamide in combination for severe neuropsychiatric lupus with catatonia. *Am J Med* **88**: 442–443.

Fricchione G, Mann SC & Caroff SN (2000). Catatonia, lethal catatonia and neuroleptic malignant syndrome. *Psychiatr Ann* **30**: 347–355.

Friedlander A (1901). *Über den Einfluss des Typhus abdominalis auf das Nervensystem.* Berlin: Karger.

Friedlander RI & Solomons K (2002). ECT: Use in individuals with developmental disabilities. *JECT* **18**: 38–42.

Fruensgaard K (1976). Withdrawal psychosis: A study of 30 consecutive cases. *Acta Psychiatr Scand* **53**: 105–118.

Fukutake T, Hirayama K & Komatsu T (1993). Transient unilateral catalepsy and right parietal lobe damage. *Jpn J Psychiatry* **47**: 647–650.

Fuster JM (1997). *The Prefrontal Cortex: Anatomy, Physiology, and Neuropsychology of the Frontal Lobe.* Philadelphia: Lippincott-Raven.

Gabris G & Muller C (1983). La catatonie dite "pernicieuse". *L'Encephale* **9**: 365–385.

Gaind GS, Rosebush PI & Mazurek MF (1994). Lorazepam treatment of acute and chronic catatonia in two mentally retarded brothers. *J Clin Psychiatry* **55**: 20–23.

Galynker II, Goldfarb R, Stefanovic M, Katsovich L & Miozzo R (2000). SPECT in the diagnosis of catatonia. *APA Meeting 2000 Abstracts*, NR432.

Galynker II, Weiss J, Ongseng F & Finestone H (1997). ECT treatment and cerebral perfusion in catatonia. *J Nuclear Med* **38**: 251–254.

Ganser S (1904). Zur lehre vom Hysterischen Dämmerzustande. *Arch Psychiatr Nervenkr* **38**: 34–46.

Ganser S & Shorter CE (Trans.) (1965). A peculiar hysterical state. *Br J Criminol* **5**: 120–126.

Gelenberg AJ (1976). The catatonic syndrome. *Lancet* **1**: 1339–1341.

Gelenberg AJ (1977). Catatonic reactions to high-potency neuroleptic drugs. *Arch Gen Psychiatry* **34**: 947–950.

Gelenberg AJ & Mandel MR (1977). Catatonic reactions to high potency neuroleptic drugs. *Arch Gen Psychiatry* **34**: 947–950.

Geller W & Mappes C (1952). Deadly catatonia. *Arch Psychiatr Nervenkr* **189**: 147–161.

Gelman S (1999). *Medicating Schizophrenia.* New Brunswick NJ: Rutgers University Press.

Geretsegger C & Rochowanski E (1987). Electroconvulsive therapy in acute life-threatening catatonia with associated cardiac and respiratory decompensation. *Convulsive Ther* **3**: 291–295.

Ghaziuddin N, Alkhouri I, Champine D, Quinlan P, Fluent T & Ghaziuddin M. (2002). ECT treatment of NMS and catatonia in an adolescent. *JECT* **18**: 95–98.

Gjedd JN, Rapoport JL, Garvey MA, Perlmutter S & Swedo SE (2000). MRI assessment of children with obsessive-compulsive disorder or tics associated with streptococcal infection. *Am J Psychiatry* **157**: 281–283.

Gillberg C & Wing L (1999). Autism: not an extremely rare disorder. *Acta Psychiatr Scand* **99**: 399–406.

Gjessing LR (1974). A review of periodic catatonia. *Biol Psychiatry* **8**: 23–45.

Gjessing LR, Harding GFA, Jenner FA & Johannessen NB (1967). The EEG in three cases of periodic catatonia. *Br J Psychiatry* **113**: 1271–1282.

Gjessing R (1932). Beiträge zur Kenntnis der Pathophysiologie des katatonen Stupors. *Arch Psychiat Nervenkr* Mitteilung I, II. **96**: 319–392, 393–473.

Gjessing R (1936). Beiträge zur Kenntnis der Pathophysiologie des katatonen Erregung. Mitteilung III. *Arch Psychiat Nervenkr* **104**: 355–416.

Gjessing R (1938). Disturbances of somatic functions in catatonia with a periodic course and their compensation. *J Ment Sci* **84**: 608–621.

Gjessing R (1939). Beiträge zur Kenntnis der Pathophysiologie periodisch-katatoner Zustände. Mitteilung IV. *Arch Psychiat Nervenkr.* **109**: 525–595.

Gjessing R (1976). *Contributions to the Somatology of Periodic Catatonia.* Oxford: Pergamon Press.

Glassman AH, Kantor SJ & Shostak M (1975). Depression, delusions, and drug response. *Am J Psychiatry* **132**: 716–719.

Gloor P (1969). *Hans Berger on the Electroencephalogram of Man. Electroenceph clin Neurophysiol*, Suppl 28, Amsterdam: Elsevier.

Goldar JC & Starkstein SE (1995). Karl Ludwig Kahlbaum's concept of catatonia. *History of Psychiatry* **VI**: 201–207.

Goldberg E (1992). The frontal lobes in neurological and psychiatric conditions. *Neuropsychiatry Neuropsychol Behav Neurol* **4**: 231–232.

Good MI (1976). Catatonia-like symptomatology and withdrawal dyskinesias. *Am J Psychiatry* **133**: 1454–1456.

Goodwin FK & Jamison KR (1990). *Manic Depressive Illness*. New York: Oxford University Press.

Gould SJ (2001). What only the embryo knows. *The New York Times*, Op-Ed (August 27).

Graham PJ & Foreman DM (1995). An ethical dilemma in child and adolescent psychiatry. *Psychiatric Bull* **19**: 84–86.

Graudins A, Stearman A & Chan B (1998). Treatment of serotonin syndrome with cyproheptadine. *J Emerg Med* **16**: 615–619.

Greden JF & Carroll BJ (1979). The dexamethasone suppression test as a diagnostic aid in catatonia. *Am J Psychiatry* **136**: 1199–1200.

Greenberg LB & Gujavarty K (1985). The neuroleptic malignant syndrome: Review and report of three cases. *Comprehens Psychiatry* **26**: 63–70.

Grinnell F (1992). *The Scientific Attitude*, 2nd edn. New York: Guilford Press.

Grisaru N, Chudakov B, Yaroslavsky Y & Belmaker RH (1998). Catatonia treated with transcranial magnetic stimulation. (Letter.) *Am J Psychiatry* **155**: 1630.

Guerrera RJ (1999). Sympathoadrenal hyperactivity and the etiology of neuroleptic malignant syndrome. *Am J Psychiatry* **156**: 169–180.

Guggenheim FG & Babigian HM (1974a). Catatonic schizophrenia: Epidemiology and clinical course. *J Nerv Ment Dis* **158**: 291–305.

Guggenheim FG & Babigian HM (1974b). Diagnostic consistency in catatonic schizophrenia. *Schiz Bull* **11**: 103–108.

Guiraud P (1924). Conception neurologique du syndrome catatonique. *Encephale* **19**: 571–579.

Guttmacher LB & Cretella H (1988). Electroconvulsive therapy in one child and three adolescents. *J Clin Psychiatry* **49**: 20–23.

Guy W (1976). Abnormal involuntary movement scale. *ECDEU Assessment Manual for Psychopharmacology*. Rockville MD: US Dept HEW, PHS, ADAMHA.

Guze SB (1967). The occurrence of psychiatric illness in systemic lupus erythematosus. *Am J Psychiatry* **123**: 1562–1570.

Häfner H & Kasper S (1982). Akute lebensbedrohliche Katatonie. *Nervenarzt* **53**: 385–394.

Hall DC & Reis RK (1983). Bipolar illness, catatonia, and the dexamethasone suppression test in adolescence: case report. *J Clin Psychiatry* **44**: 222–224.

Hansen ES & Bolwig TG (1988). Cotard syndrome: an important manifestation of melancholia. *Nord Psykiatr Tidsskr* **52**: 459–464.

Hansen M (1908). *Zur Lehre der Katatonie mit Stupor*. Thesis, Kiel University. Kiel: AF Jensen.

Hasan S & Buckley P (1998). Novel antipsychotics and the neuroleptic malignant syndrome: a review and critique. *Am J Psychiatry* **155**: 1113–1116.

Haskovec L (1925). Le psychisme sous-cortical. *Rev Neurol* **1**: 976–978.

Hauber W (1998). Involvement of basal ganglia transmitter systems in movement inactivation. *Proc Neurobiol* **56**: 507–540.

Hauser P, Devinsky O, De Bellis M, Theodore WH & Post RM (1989). Benzodiazepine withdrawal delirium with catatonic features. Occurrence in patients with partial seizure disorders. *Arch Neurology* **46**: 696–699.

Hawkins JM, Archer KJ, Strakowski SM & Keck PE (1995). Somatic treatment of catatonia. *Intl J Psychiatry Med* **25**: 345–369.

HCIA (1998). *Length of Stay By Diagnosis.* Baltimore: HCIA Inc.

Healy D (2002). *The Creation of Psychopharmacology.* Cambridge, MA: Harvard University Press.

Hearst ED, Munoz RA & Tuason VB (1971). Catatonia: Its diagnostic validity. *Dis Nerv Syst* **32**: 453–456.

Heckl RW (1987). Das Stiff-man-Syndrom. In H Hippius, E Rüther & M Schmauß (Eds). *Katatone und dyskinetische Syndrome.* pp. 145–148. Berlin: Springer-Verlag.

Hegerl U, Bottlender R, Gallinat J, Kuss HJ, Ackenheil M & Moller HJ (1998). The serotonin syndrome scale: first results on validity. *Eur Arch Psychiatry Clin Neurosci.* **248**: 96–103.

Heinroth JC (J Schmorak, Trans.) (1975). *Textbook of Disturbances of Mental Life*, vol. 1 and 2. Baltimore: Johns Hopkins Press.

Hermann RC, Dowart RA, Hoover CW & Brody J (1995). Variation in ECT use in the United States. *Am J Psychiatry* **152**: 869–875.

Hermesh H, Aizenberg D & Weizman A (1987). A successful electroconvulsive treatment of neuroleptic malignant syndrome. *Acta Psychiatr Scand* **75**: 237–239.

Hermesh H, Aizenberg D, Weizman A., Lapidot M, Mayor C & Munitz H (1992). Risk for definite neuroleptic malignant syndrome. A prospective study in 223 consecutive in-patients. *Br J Psychiatry* **161**: 722–723.

Hermesh H, Hoffnung RA, Aizenberg D, Molcho A & Munitz H (1989a). Catatonic signs in severe obsessive compulsive disorder. *J Clin Psychiatry* **50**: 303–305.

Hermesh H, Sirota P & Eviatar J (1989b). Recurrent neuroleptic malignant syndrome due to haloperidol and amantadine. *Biol Psychiatry* **25**: 962–965.

Hermle L & Oepen G (1986). Zur differential diagnose der akut lebensbedrohlichen Katatonie und des malignen Neuroleptikasyndrome – ein kasuistischer Beitrag. *Fortschr Neurol Psychiatr* **54**: 189–195.

Hill D & Parr G (Eds) (1963). *Electroencephalography.* New York: Macmillan Co.

Hinsie LE (1932a). The catatonic syndrome in dementia praecox. *Psychiatric Quart* **6**: 457–468.

Hinsie LE (1932b). Clinical manifestations of the catatonic form of dementia praecox. *Psychiatric Quart* **6**: 469–474.

Hinsie LE & Campbell RJ (1970). *Psychiatric Dictionary*, 4th edn. New York: Oxford University Press.

Hippius H, Rüther E & Schmauß M (1987). *Katatone und dyskinetische Syndrome.* Berlin: Springer-Verlag.

Hirose S & Ashby CR (2002). Immediate effect of intravenous diazepam in neuroleptic-induced acute akathisia: An open-label study. *J Clin Psychiatry* **63**: 524–527.

Hirschfeld RM, Allen MH, McEvoy PJ, Keck PE & Russell JM (1999). Safety and tolerability of oral loading divalproex sodium in acutely manic bipolar patients. *J Clin Psychiatry* **60**: 815–818.

Ho SS, Berkovic SF, Newton MR, Austin MC, McKay WJ & Bladin PF (1994). Parietal lobe epilepsy: Clinical features and seizure localization by ictal SPECT. *Neurology* **44**: 2277–2284.

Hoch A (1921). *Benign Stupors.* New York: Macmillan Co.

Höfler J & Bräunig P (1995). Abnahme der Häufigkeit katatoner Schizophrenien im Epochenvergleich. In P Bräunig (Ed.). *Differenzierung katatoner und neuroleptika-induzierter Bewegungsstörungen*, pp. 32–35. Stuttgart: Georg Thieme Verlag.

Hofmann M, Seifritz E, Botschev C, Krauchi K & Muller-Spahn F (2000). Serum iron and ferritin in acute neuroleptic akathisia. *Psychiatry Res* **93**: 201–207.

Hogarty G & Gross M (1966). Pre-admission symptom difference between first-admitted schizophrenics in the predrug and postdrug era. *Comprehens Psychiatry* **7**: 134–140.

Holm VA, Cassidy SB, Butler MG, Hanchett JM, Greensway LR, Whitman BY & Greenberg F (1993). Prader-Willi syndrome: Consensus diagnostic criteria. *Pediatrics* **91**: 398–402.

Hornstein GA (2000). *To Redeem One Person Is To Redeem the World.* New York: Free Press.

Huber G (1954). Zur nosologischen Differenzierung lebensbedrohlicher katatoner Psychosen. *Schweiz Arch Neurol Psychiat* **78**: 216–222.

Hunter R (1973). Psychiatry and neurology. *Proc Royal Soc Medicine* **66**: 359–364.

Hunter R & Macalpine I (1982). *Three Hundred Years of Psychiatry 1535–1860.* Hartsdale, NY: Carlisle Publishing Co.

Hynes AF & Vickar EL (1996). Case Study: Neuroleptic malignant syndrome without pyrexia. *J Am Acad Child Adolesc Psychiatry* **35**: 959–962.

Ilbeigi MS, Davidson ML & Yarmush JM (1998). An unexpected arousal effect of etomidate in a patient on high-dose steroids. *Anesthesiology* **89**: 1587–1589.

Insel TR, Roy BF, Cohen RM & Murphy DL (1982). Possible development of the serotonin syndrome in man. *Am J Psychiatry* **139**: 954–955.

Jasper HH, Riggio S & Goldman-Rakic PS (Eds) (1995). *Epilepsy and the Functional Neuroanatomy of the Frontal Lobe, Advances in Neurology*, vol. 66. New York: Raven Press.

Jaspers K, Hoenig J & Hamilton MW (Trans.) (1963). *General Psychopathology.* Chicago: University of Chicago Press.

Jefferson J W, Greist JH & Ackerman DL (1983). *Lithium Encyclopedia for Clinical Practice.* Middleton WI: Lithium Information Center.

Jelliffe SE (1940). The parkinsonian body posture. Some considerations of unconscious hostility. *Psychoanalytic Rev* **27**: 467–79.

Jelliffe SE & White WA (1917). *Disease of the Nervous System. A Textbook of Neurology and Psychiatry.* Philadelphia: Lea & Febiger.

Jellinger KA (1999). Post-mortem studies in Parkinson's disease. Is it possible to detect brain areas for specific symptoms? *J Neural Transm Suppl* **56**: 1–29.

Johnson J (1984). Stupor: A review of 25 cases. *Acta Psychiatr Scand* **70**: 370–377.

Johnson J (1993). Catatonia: the tension insanity. *Br J Psychiatry* **162**: 733–738.

Johnson J & Lucey PA (1987). Encephalitis lethargica, a contemporary cause of catatonic stupor. *Br J Psychiatry* **151**: 550–552.

Johnson V & Bruxner G (1998). Neuroleptic malignant syndrome associated with olanzapine. *Aust NZ J Psychiatry* **32**: 884–886.

Jong HH de (1945). *Experimental Catatonia, a General Reaction-Form of the Central Nervous System, and its Implications for Human Pathology.* Baltimore: Williams & Wilkins.

Jong HH de & Baruk H (1930). *La catatonie expérimentale par la bulbocapnine: étude physiologique et clinique.* Paris: Masson, 1930.

Joseph AB, Anderson WA & O'Leary DH (1991). Brainstem and vermis atrophy in catatonia. *Am J Psychiatry* **29**: 730–734.

Joseph R (1999). Frontal lobe psychopathology, mania, depression, confabulation, catatonia, perseveration, obsessive compulsions, and schizophrenia. *Psychiatry* **62**: 138–172.

Kahlbaum KL (1863). *Die Gruppierung der psychischen Krankheiten und die Einteilung der Seelenstörungen.* Danzig: A W. Kafemann.

Kahlbaum KL (1863; translated 1996). Die Beziehungen der neuen Gruppirung zu früheren Eintheilungen und zu einer allgemeinen Pathologie der psychischen Krankheiten. [The relationships of the new groupings to old classifications and to a general pathology of mental disorder]. Part 3 from Kahlbaum, 1863; translated by G.E. Berrios. *History of Psychiatry* **7**: 167–181.

Kahlbaum KL (1874; translated 1973). *Die Katatonie oder das Spannungsirresein.* Berlin: Verlag August Hirshwald, 1874. Translated: Kahlbaum, K: *Catatonia.* Translated by Y Levis & T Pridon Baltimore: Johns Hopkins University Press, 1973.

Kalinowsky LB, Hippius H & Klein HE (1982). *Biological Treatments in Psychiatry.* New York: Grune & Stratton.

Kalinowsky LB & Hoch PH (1952). *Shock Treatments, Psychosurgery and Other Somatic Treatments in Psychiatry.* New York: Grune & Stratton.

Kanemoto K, Miyamoto T & Abe R (1999). Ictal catatonia as a manifestation of a de novo absence status epilepticus following benzodiazepine withdrawal. *Seizure* **8**: 364–366.

Kanner L (1943). Autistic disturbances in affective contact. *Nervous Child* **2**: 217–250.

Kantor SJ & Glassman AH (1977). Delusional depressions: Natural history and response to treatment. *Br J Psychiatry* **131**: 351–360.

Kantrovich NV & Constantinovich SK (1937). The effect of alohol in catatonic syndromes. *Am J Psychiatry* **92**: 651–654.

Kapstan A, Miodownick C & Lerner V (2000). Oneiroid syndrome: a concept of use for western psychiatry. *Isr J Psychiatry Relat Sci* **37**: 278–85.

Karagianis JL, Phillips LC, Hogan KP & LeDrew KK (1999). Clozapine-associated neuroleptic malignant syndrome: Two new cases and a review of the literature. *Ann Pharmacother* **33**: 623–630.

Karagianis JL, Phillips L, Hogan K & LeDrew K (2001). Neuroleptic malignant syndrome associated with quetiapine. *Can J Psychiatry* **46**: 370–371.

Kardos J (1999). Recent advances in GABA research. *Neurochem Int* **34**: 353–358.

Kasture SB, Mandhene SN & Chopde CT (1996). Baclofen induced catatonia: modification by serotonergic agents. *Neuropharmacology* **35**: 595–596.

Katzenstein R (1963). Karl Ludwig Kahlbaum und sein Beitrag zur Entwicklung der Psychiatrie. *Med Dissert*, pp. 1–42. Zurich: Juris-Verlag.

Keck PE & Arnold LM (2000). The serotonin syndrome. *Psychiatric Annals* **30**: 333–343.

Keck PE, McElroy SL & Pope Jr HG (1991). Epidemiology of neuroleptic malignant syndrome. *Psychiatric Annals* **21**: 148–151.

Keck PE, McElroy SL, Tugrul KC & Bennet JA (1993). Valproate oral loading in the treatment of acute mania. *J Clin Psychiatry* **54**: 305–308.

Keck PE, Pope HG, Cohen BM, McElroy SL & Nierenberg AA (1989). Risk factors for neuroleptic malignant syndrome. *Arch Gen Psychiatry* **46**: 914–918.

Keepers GA (1990). Neuroleptic malignant syndrome associated with withdrawal from carbamazepine. *Am J Psychiatry* **147**: 1687.

Kellam AMP (1987). The neuroleptic malignant syndrome, so-called. A survey of the world literature. *Br J Psychiatry* **150**: 752–759.

Kennard MA, Rabinovitch MS & Fister WP (1955). The use of frequency analysis in the interpretation of the EEG's of patients with psychological disorders. *EEG clin Neurophysiol* **7**: 29–41.

Kennard MA & Schwartzman AE (1957). A longitudinal study of electroencephalographic frequency patterns in mental hospital patients and normal controls. *EEG clin Neurophysiol* **9**: 263–274.

Kiernan JG (1877; reprinted 1994). Katatonia, a clinical form of insanity. Original April 2, 1877 (Reprinted *Am J Psychiatry* **151**: 103–111.)

Kilzieh N & Akiskal H (1999). Rapid-cycling bipolar disorder: An overview of research and clinical experience. *Psych Clin North Am* **22**: 585–607.

Kindt H (1980). *Katatonie. Ein Modell psychischer Krankheit*. Stuttgart: Ferdinand Enke Verlag.

Kinross-Wright VJ (1958). Trifluoperazine and schizophrenia. In Bull H (Ed.). *Trifluoperazine: Clinical and Pharmacologic Aspects*, pp. 62–70. Philadelphia: Lea and Febiger.

Kinrys PF & Logan KM (2001). Periodic catatonia in an adolescent. (Letter.) *J Am Acad Child Adolesc Psychiatry* **40**: 741–742.

Kirby G (1913). The catatonic syndrome and its relation to manic-depressive insanity. *J Nerv Ment Dis* **40**: 694–704.

Kirby GH & Davis TK (1921). Psychiatric aspects of epidemic encephalitis. *Arch Neurol Psychiatry* **5**: 491–551.

Kish SJ, Kleinert R, Minauf M, Gilbert J, Walter GF, Slimovitch C, Maurer E, Rezvani Y, Myers R & Hornykiewicz O (1990). Brain neurotransmitter changes in three patients who had a fatal hyperthermia syndrome. *Am J Psychiatry* **147**: 1358–1363.

Klaesi J (1945). Über die therapeutische Anwendung der "Daucrnarkose" mittels Somnifen bei Schizophrenen. *Ztschr. F. d. ges. Psychiat. u. Neurol.* **74**: 557–592.

Klee A (1961). Akinetic mutism: Review of the literature and report of a case. *JNMD* **133**: 536–553.

Klein DF (1964). Delineation of two drug-responsive anxiety syndromes. *Psychopharmacologia* **5**: 397–408.

Klein DF (1968). Psychiatric diagnosis and a typology of clinical drug effects. *Psychopharmacologia* **13**: 359–386.

Klein DF & Fink M (1962a). Psychiatric reaction patterns to imipramine. *Am J Psychiatry* **119**: 432–438.

Klein DF & Fink M (1962b). Behavioral reaction patterns with phenothiazines. *Arch Gen Psychiatry* **7**: 449–459.

Kleist K (1928). Über zykloide, paranoide und epileptoide Psychosen und über die Frage der Degenerationspsychosen. *Schweiz Archiv Neurol Psychiat* **23**: 1–35.

Kleist K (1943). Die Katatonien. *Nervenarzt* **16**: 1–10.

Kleist K (1960). Schizophrenic symptoms and cerebral pathology. *J Ment Sci* **106**: 246–255.

Kleist K, Leonhard K & Schwab H (1940). Die Katatonie auf Grund katamnestischer Untersuchungen. III Teil. Formen und Verläufe der eigentlichen Katatonie. *Zeit Neurol* **168**: 538–586.

Klerman GL (1981). The spectrum of mania. *Comprehens Psychiatry* **22**: 11–20.

Koch M, Chandragiri S, Rizvi S, Petrides G & Francis A (2000). Catatonic signs in neuroleptic malignant syndrome. *Comprehens Psychiatry* **41**: 73–75.

Koek RJ & Mervis JR (1999). Treatment refractory catatonia, ECT, and parenteral lorazepam. *Am J Psychiatry* **156**: 160–161.

Kolb B & Whishaw IQ (1996). *Fundamentals of Human Neuropsychology,* 4th edn. New York: WH Freeman.

Komori T, Nomaguchi M, Kodama S, Takigawa M & Nomura J (1997). Thyroid hormone and reserpine abolished periods of periodic catatonia: a case report. *Acta Psychiatr Scand* **96**: 155–156.

Koponen H, Repo E & Lepole U (1991). Long-term outcome after neuroleptic malignant syndrome. *Acta Psychiatr Scand* **84**: 550–551.

Kornhuber J & Weller M (1993). Amantadine and the glutamate hypothesis of schizophrenia. Experiences in the treatment of the neuroleptic malignant syndrome. *J Neural Transmission* **92**: 57–65.

Kornstein SG, Schatzberg AF, Thase ME, Yonkers KA, McCullough JP, Keitner GI, Gelenberg AJ, Davis SM, Harrison WM & Keller MB (2000). Gender differences in treatment response to sertraline versus imipramine in chronic depression. *Am J Psychiatry* **157**: 1445–1452.

Kosten TR & Kleber ND (1988). Rapid death during cocaine abuse: A variant of the neuroleptic malignant syndrome? *Am J Drug Alcohol Abuse* **14**: 335–346.

Kraepelin E (1896; reprinted 1902). *Psychiatrie: ein Lehrbuch für Studierende und Ärzte*, 6th edn. Leipzig: J Ambrosius Barth. (Abstracted and reprinted. *Clinical Psychiatry: A Textbook for Students and Physicians*. New York: Macmillan.)

Kraepelin E (1903; reprinted 1907). *Psychiatrie: ein Lehrbuch für Studierende und Ärzte*, 7th edn. Leipzig: J Ambrosius Barth. (Abstracted and reprinted *Clinical Psychiatry: A Textbook for Students and Physicians*. New York: Macmillan.)

Kraepelin E (1913). *Psychiatrie*, 8th edn. Leipzig: J Ambrosius Barth. (Reprinted and translated T Johnstone, 1913. Bailliere, Tindall and Cox.)

Kraepelin E (1919). *Dementia Praecox and Paraphrenia*. RM Barclay (trans.) & GM Robertson (Ed). Edinburgh: Livingstone.

Kraepelin E (1921; reprinted 1976). *Manic-Depressive Insanity and Paranoia*. RM Barclay (trans.) & GM Robertson (Ed). Edinburgh: ES Livingstone. (Reprinted New York: Arno Press.)

Kraepelin E (1962). *One Hundred Years of Psychiatry*. W. Baskin (trans.). New York: Philosophical Library. (Original *Hundert Jahre Psychiatrie*. Berlin: Julius Springer Verlag, 1918.)

Kraepelin E (1971). *Dementia Praecox and Paraphrenia*. RM Barclay (trans.) & GM Robertson (Ed.). Huntington, NY: Krieger Publishing Co.

Kramer MS (1977). Menstrual epileptoid psychosis in an adolescent girl. *Am J Dis Child* **131**: 316–317.

Kramp P & Bolwig TG (1981). Electroconvulsive therapy in acute delirious states. *Comprehens Psychiatry* **22**: 368–371.

Kritzinger PR & Jordaan GP (2001). Catatonia: an open prospective series with carbamazepine. *Int J Neuropsychopharmacol* **4**: 251–157.

Kroessler D (1985). Relative efficacy rates for therapies of delusional depression. *Convulsive Ther.* **1**: 173–182.

Krüger S & Bräunig P (2000a). Catatonia in affective disorder: New findings and a review of the literature. *CNS Spectrums* **5**: 48–53.

Krüger S & Bräunig P (2000b). Ewald Hecker. *Am J Psychiatry* **157**: 1220.

Krüger S & Bräunig P (2001). Intravenous valproic acid in the treatment of severe catatonia. *J Neuropsychiatry Clin Neurosci* **13**: 303–304.

Krüger S, Bräunig P & Cooke RG (2000a). Comorbidity of obsessive-compulsive disorder in recovered inpatients with bipolar disorder. *Bipolar Disord* **2**: 71–74.

Krüger S, Bräunig P, Hoffler J, Shugar G, Borner I & Langkar J (2000b). Prevalence of obsessive-compulsive disorder in schizophrenia and significance of motor symptoms. *J Neuropsychiatry Clin Neurosci* **12**: 16–24.

Krüger S, Cooke RG, Hasey GM, Jorna T & Persad E (1995). Comorbidity of obsessive compulsive disorder in bipolar disorder. *J Affective Disorders* **34**: 117–120.

Kukleta M & Lamarche M (2000). Synchronizing effect of clock rhythm on the 'when to move' decision in repeated voluntary movements. *Int J Psychophysiol* **39**: 31–38.

Kurlan R, Hamill R & Shoullson I (1984). Neuroleptic malignant syndrome. *Clin Neuropharmacol* **7**: 109–120.

Kushner HI (1999). *A Cursing Brain? The Histories of Tourette Syndrome.* Boston: Harvard University Press.

Lanczik M (1922). Karl Ludwig Kahlbaum (1828–1899) and the emergence of psychopathological and nosological research in German psychiatry. *History of Psychiatry* **3**: 53–58.

Lange J (1992). *Katatonische Erscheinungen im Rahmen manischer Erkrankungen. Monographien aus dem Gesamtgebiete der Neurologie und Psychiatrie,* vol. 31. Berlin: Julius Springer.

Lanham JG, Brown MM & Hughes GRV (1985). Cerebral systemic lupus erythematosus presenting with catatonia. *Postgrad Med J* **61**: 329–330.

Lappin RI & Auchincloss EL (1994). Treatment of the serotonin syndrome with cyproheptadine. *Lancet* **331**: 1021–1022.

Lask B, Britten C, Kroll L, Magagna J & Tranter M (1991). Children with pervasive refusal. *Arch Dis Childhood* **66**: 866–889.

Laskowska D (1967). Attempted explanation of the pathophysiological mechanisms leading to the development of the acute confusocatatonic syndrome (Stauder's "mortal catatonic" syndrome) during schizophrenia. *Ann Medicopsychol* **125**: 549–559.

Lauter H & Sauer H (1987). Zur elektrokrampftherapie bei Katatone. In H Hippius, E Rüther & M Schmauß (Eds). *Katatone und dyskinetische Syndrome,* pp. 165–170. Berlin: Springer-Verlag.

Lauterbach E (1995). Bipolar disorders, dystonia and compulsion after dysfunction of the cerebellum, dentatorubrothalamic tract, and substantia nigra. *Biol Psychiatry* **40**: 726–730.

Lavie CJ, Ventura HO & Walker G (1986). Neuroleptic malignant syndrome: three episodes with different drugs. *Southern Med J* **79**: 1571–1573.

Lazarus A (1986). Therapy of neuroleptic malignant syndrome. *Psychiatr Develop* **1**: 19–30.

Lazarus A, Mann SC & Caroff SN (1989). *The Neuroleptic Malignant Syndrome and Related Conditions.* Washington D.C.: American Psychiatric Press, Inc.

Lebensohn ZM (1984). Electroconvulsive therapy: Psychiatry's villain or hero? *Am J Soc Psychiatry* **4**: 39–43.

Lebensohn ZM (1999). The history of electroconvulsive therapy (ECT) in the United States and its place in American psychiatry. A personal memoir. *Comprehens Psychiatry* **40**: 173–81.

Lee JW (1998). Serum iron in catatonia and neuroleptic malignant syndrome. *Biol Psychiatry* **44**: 499–507.

Lee JW, Schwartz DL & Hallmayer J (2000). Catatonia in a psychiatric intensive care facility: incidence and response to benzodiazepines. *Ann Clin Psychiatry* **12**: 89–96.

Leis AA, Stokic DS, Fuhr P, Kofler M, Kronenberg MF, Wissel J, Glocker FX, Seifert C & Stetkarova I (2000). Nociceptive fingertip stimulation inhibits synergistic motorneuron pools in the human upper limb. *Neurology* **55**: 1305–1309.

Leonhard K (1942a). Zur Unterteilung und Erbbiologie der Schizophrenien. 1. Mitteilung. Die typischen Unterformen der Katatonie. *Allg Z Psychiatr* **120**: 1–27.

Leonhard K (1942b). Zur Unterteilung und Erbbiologie der Schizophrenien. 2. Mitteilung. Kombiniert-systematische und periodische Katatonien. *Allg Z Psychiatr* **121**: 1–35.

Leonhard K (1961). Cycloid psychoses – endogenous psychoses which are neither schizophrenic nor manic depressive. *J Mental Sci* **197**: 632–648.

Leonhard K (1979). *The Classification of Endogenous Psychoses.* 5th edn. E Robins (Ed) & R Berman (trans.). New York: Irvington Publications.

Leonhard K (1995). *Aufteilung der endogenen Psychoses und ihre differnzierte Ätiologie.* H. Beckmann (Ed.). Stuttgart: Georg Tieme Verlag. (Original published 1957; Jena: Akademie Press.)

Levenson JL (1985). Neuroleptic malignant syndrome. *Am J Psychiatry* **142**: 1137–1145.

Levin T, Petrides G, Weiner J, Saravay S, Multz AS & Bailine S (2002). Intractable delirium successfully treated with ECT. *Psychosomatics* **43**: 63–66.

Levinson DF & Simpson GM (1986). Neuroleptic-induced extrapyramidal symptoms with fever. *Arch Gen Psychiatry* **43**: 839–848.

Levy AB (1984). Delirium and seizures due to abrupt alprazolam withdrawal: case report. *J Clin Psychiatry* **45**: 38–39.

Lieberman AA (1954). The Ganser syndrome: a case study. *J Nerv Ment Dis* **88**: 10–16.

Lim J, Yagnik P, Schraeder P & Wheeler S (1986). Ictal catatonia as a manifestation of nonconvulsive status epilepticus. *J Neurol Neurosurg Psychiatry* **49**: 833–836.

Lindsay JSB (1948). Periodic catatonia. J Ment Sci **94**: 590–602.

Linkowski P, Desmedt D, Hoffmann G, Kerkhofs M & Mendelewicz J (1984). Sleep and neuroendocrine disturbances in catatonia. A case report. *J Affective Dis* **7**: 87–92.

Lipowski ZJ (1990). *Delirium: Acute Confusional States.* New York: Oxford University Press.

Lishman WA (1978). *Organic Psychiatry*. Oxford: Blackwell Scientific Publications.

Lohr JB & Wisniewski AA (1987). *Movement Disorders: A Neuropsychiatric Approach*. New York: Guilford Press.

Looper KJ & Milroy TM (1997). Catatonia 20 years later. *Am J Psychiatry* **154**: 883.

Louis ED & Pflaster NL (1995). Catatonia mimicking nonconvulsive status epilepticus. *Epilepsia* **36**: 943–945.

Luchins DJ, Metz JT, Marks RC & Cooper MD (1989). Basal ganglia regional glucose metabolism asymmetry during a catatonic episode. *Biol Psychiatry* **26**: 725–728.

Lund CE, Mortimer AM, Rogers D & McKenna PJ (1991). Motor, volitional and behavioural disorders in schizophrenia. 1: Assessment using the modified Rogers scale. *Br J Psychiatry* **158**: 323–327.

Lugaresi E, Pazzaglia P & Tassinari CA (1971). Differentiation of "absence status" and "temporal lobe status." *Epilepsia* **12**: 63–76.

Luria AR (1973). *The Working Brain*. New York: Basic Books.

MacDonald III AW, Cohen JD, Stenger VA & Carter CS (2000). Dissociating the role of the dorsolateral prefrontal cortex and anterior cingulate cortex in cognitive control. *Science* **288**: 1835–1838.

Magrinat G, Danziger JA, Lorenzo IC & Flemenbaum A (1983). A reassessment of catatonia. *Comprehens Psychiatry* **24**: 218–228.

Mahendra B (1981). Editorial: Where have all the catatonics gone? *Psychol Med* **11**: 669–671.

Maisel T (1936). *Zur Frage der akuten Todesfälle bei Katatonie*. Thesis, University of Breslau. Breslau: M Bermann.

Malur C, Cabahug C & Francis AJ (2000). SPECT brain imaging in catatonia. *APA Meeting 2000 Abstracts*, NR142.

Malur C, Fink M & Francis A (2000). Can delirium relieve psychosis? *Comprehens Psychiatry* **41**: 450–453.

Mann SC, Auriocombe M, Macfadden W, Caroff SN, Campbell EC & Tignol J (2001). La catatonie léthale: aspects cliniques et conduite thérapeutique. Une revue de la littérature. *L'Encéphale* **27**: 213–216.

Mann SC, Caroff SN, Bleier HR, Antelo E & Un H (1990). Electroconvulsive therapy of the lethal catatonia syndrome. *Convulsive Ther* **6**: 239–247.

Mann SC, Caroff SN, Bleier HR, Welz WKR, Kling MA & Hayashida M (1986). Lethal catatonia. *Am J Psychiatry* **143**: 1374–1381.

Marneros A & Jäger A (1993). Treatment of catatonic stupor with oral lorazepam in 14-year-old psychotic boy. *Pharmacopsychiat* **26**: 259–260.

Mártényi F, Metcalfe S, Schausberger B & Dossenbach MRK (2001). An efficacy analysis of olanzapine treatment data in schizophrenia patients with catatonic signs and symptoms. *J Clin Psychiatry* **62** (Suppl 2): 25–27.

Mashimo K, Kanaya M & Yamauchi T (1995). Electroconvulsive therapy for a schizophrenic patient in a catatonic stupor with joint contracture. *Convulsive Ther* **11**: 216–219.

Mason PJ, Morris VA & Balcezak TJ (2000). Serotonin syndrome. Presentation of 2 cases and review of the literature. *Medicine* **79**: 201–209.

Mastain B, Vaiva G, Guerouaou D, Pommery J & Thomas P (1995). Dramatic improvement of catatonia with zolpidem. *Rev Neurol* **151**: 52–56.

Masuda Y, Imaizumi H, Satoh M, Aimono M, Chaki R, Nakamura M, Asai Y & Namiki A (in press). Electroconvulsive therapy following resolution of neuroleptic malignant syndrome. *Anesthesiology*.

Mathews T & Aderibigbe YA (1999). Proposed research diagnostic criteria for neuroleptic malignant syndrome. *Int J Neuropsychopharmacol* **2**: 129–144.

May JV (1922). *Mental Diseases: A Public Health Problem*. Boston: RG Badger.

Mayer-Gross W (1924). Selbstschilderungen der Verwirrtheit. Die oneroide. *Erlebens-form: psychopathologish-Klinische Untersuchungen*. Berlin: Springer Verlag.

Mayer-Gross W, Slater E & Roth M (1960). *Clinical Psychiatry*. London: Cassell & Co.

McCall WV (1989). Neuroendocrine markers in periodic catatonia. (Letter.) *J Clin Psychiatry* **50**: 109.

McCall WV (1992). The response to an amobarbital interview as a predictor of therapeutic outcome in patients with catatonic mutism. *Convulsive Ther* **8**: 174–178.

McCall WV, Mann SC, Shelp FE & Caroff SN (1995). Fatal pulmonary embolism in the catatonic syndrome: Two case reports and a literature review. *J Clin Psychiatry* **56**: 21–25.

McCall WV, Shelp FE & McDonald WM (1992). Controlled investigation of the amobarbital interview in catatonic mutism. *Am J Psychiatry* **149**: 202–206.

McCarron MM, Boettger ML & Peck JJ (1982). A case of neuroleptic malignant syndrome successfully treated with amantadine. *J Clin Psychiatry* **43**: 381–382.

McCarron MM, Schulze BW, Thompson GA, Conder MC & Goetz WA (1981). Acute phencyclidine intoxication: Clinical patterns, complications, and treatment. *Ann Emerg Med* **10**: 290–297.

McDonald LV & Liskow BI (1992). Reversal of catatonia with midazolam. *Jefferson Jrl Psychiatry* **10**: 50–51.

McEvoy JP & Lohr JB (1983). Diazepam for catatonia. *Am J Psychiatry* **141**: 284–285.

McHugh PR & Slavney PR (1998). The *Perspectives of Psychiatry*, 2nd edn. Baltimore: Johns Hopkins University Press.

McKenna K, Gordon C & Rapoport J (1994). Childhood-onset schizophrenia: timely neurobiological research. *J Am Acad Child Adolesc Psychiatry* **33**: 771–781.

McKenna PJ, Lund CE, Mortimer AM & Biggins CA (1991). Motor, volitional and behavioural disorders in schizophrenia. 2. The 'conflict of paradigms' hypothesis. *Br J Psychiatry* **158**: 328–336.

Meduna L (1935). Versuche über die biologische Beeinflussung des Ablaufes der Schizophrenie: Camphor und Cardiozolkrampfe. *Z ges Neurol Psychiatr* **152**: 235–62.

Meduna L (1937). *Die Konvulsionstherapie der Schizophrenie*. Halle A.S.: Carl Marhold Verlagsbuchhandlung.

Meduna L (1950). *Oneirophrenia*. Urbana, IL: University Illinois Press.

Meduna L (1985). Autobiography. *Convulsive Ther.* **1**: 43–57, 121–38.

Meltzer HY (1973). Rigidity, hyperpyrexia and coma following fluphenazine enanthate. *Psychopharmacologia* **29**: 337–346.

Meltzer HY (2000). Massive serum creatine kinase increases with atypical antipsychotic drugs: What is the mechanism and the message? *Psychopharmacology* **150**: 349–350.

Menza MA & Harris D (1989). Benzodiazepines and catatonia: an overview. *Biol Psychiatry* **26**: 842–846.

Meterissian GB (1996). Risperidone-induced neuroleptic malignant syndrome: a case report and review. *Can J Psychiatry* **41**: 52–54.

Meyer J, Huberth A, Ortega G, Syagailo YV, Jatzke S, Mossner R, Strom TM, Ulzheimer-Teurber I, Stöber G, Schmitt A & Lesch KP (2001). A missense mutation in a novel gene encoding putative cation channel is associated with catatonic schizophrenia in a large pedigree. *Mol Psychiatry* **6**: 302–306.

Miller BC & Cummings J (Eds) (1999). *The Human Frontal Lobes, Function and Disorders*, New York: Guilford Press.

Miller LJ (1994). Use of electroconvulsive therapy during pregnancy. *Hosp Commun Psychiatry* **45**: 444–450.

Milner B (1982). Some cognitive effects of frontal lobe lesions in man. In DE Broadbent, L Weiskrantz (Eds). *The Neuropsychology of Cognitive Function*, pp. 211–226. London: The Royal Society.

Mimica N, Folnegovi-Šmalc V & Folnegovi Z (2001). Catatonic schizophrenia in Croatia. *Eur Arch Psychiatry Clin Neurosci* **251**(Suppl1): 17–20.

Minde K (1966). Periodic catatonia: A review with special reference to Rolv Gjessing. *Canad Psych Assoc J* **11**: 421–425.

Miozzo RA, Ruben E, Stefanovic M, Belman L, Galynker II & Cohen LJ (2001). State specific rCBF changes in acute catatonia. *APA, Abstracts* 2001, NR33.

Miyata H, Kubota F, Shibata N & Kifune A (1997). Non-convulsive status epilepticus induced by antidepressants. *Seizure* **6**: 405–407.

Modell JG (1997). Protracted benzodiazepine withdrawal syndrome mimicking psychotic depression. *Psychosomatics* **38**: 160–161.

Moise FN & Petrides G (1996). Case study: Electroconvulsive therapy in adolescents. *J Am Acad Child Adolesc Psychiatry* **35**: 312–318.

Moniz E (1936; trans. 1964). Essai d'un traitement chirurgical de certaines psychoses. *Bull de l'Académie de Médecine* **115**: 385–392. (English translation: *J Neurosurgery* **21**: 1108–1114.)

Mora G (1973). Introduction to the English translation: *Catatonia*, pp. vii–xviii. Baltimore: Johns Hopkins University Press.

Morinaga K, Hayashi S, Matsumoto Y, Omiya N, Mikami J, Ueda M, Sato H, Inoue Y & Okawara S (1991). CT and 1231-IMP SPECT findings of head injuries with hyponatremia. *No To Shinkei* **43**: 891–894.

Morishita S & Aoki S (1999). Clonazepam in the treatment of prolonged depression. *J Affective Dis.* **53**: 275–278.

Morrison JR (1973). Catatonia: Retarded and excited types. *Arch Gen Psychiatry* **28**: 39–41.

Morrison JR (1974a). Karl Kahlbaum and catatonia. *Comprehens Psychiatry* **15**: 315–316.

Morrison JR (1974b). Catatonia: Prediction of outcome. *Comprehens Psychiatry* **15**: 317–324.

Morrison JR (1975). Catatonia: Diagnosis and treatment. *Hosp Community Psychiatry* **26**: 91–94.

Morrison JR, Winokur G, Crowe R & Clancy J (1973). The Iowa 500: A first follow-up. *Arch Gen Psychiatry* **29**: 57–63.

Mosolov SN & Moschchevitin SI (1990). [Use of electroconvulsive therapy to break the continual course of drug-resistant affective and schizoaffective psychoses.] *Zh Nevropatol Psikhiatr Im S S Korsakova* **90**: 121–125.

Mullen PE (1986). The mental state and states of mind. In P Hill, R Murray & A Thorley (Eds). *Essentials of Postgraduate Psychiatry*, 2nd edn., vol. 1, p. 28. New York: Grune & Stratton.

Munoz A, Huntman MM & Jones EG (1998). GABA(B) receptor gene expression in monkey thalamus. *J Comp Neurol* **394**: 118–126.

Nasar S (1998). *A Beautiful Mind*. New York: Simon & Schuster.

Nazoe S, Naruo T, Yonikura R, Nakabeppu Y, Nagai N, Nakajo M & Tanaka H (1995). Comparison of regional cerebral blood flow in patients with eating disorders. *Brain Res Bull* **36**: 251–255.

Neisser C (1887). *Über die Katatonie. Ein Beitrag zur Klinischen Psychiatrie*. Stuttgart: Ferdinand Enke Verlag.

Neisser C (1924). Karl Ludwig Kahlbaum (1828–1899). In TH Kirchhoff (ed.). *Deutsche Irrenärzte. Einzelbilder ihres Lebens und Wirkens*, Bd 2, pp. 87–96. Berlin: Springer.

Nelson JC & Davis JM (1997). DST studies in psychotic depression. *Am J Psychiatry* **154**: 1497–1503.

Nemeroff CB & Loosen PT (Eds) (1987). *Handbook of Clinical Psychoneuroendocrinology*. New York: Guilford Press.

Neuman E, Rancurel G, Lecrubier Y, Fohanno D & Boller F (1996). Schizophreniform catatonia in 6 cases secondary to hydrocephalus with subthalamic mesencephalic tumor associated with hypodopaminergia. *Neuropsychobiology* **34**: 76–81.

Neveu P, Morrel P, Marchandon AM & Pautet P (1973). Malignant catatonia treatment using hibernation. *Ann Med Psychol (Paris)* **2**: 267–274.

Nisijima K & Ishiguro T (1999). Electroconvulsive therapy for the treatment of neuroleptic malignant syndrome with psychotic symptoms: a report of five cases. *JECT* **15**: 158–163.

Nisijima K, Kusakabe Y, Ohtuka K & Ishiguro T (1998). Addition of carbamazepine to long-term treatment with neuroleptics may induce neuroleptic malignant syndrome. *Biol Psychiatry* **44**: 930–931.

Nordahl E, Benkelfat C, Semple WE, Gross M, King AC & Cohen RM (1989). Cerebral glucose metabolic rates in obsessive compulsive disorder. *Neuropsychopharmacology* **2**: 23–28.

Normann C, Brandt, Berger M & Walden J (1998). Delirium and persistent dyskinesia induced by a lithium-neuroleptic interaction. *Pharmacopsychiat* **31**: 201–204.

Northoff G (2000). Brain imaging in catatonia: Current findings and pathophysiologic model. *CNS Spectrums* **5**: 34–46.

Northoff G, Braus D, Sartorius A, Khoram-Sefat D, Russ M, Eckert J, Herrig H, Leschinger A & Henn FA (1999a). Reduced activation and altered laterality in two neuroleptic-naive catatonic patients during motor task in functional MRI. *Psychological Med* **29**: 997–1002.

Northoff G, Eckert J & Fritze J (1997). Glutamatergic dysfunction in catatonia? Successful treatment of three acute akinetic catatonic patients with the NMDA antagonist amantadine. *J Neurol Neurosurg Psychiatry* **62**: 404–406.

Northoff G, Kock A, Wenke J, Eckert J, Boker H, Pflug B & Bogerts B (1999b). Catatonia as a psychomotor syndrome: a rating scale and extrapyramidal motor symptoms. *Mov Disord* **14**: 404–416.

Northoff G, Lins H, Böker H, Danos P & Bogerts B (1999c). Therapeutic efficacy of n-methyl d-aspartate antagonist amantadine in febrile catatonia. *J Clin Psychopharmacol* **19**: 484–486.

Northoff G, Nagel D, Danos P, Leschinger A, Lesche J & Bogerts B (1999d). Impairment in visual-spatial function in catatonia: A neuropsychological investigation. *Schizophrenia Res* **37**: 133–147.

Northoff G, Pfenning A, Krug M, Danos P, Leschinger A, Schwarz A & Bogerts B (2000). Delayed onset of late movement-related cortical potentials and abnormal response to lorazepam in catatonia. *Schizophr Res* **44**: 193–211.

Northoff G, Steinke R, Czcervenka C, Krause R, Ulrich S, Danos P, Kropf D, Otto H-J & Bogerts B (1999e). Decreased density of GABA-A receptors in the left sensorimotor cortex in akinetic catatonia: investigation of in vivo benzodiazepine receptor binding. *J Neurol Neurosurg Psychiatry* **67**: 445–450.

Northoff G, Wenke J, Demisch L, Eckert J, Gille B & Pflug B (1995). Catatonia: Short-term response to lorazepam and dopaminergic metabolism. *Psychopharmacology* **122**: 182–186.

O'Connor MK, Knapp R, Husain M, Rummans TA, Petrides G, Smith G, Mueller M, Snyder K, Bernstein H, Rush AJ, Fink M & Kellner C (2001). The influence of age on the response of major depression to electroconvulsive therapy. A CORE report. *Am J Geriatr Psychiatry* **9**: 382–390.

O'Gorman G (1970). *The Nature of Childhood Autism*, 2nd edn. London: Butterworths.

O'Griofa FM & Voris JC (1991). Neuroleptic malignant syndrome associated with carbamazepine. *Southern Med J* **84**: 1378–1380.

Osman AA & Khurasani MH (1994). Lethal catatonia and neuroleptic malignant syndrome. A dopamine receptor shut-down hypothesis. *Br J Psychiatry* **165**: 548–550.

Overshett DH, Janowsky DS, Gillin JC, Shiromani PJ & Suten EL (1986). Stress induced immobility in rats with cholinergic supersensitivity. *Biol Psychiatry* **21**: 657–664.

Pakkenberg B (1992). The volume of the mediodorsal thalamic nucleus in treated and untreated schizophrenics. *Schizophr Res* **7**: 95–100.

Palmieri MG, Iani C, Scalise A, Desiato MT, Loberti M, Telera S & Caramia MD (1999). The effect of benzodiazepines and flumazenil on motor cortical excitability in the human brain. *Brain Res* **81**: 192–199.

Pantelis C, Barnes TRE & Nelson HE (1992). Is the concept of frontal-subcortical dementia relevant to schizophrenia? *Brit J Psychiatry* **160**: 442–460.

Panzer M, Tandon R & Greden JF (1990). Benzodiazepine and catatonia. *Biol Psychiatry* **28**: 177–179.

Pataki J, Zervas IM & Jandorf L (1992). Catatonia at a university in-patient service (1985–1990). *Convulsive Ther.* **8**: 163–173.

Patterson JF (1986). Akinetic Parkinsonism and the catatonic syndrome: An overview. *Southern Med J* **79**: 682–685.

Pauleikhoff B (1969). Die Katatonie (1868–1968). *Fortschr Neurol Psychiatr Grenzgebiete* **37**: 461–496.

Pavlovsky P, Kukanova P, Pietrucha S & Zvolsky P (2001). Lethal catatonia. *Cesk Slov Psychiatr* **97**: 8–12.

Pearlman CA (1986). Neuroleptic malignant syndrome: A review of the literature. *J Clin Psychopharmacol* **6**: 257–273.

Peele R & von Loetzen IS (1973). Phenothiazine deaths: A critical review. *Am J Psychiatry* **130**: 306–309.

Peet M & Collier J (1990). Use of carbamazepine in psychosis after neuroleptic malignant syndrome. *Br J Psychiatry* **156**: 579–81.

Pelonero AL, Levenson JL & Pandurangi AK (1998). Neuroleptic malignant syndrome: A review. *Psychiatr Serv* **49**: 1163–1172.

Penatti CA, Gurgneira SA, Bechara EJ & Demasi M (1998). Neuroleptic drug-stimulated iron uptake by synaptosome preparations of rat cerebral cortex. *Biochem Biophys Acta* **1407**: 61–68.

Penn H, Racy J, Lapham L, Mandel M & Sandt J (1972). Catatonic behavior, viral encephalopathy and death. The problem of fatal catatonia. *Arch Gen Psychiatry* **27**: 758–761.

Peralta V & Cuesta MJ (2001a). Motor features in psychotic disorders. I. Factor structure and clinical correlates. *Schizophr Res* **47**: 107–116.

Peralta V & Cuesta MJ (2001b). Motor features in psychotic disorders. II. Development of diagnostic criteria for catatonia. *Schizophr Res* **47**: 117–126.

Peralta V, Cuesta MJ, Mata I, Serrano JF, Perez-Nieves F & Natividad MC (1999). Serum iron in catatonic and non-catatonic psychotic patients. *Biol Psychiatry* **45**: 788–90.

Peralta V, Cuesta MJ, Serrano JF & Mata I (1997). The Kahlbaum syndrome: A study of its clinical validity, nosological status, and relationship with schizophrenia and mood disorder. *Comprehens Psychiatry* **38**: 61–67.

Perris C (1995). Leonhard and the cycloid psychoses. In GE Berrios & R Porter (Eds). *A History of Clinical Psychiatry*, vol. 16, pp. 421–430. London: Athlone Press.

Petrides G, Divadeenam K, Bush G & Francis A (1997). Synergism of lorazepam and ECT in the treatment of catatonia. *Biol Psychiatry* **42**: 375–81.

Petrides G & Fink M (1996). The "half-age" stimulation strategy for ECT dosing. *Convulsive Ther.* **12**: 138–146.

Petrides G & Fink M (2000). Catatonia. In C Andrade (Ed.). *Advances in Psychiatry*, pp. 26–44. Oxford: Oxford University Press.

Pettinati HM, Stephens RN, Willis KM & Robin S (1990). Evidence for less improvement in depression in patients taking benzodiazepines during unilateral ECT. *Am J Psychiatry* **147**: 1029–1035.

Pfuhlmann B, Franzek E, Stöber G, Cetkovich-Bakmas M & Beckman H (1997). On interrater reliability for Leonhard's classification of endogenous psychoses. *Psychopathology* **30**: 100–150.

Pfuhlmann B & Stöber G (2001). The different conceptions of catatonia: historical overview and critical discussion. *Eur Archiv Psychiatry Clin Neurosci* **251**: (Suppl 1): 4–7.

Philbrick KL & Rummans TA (1994). Malignant catatonia. *J Neuropsychiatry Clin Neurosci* **6**: 1–13.

Plum F & Posner JB (1980). *The Diagnosis of Stupor and Coma*, 3rd edn. Philadelphia: FA Davis.

Pollack M, Fink M, Klein DF, Willner A & Blumberg AG (1965). Imipramine-induced behavioral disorganization in schizophrenic patients: Physiological and psychological correlates. In J Wortis (Ed.). *Biological Psychiatry*, New York: Plenum Press. vol. 7, pp. 53–61.

Pope HG, Keck PE & McElroy SL (1986). Frequency and presentation of neuroleptic malignant syndrome in a large psychiatric hospital. *Am J Psychiatry* **143**: 1227–1233.

Post RM, Rubinow DM & Ballenger JC (1984). Conditioning, sensitization, and kindling: Implications for the course of affective illness. In RM Post & JC Ballenger (Eds). *The Neurobiology of Mood Disorders*, pp. 432–466. Baltimore: Williams & Wilkins.

Postman, N (1992). *Technopoly: The Surrender of Culture to Technology.* New York: Knopf.

Powell JC, Silviera WR & Lindsay R (1988). Pre-pubertal depressive stupor: A case report. *Br J Psychiatry* **153**: 689–692.

Primavera A, Fonti A, Novello P, Roccatagliata G & Cocito L (1994). Epileptic seizures in patients with acute catatonic syndrome. *J Neurol, Neurosurg, Psychiatry* **57**: 1419–1422.

Quétel C (1990). *History of Syphilis.* Cambridge: Polity Press.

Rachlin HL, Goldman GS, Gurvitz M, Lurie A & Rachlin L (1956). Follow-up study of 317 patients discharged from Hillside Hospital in 1950. *J Hillside Hosp* **5**: 17–40.

Raeva SN, Vainberg NA, Dubynin VA, Tsetlin IM, Tikhonov YN & Lashin AP (1999). Changes in the spike activity of neurons in the ventrolateral nucleus of the thalamus in humans during performance of a voluntary movement. *Neurosci Behav Physiol* **29**: 505–513.

Raja M, Altavista MC, Cavallari S & Lubich L (1994). Neuroleptic malignant syndrome and catatonia. A report of three cases. *Eur Arch Psychiatry Clin Neuroscience* **243**: 299–303.

Rankel HW & Rankel LE (1988). Carbamazepine in the treatment of catatonia. *Am J Psychiatry* **145**: 361–362.

Rapoport M, Feder V & Sandor P (1998). Response of major depression and Tourette's syndrome to ECT: A case report. *Psychosom Med* **60**: 528–529.

Rauch J (1906). *Über die katatonen symptome.* Thesis, Leipzig University.

Realmuto GM & August GJ (1991). Catatonia in autistic disorder: A sign of comorbidity or variable expression? *J Autism Develop Disord* **21**: 517–528.

Realmuto GM & Main B (1982). Coincidence of Tourette's disorder and infantile autism. *J Autism Develop Disord* **12**: 367–372.

Regestein QR, Alpert JS & Reich P (1977). Sudden catatonic stupor with disastrous outcome. *JAMA* **238**: 618–620.

Regis E (1901). *Le delire onirique des intoxications et des infections.* Paris: Academie de Medicine.

Reiter PJ (1926). Extrapyramidal disturbances in dementia praecox. *Acta Psychiatr Neurol* **1**: 287–305.

Revuelta E, Bordet R, Piquet T, Ghawche F, Destee A & Goudemand M (1994). Catatonie aiguë et syndrome malin des neuroleptiques: un cas au cours d'une psychose infantile. *Encephale* **20**: 351–354.

Richard IH (1998). Acute, drug-induced, life-threatening neurological syndromes. *Neurologist* **4**: 196–210.

Riederer P. (Ed.) (2001). Biological psychiatry. *J Neural Transm* **108**: 617–716.

Rinkel M (1966). *Biological Treatment of Mental Illness.* New York: LC Page & Co.

Rinkel M & Himwich HE (1959). *Insulin Treatment in Psychiatry*. New York: Philosophical Library.

Robb AS, Chang W, Lee HK & Cook MS (2000). Case study: Risperidone-induced neuroleptic malignant syndrome in adolescent. *J Child Adolesc Psychopharmacol* **10**: 327–330.

Roberts DR (1965). Catatonia in the brain: A localization study. *Int J Neuropsychiatry* **1**: 395–403.

Robins E & Guze SB (1970). Establishment of diagnostic validity in psychiatric illness: Its application to schizophrenia. *Am J Psychiatry* **126**: 983–987.

Rogers D (1990). Psychiatric consequences of basal ganglia disease. *Sem Neurol* **10**: 262–266.

Rogers D (1991). Catatonia: A contemporary approach. *J Neuropsychiatry Clin Neurosci* **3**: 334–340.

Rogers D (1992). *Motor Disorder in Psychiatry: Towards a Neurological Psychiatry*. Chichester: John Wiley & Sons.

Rogers D, Karki C, Bartlett C & Pocock P (1991). The motor disorders of mental handicap. An overlap with the motor disorders of severe psychiatric illness. *Br J Psychiatry* **158**: 97–102.

Rohland BM, Carroll BT & Jacoby RG (1993). ECT in the treatment of the catatonic syndrome. *J Affect Disord* **29**: 255–61.

Romano J & Engel GL (1994). Delirium. I: EEG data. *Arch Neurol Psychiatry* **51**: 356–377.

Rosebush PI, Hildebrand AM, Furlong BG & Mazurek MF (1990). Catatonic syndrome in a general psychiatric population: Frequency, clinical presentation, and response to lorazepam. *J Clin Psychiatry* **51**: 357–362.

Rosebush P, MacQueen GM & Mazurek MF (1999). Catatonia following gabapentin withdrawal. *J Clin Psychopharmacol* **19**: 188–189.

Rosebush P & Mazurek MF (1991a). Serum iron and neuroleptic malignant syndrome. *Lancet* **338**: 149–151.

Rosebush PI & Mazurek MF (1991b). Lorazepam and catatonic immobility. *J Clin Psychiatry* **52**: 187–188.

Rosebush P & Stewart T (1989). A prospective analysis of 24 episodes of neuroleptic malignant syndrome. *Am J Psychiatry* **146**: 717–725.

Rosenberg MR & Green M (1989). Neuroleptic malignant syndrome. Review of response to therapy. *Arch Inten Med* **149**: 1927–1931.

Rummans T & Bassingthwaighte ME (1991). Severe medical and neurologic complications associated with near-lethal catatonia treated with electroconvulsive therapy. *Convulsive Ther* **7**: 121–24.

Sachdev P (1993). The neuropsychiatry of brain iron. *J Neuropsychiatry Clin Neurosci* **5**: 18–29.

Sachdev P (1995). *Akathisia and Restless Legs.* Cambridge: Cambridge University Press.

Sachdev P, Kruk J, Kneebone M & Kissane D (1995). Clozapine-induced neuroleptic malignant syndrome: review and report of new cases. *J Clin Psychophamacol* **15**: 365–371.

Sackeim HA, Decina P, Portnoy S, Neeley P & Malitz S (1987). Studies of dosage, seizure threshold, and seizure duration in ECT. *Biol Psychiatry* **22**: 249–268.

Sackeim HA, Luber B, Katzman GP, Moeller JR, Prudic J, Devanand DP & Nobler MS (1996). The effects of electroconvulsive therapy on quantitative electroencephalograms. *Arch gen Psychiatry* **53**: 814–824.

Sackeim HA, Hasket RF, Mulsant BH et al. (2001). Continuation pharmacotherapy in the prevention of relapse following electroconvulsive therapy. *JAMA* **285**: 1299–1307.

Sackeim HA, Prudic J, Devanand DP, et al. (1993). Effects of stimulus intensity and electrode placement on the efficacy and cognitive effects of electroconvulsive therapy. *N Engl J Med* **328**: 839–846.

Sackeim HA, Prudic J, Devanand DP, et al. (2000). A prospective, randomised, double-blind comparison of bilateral and right unilateral electroconvulsive therapy at different stimulus intensities. *Arch Gen Psychiatry* **57**: 425–434.

Sacks O (1974). Awakenings. Garden City NY: Doubleday & Co. (The film from the book: Columbia Pictures, 1991.)

Sakel M (1935). *Neue Behandlungsmethode der Schizophrenie.* Vienna: Moritz Perles Verlag.

Sakel M (1938). *The Pharmacological Shock Treatment of Schizophrenia.* (Trans. J. Wortis.) New York: Nervous and Mental Disease Publishing Co.

Sakkas P, Davis JM, Janicak PG & Wang ZY (1991). Drug treatment of the neuroleptic malignant syndrome. *Psychopharm Bull* **27**: 381–384.

Satoh K, Suzuki T, Narita M, Ishikura S, Shibasaki M, Kato T, Takahashi S, Fukuyama H, Ohnishi H & Morita R (1993a). Regional cerebral blood flow in catatonic schizophrenia. *Psychiatry Res* **50**: 203–216.

Satoh K, Narita M, Someya T, Fukuyama H & Yonekura Y (1993b). Functional brain imaging of a catatonic type of schizophrenia. PET and SPECT studies. *Jpn J Psychiatry Neurol* **47**: 881–885.

Saver JL, Greenstein P, Ronthal M & Mesulam M (1993). Asymmetric catalepsy after right hemisphere stroke. *Mov Disord* **8**: 69–73.

Scheibel AB (1997). The thalamus and neuropsychiatric illness. *J Neuropsychiatry and Clin Neurosciences* **9**: 342–353.

Scheid KF (1937). *Febrile Episoden bei schizophenen Psychosen. Eine klinische und pathologische Studie.* Leipzig: Thieme.

Scheidegger W (1929). Katatone Todesfälle in der Psychiatrischen Klinik von Zürich von 1900 bis 1928. *Z. Neurologie* **120**: 587–600.

Schmider J, Standhart H, Deuschle M, Drancoli J & Heuser J (1999). A double-blind comparison of lorazepam and oxazepam in psychomotor retardation and mutism. *Biol Psychiatry* **46**: 437–441.

Schmuecker JD, Reid MJ & Williams DJ (1992). Disulfiram toxicity and catatonia in a forensic outpatient. *Am J Psychiatry* **149**: 1275–1276.

Schott K, Bartels M, Heimann H & Buchkremer G (1992). Ergebnisse der Elektrokrampf-therapie unter restriktiver Indikation. Eine retrospektive Studie uber 15 Jahre. [Results of electroconvulsive therapy in restrictive conditions. A retrospective study of 15 years.] *Nervenarzt* **63**: 422–425.

Schüle von H (1898). Zur Katatonie-Frage: Eine klinische Studie. *Allgemeine Zeitschrift für Psychiatrie* **54**: 515–552.

Sechi G, Manca S, Deiana GA, Corda DG, Pisu A & Rosati G (1996). Acute hyponatremia and neuroleptic malignant syndrome in Parkinson's disease. *Prog Neuro-Psychopharm Biol Psychiatry* **20**: 533–542.

Sedivec V (1981). Psychoses endangering life. *Cesk Psychiatr* **77**: 38–41.

Sedler MJ (1985). The legacy of Ewald Hecker: A new translation of "Die Hebephrenie". *Am J Psychiatry* **142**: 1265–1271.

Segarra JM & Angelo JN (1970). Presentation 1. In AL Benton (ed.). *Behavioral Change in Cerebrovascular Disease*, pp. 3–14. New York: Harper and Row.

Sengoku A & Takagi S (1998). Electroencephalographic findings in functional psychoses: state or trait indicators? *Psychiatry and Clinical Neurosciences* **52**: 373–381.

Senser RN, Alper H, Yunten N & Dundar C (1993). Bilateral acute thalamic infarcts causing thalamic dementia. *AJR* **161**: 678–679.

Shagass C (1954). The sedation threshold. A method for estimating tension in psychiatric patients. *Electroencephalog Clin Neurophysiol* **6**: 221–223.

Shalev A, Hermesh H & Munitz H (1989). Mortality from neuroleptic malignant syndrome. *J Clin Psychiatry* **50**: 18–25.

Shalev A & Munitz H (1986). The neuroleptic malignant syndrome: agent and host interaction. *Acta Psychiatr Scand* **73**: 337–347.

Shapiro A, Shapiro E, Young JG & Feinberg TE (1988). *Gilles de la Tourette Syndrome*, 2nd edn. New York: Raven Press.

Sharma R, Trappler B, Ng YK & Leeman CP (1996). Risperidone-induced neuroleptic malignant syndrome. *Ann Pharmacother* **30**: 775–778.

Sheftner WA & Shulman RB (1992). Treatment choice in neuroleptic malignant syndrome. *Convulsive Ther* **8**: 267–279.

Silva H, Jerez S, Catenacci M & Mascaro J (1989). Disminucion de la esquizofrenia catatonica en pacientes hospitalizados en 1984 respecto de 1964 [Decrease of catatonic schizophrenia in patients hospitalized in 1984 compared to 1964]. *Acta Psiquiatr Psicol Am Lat* **35**(3–4): 132–138.

Simpson DM & Davis GC (1984). Case report of neuroleptic malignant syndrome associated with withdrawal from amantadine. *Am J Psychiatry* **141**: 796–797.

Sing KJ, Ramaekers GM & van Harten PN (2002). Neuroleptic malignant syndrome and quetiapine. *Am J Psychiatry* **159**: 149–150.

Siroth L (1914). *Katatonie und organischnervöse Begleiterscheinungen.* Thesis, Berlin University. Berlin: C. Siebert.

Sours JA (1962). Akinetic mutism simulating catatonic schizophrenia. *Am J Psychiatry* 451–455.

Spear J, Ranger M & Herzberg J (1997). The treatment of stupor associated with MRI evidence of cerebrovascular disease. *Int J Geriatric Psychiatry* **12**: 791–794.

Spiess-Kiefer C (1989). Malignes neuroleptisches Syndrom. In H Hippius, E Rüther & M Schmauss (Eds). *Katatone und dyskinetische Syndrome*, pp. 171–195. Berlin: Springer-Verlag.

Spitzka EC (1883). *Insanity. Its Classification, Diagnosis and Treatment.* New York: Bermingham & Co. (Also reprinted by EB Treat, New York 1887 and by Arno Press, New York, 1973.)

Spivak B, Gonen N, Mester R, Averbuck E, Adlersberg S & Weizman A (1996). Neuroleptic malignant syndrome associated with abrupt withdrawal of anticholinergic agents. *Int Clin Psychopharm* **11**: 207–209.

Spivak B, Weizman A, Wolovick L, Hermesh H, Tyano S & Munitz H (1990). Neuroleptic malignant syndrome during abrupt reduction of neuroleptic treatment. *Acta Psychiatr Scand* **81**: 168–169.

Staal WG, Hulshoff HE, Schnack H, van der Schot AC & Kahn RS (1998). Partial volume decrease of the thalamus in relatives of patients with schizophrenia. *Am J Psychiatry* **155**: 1784–1786.

Stauder KH (1934). Die tödliche Katatonie. *Arch Psychiatr Nervenkrank* **102**: 614–634.

Steck H (1926). Les syndromes extrapyramidaux dans les maladies mentales. *Arch Suisses Neurol Psychiatr* **19**: 195–233.

Steck H (1927). Les syndromes extrapyramidaux dans les maladies mentales. *Arch Neurol Psychiatr* **20**: 92–136.

Steck H (1931). Les syndromes mentaux post encephalitiques. *Arch Suisses Neurol Psychiatr* **27**: 137–173.

Steinberg H (1999). Karl Ludwig Kahlbaum – Leben und Werk bis zur Zeit seines Bekanntwerdens. *Fortschr Neurol Psychiat* **67**: 367–372.

Sternbach H (1991). The serotonin syndrome. *Am J Psychiatry* **148**: 705–713.

Still J, Friedman B, Law E, Deppe S, Epperly N & Orlet H (1998). Neuroleptic malignant syndrome in a burn patient. *Burns* **24**: 573–575.

Stöber G (2001). Genetic predisposition and environmental causes in periodic and systematic catatonia. *Eur Arch Clin Neurosci* **2** (Suppl 1): 21–24.

Stöber G, Franzek E, Lesch KP & Beckmann H (1995). Periodic catatonia: a schizophrenic subtype with major gene effect and anticipation. *Eur Arch Psychiatry Clin Neurosci* **245**: 135–141.

Stöber G, Meyer J, Nanda I, Wienker TF, Saar K, Knapp M, Jatzke S, Schmid M, Lesch KP & Beckmann H (2000a). Linkage and family-based association study of schizophrenia and the synapsin III locus that maps chromosome 22q13. *Am J Med Genetics* **93**: 392–397.

Stöber G, Meyer J, Nanda I, Wienker TF, Saar K, Jatzke S, Schmid M, Lesch KP & Beckmann H (2000b). hKCNN3 which maps chromosome Iq21 is not the causative gene in periodic catatonia, a familial subtype of schizophrenia. *Eur Arch Psychiatry Clin Neuroscience* **250**: 163–168.

Stöber G, Pfuhlmann B, Nürnberg G, Schmidke A, Reis A, Franzek E & Wienker TF (2001). Towards a genetic basis of periodic catatonia: pedigree sample for genome scan I and II. *Eur Arch Clin Neurosci* **2** (Suppl 1): 25–30.

Stöber G, Saar K, Ruschendorf F, Meyer J, Nurnberg G, Jatzke S, Franzek E, Reis A, Lesch KP, Wienker TF & Beckmann H (2000c). Splitting schizophrenia: Periodic catatonia susceptibility locus on chromosome 15q15. *Am J Hum Genetics* **67**: 1201–1207.

Stöber G & Ungvari G (Eds) (2001). Catatonia: A new focus of research. *Eur Arch Psychiatry Clin Neurosci* **2** (Suppl 1): 1–34.

Strömgren LS (1997). ECT in acute delirium and related clinical states. *Convulsive Ther* **13**: 10–17.

Stompe T, Ontwein-Swoboda G, Ritter K, Schanda H & Friedmann A (2002). Are we witnessing the disappearance of catatonic schizophrenia? *Comprehens Psychiatry* **43**: 167–174.

Swanson LW (2000). Cerebral hemisphere regulation of motivated behavior. *Brain Res* **886**: 113–164.

Swartz CM (1985a). Time course of post-electroconvulsive therapy prolactin levels. *Convulsive Ther* **1**: 81–88.

Swartz CM (1985b). Characterization of the total amount of prolactin released by electroconvulsive therapy. *Convulsive Ther* **1**: 252–257.

Swartz CM & Galang RL (2001). Adverse outcome with delay in identification of catatonia in elderly patients. *Am J Geriatric Psychiatry* **9**: 78–80.

Swartz CM, Morrow V, Surles L & James MF (2001). Long-term outcome after ECT for catatonic depression. *JECT* **17**: 180–183.

Taieb O, Flament MF, Corcos M, Jeammet P, Basquin M, Mazet P & Cohen D (2001). Electroconvulsive therapy in adolescents with mood disorder: patients' and parents' attitudes. *Psychiatry Res* **104**: 183–190.

Takeuchi H (1996). A case of neuroleptic malignant syndrome treated with intermittent intravenous injections of diazepam. *Hiroshima J Anesthsesia* **32** (Suppl): 31–34.

Tandon R & Greden JF (1989). Cholinergic hyperactivity and negative schizophrenic symptoms: a model of dopaminergic/cholinergic interactions in schizophrenia. *Arch Gen Psychiatry* **46**: 745–753.

Taylor MA (1981). *The Neuropsychiatric Mental Status Examination.* New York: Spectrum Publications.

Taylor MA (1990). Catatonia: A review of a behavioral neurologic syndrome. *Neuropsychiatry Neuropsychol Behav Neurol* **3**: 48–72.

Taylor MA (1992). Are schizophrenia and affective disorder related? A selective literature review. *Am J Psychiatry* **149**: 22–32.

Taylor MA (1993). *The Neuropsychiatric Guide to Modern Everyday Psychiatry.* New York: Free Press.

Taylor MA (1999). *The Fundamentals of Clinical Neuropsychiatry.* New York: Oxford University Press.

Taylor MA (2001). Confessions of a drug user. *Neuropsychiatry Neuropsychol Behav Neurol* **14**: 81–82.

Taylor MA & Abrams R (1973). The phenomenology of mania: a new look at some old patients. *Arch Gen Psychiatry* **29**: 520–522.

Taylor MA & Abrams R (1977). Catatonia: prevalence and importance in the manic phase of manic-depressive illness. *Arch Gen Psychiatry* **34**: 1223–1225.

Terao T (1999). Carbamazepine in the treatment of neuroleptic malignant syndrome. *Biol Psychiatry* **45**: 381.

Terry GC (1939). *Fever and Psychoses.* New York: Paul B. Hoeber Inc.

Thickbroom GW, Byrnes ML, Sacco P, Ghosh S, Morris IT & Mastaglia FL (2000). The role of the supplementary motor area in externally timed movement; the influence of predictability of movement timing. *Brain Res* **874**: 233–241.

Thomas P, Maron M, Rascle C, Cottencin O, Vaiva G & Goudemand M (1998). Carbamazepine in the treatment of neuroleptic malignant syndrome. *Biol Psychiatry* **43**: 303–305.

Thomas P, Rascle C, Mastain B, Maron M & Vaiva G (1997). Test for catatonia with zolpidem. (Letter.) *Lancet* **349**: 702.

Thompson JW, Weiner RD & Mayers CP (1994). Use of ECT in the United States in 1975, 1980, 1986. *Am J Psychiatry* **151**: 1657–1661.

Thompson SW & Greenhouse AH (1968). Petit mal status in adults. *Ann Int Med* **6**: 1271–1279.

Thuppal M & Fink M (1999). Electroconvulsive therapy and mental retardation. *JECT* **15**: 140–149.

Tinuper P, Montagna P, Cortelli P, Avoni P, Lugaresi A, Schoch P, Bonetti EP, Gallassi R, Sforza E & Lugaresi E (1992). Idiopathic recurring stupor: a case with possible involvement of the gamma-aminobutyric acid (GABA)ergic system. *Ann Neurol* **31**: 503–506.

Tinuper P, Montagna P, Plazzi G, Avoni P, Cerullo A, Cortelli P, Sforza E, Bonetti EP, Schoch P & Rothstein JD (1994). Idiopathic recurring stupor. *Neurology* **44**: 621–625.

Tolsma FJ (1967). The syndrome of acute pernicious psychosis. *Psychiatr Neurol Neurochirurg* **70**: 1–21.

Tormey WP, Cronin T & Devlin JD (1987). Hyponatraemia masquerading as malignant neuroleptic syndrome. *Brit J Psychiatry* **150**: 412.

Trigo MK, Crippa JAS, Hallak JEC, Vale FAC, Sakamoto AC & Zuardi AW (2001). The complexity of the differential diagnosis in psychiatry exemplified by a catatonic syndrome. *Rev Psiquiatr Clin* **28**: 144–147.

Trimble MR (1978). Serum prolactin in epilepsy and hysteria. *BMJ* **2**: 1682.

Trimble MR (1991). *The Psychoses of Epilepsy*. New York: Raven Press.

Trivedi HK, Mendelowitz AJ & Fink M (in press). A Gilles de la Tourette form of catatonia: Response to ECT. *JECT*.

Troller JN & Sachdev PS (1999). Electroconvulsive treatment of neuroleptic malignant syndrome: a review and report of cases. *Aust NZ J Psychiatry* **33**: 650–659.

Turek IS & Hanlon TE (1977). The effectiveness and safety of electroconvulsive therapy (ECT). *J Nerv Ment Dis* **164**: 419–431.

Turner TH (1989). Schizophrenia and mental handicap: a historical review, with implications for further research. *Psychol Med* **19**: 301–314.

Üçok A & Üçok G (1996). Maintenance ECT in a patient with catatonic schizophrenia and tardive dyskinesia. *Convulsive Ther* **12**: 108–112.

Ungvari GS, Chiu HFK, Chow LY, Lau BST & Tang WK (1999). Lorazepam for chronic catatonia: a randomized, double-blind, placebo-controlled cross-over study. *Psychopharmacology* **142**: 393–398.

Ungvari GS, Kau LS, Wai-Kwong T & Shing NF (2001a). The pharmacological treatment of catatonia: an overview. *Eur Arch Psychiatry Clin Neurosci* **251** (Suppl 1): 31–34.

Ungvari GS, Leung CM & Lee TS (1994a). Benzodiazepines and the psychopathology of catatonia. *Pharmacopsychiatry* **27**: 242–245.

Ungvari GS, Leung CM, Wong MK & Lau J (1994b). Benzodiazepines in the treatment of catatonic syndrome. *Acta Psychiatr Scand* **89**: 285–88.

Ungvari GS, Leung SK & Ng FS (2001b). Catatonia in Chinese patients with chronic schizophrenia. *New Research abstracts, Annual Meeting American Psychiatric Association*, p. 83. (Full text, personal communication July, 2001.)

Ungvari GS & Rankin JAF (1990). Speech-prompt catatonia: a case report and review of the literature. *Comprehens Psychiatry* **30**: 56–61.

Ungvari GS, White E & Pang AHT (1995). Psychopathology of catatonic speech disorders and the dilemma of catatonia: a selective review. *Aust NZ J Psychiatry* **29**: 653–660.

Urstein M (1912). *Manisch-depressives und Periodisches Irresein als erscheinungsform der Katatonie*. Berlin: Urban & Schwartzberg.

van Dael F (2001). Lethal catatonia: a case report and review of the literature. *Tijdschrift voor Geneeskunde* **57**: 1192–1198.

van Waarde JA, Stolker JJ & van der Mast RC (2001). Electroconvulsive therapy in mental retardation: A review. *JECT* **17**: 236–243.

Velasco M, Velasco F, Velasco AL, Jimenez F, Brito F & Marquez I (2000). Acute and chronic electrical stimulation of the centromedian thalamic nucleus. Modulation of reticulo-cortical systems and predictor factors for generalized seizure control. *Arch Med Res* **31**: 304–319.

Von Economo C (1931). *Encephalitis Lethargica.* London: Oxford University Press.

Wade JB, Taylor MA, Kasprisin A, Rosenberg S & Fiducia D (1987). Tardive dyskinesia and cognitive impairment. *Biol Psychiatry* **22**: 393–395.

Wagner-Jauregg J (1918). Über die Einwirkung der Malaria auf die Progressive Paralyse. *Psychiatr-Neurol. Wchnschr* **20**: 132–151.

Walker R & Swartz CM (1994). Electroconvulsive therapy during high-risk pregnancy. *General Hosp Psychiatry* **16**: 348–353.

Walter GJ (2002). *The Use of Electroconvulsive Therapy in Young People.* PhD thesis, University of Sydney, Australia.

Walter WG (1944). Electroencephalography in cases of mental disorder. *J Ment Sci* **90**: 64–73.

Webster DD (1968). Clinical analysis of the disability in Parkinson's disease. *Mod Treat* **5**: 257–282.

Weinberger DR (1987). Implications for normal brain development for the pathogenesis of schizophrenia. *Arch Gen Psychiatry* **44**: 660–669.

Weinberger DR, Aloia MS, Goldberg TE & Berman KF (1994). The frontal lobes in schizophrenia. *J Neuropsychiatry Clin Neurosci* **6**: 419–427.

Weinberger DR & Kelly MJ (1977). Catatonia and malignant syndrome: a possible complication of neuroleptic administration. *J Nerv Ment Dis* **165**: 263–268.

Weintraub MI (1977). Hysteria. A clinical guide to diagnosis. *Clin Symp* **29**: 27–28.

Weller M & Kornhuber J (1992a). A rationale for NMDA receptor antagonist therapy of the neuroleptic malignant syndrome. *Med Hypoth* **38**: 329–333.

Weller M & Kornhuber J (1992b). Lyell syndrome and lethal catatonia: a case for ECT. *Am J Psychiatry* **149**: 1114.

Weller M, Kornhuber J & Beckmann H (1992). Elektrokonvulsionstherapie zur Behandlung der akuten lebensbedrohlichen Katatonie bei toxischer epidermaler Nekrolyse (Lyell-Syndrom). [Electroconvulsive therapy in treatment of acute life-threatening catatonia in toxic epidermal necrolysis (Lyell Syndrome)]. *Nervenarzt* **63**: 308–310.

Wenzel J & Kuschinsky K (1990). Effects of morphine on gamma-aminobutyric acid turnover in the basal ganglia. Possible correlation with its biphasic action on motility. *Arzeimittelforschung* **40**: 811–813.

Wetzel H, Heuser I & Benkert O (1988). Benzodiazepines for catatonic symptoms, stupor, and mutism. *Pharmacopsychiat* **21**: 394–395.

Wetzel H, Heuser I & Benkert O (1987). Stupor and affective state: Alleviation of psychomotor disturbances by lorazepam and recurrence of symptoms after Ro 15-1788. *J Nerv Ment Dis* **175**: 240–242.

White DAC (1992). Catatonia and the neuroleptic malignant syndrome – a single entity? *Br J Psychiatry* **161**: 558–560.

White DAC & Robins AH (1991). Catatonia: Harbinger of the neuroleptic malignant syndrome. *Br J Psychiatry* **158**: 419–421.

Whitlock FA (1967). The Ganser syndrome. *Br J Psychiatry* **113**: 19–29.

Widlocher DJ (1983). Psychomotor retardation: clinical, theoretical, and psychometric aspects. *Psychiatric Clin North America* **6**: 27–40.

Wilcox A (1986). Perinatal distress and infectious disease as risk factors for catatonia. *Psychopathology* **19**: 196–199.

Wilkinson R, Meythaler JM & Guin-Renfroe S (1999). Neuroleptic malignant syndrome induced by haloperidol following traumatic brain injury. *Brain Injury* **13**: 1025–1031.

Wing L (1987). Autism: possible clues to the underlying pathology – 1. Clinical facts. In L Wing (Ed.). *Aspects of Autism: Biological Research*, pp. 1–10. London: Gaskell.

Wing L & Atwood A (1987). Syndromes of autism and atypical development. In DL Cohen & AM Donnellan (Eds). *Handbook of Autism and Pervasive Developmental Disorders*, vol. 1, pp. 3–19. Silver Spring, MD: VH Winston & Sons.

Wing L & Shah A (2000a). Catatonia in autistic spectrum disorders. *Br J Psychiatry* **176**: 357–362.

Wing L & Shah A (2000b). Possible causes of catatonia in autistic spectrum disorders. (Reply to Chaplin.) *Br J Psychiatry* **177**: 180–181.

Winkel PHE (1925; published 1929). *Über die katatonie; eine Beitrag zur Frage der endogenen psychosen nebst Mitteilung zweier geheilter und vier weiterer Fälle*. Thesis, Kiel University, 1925. Kiel: CH Jebens. 1929.

Wirshing DA, Bartzokis G, Pierre JM, Wirshing WC, Sun A, Tishler TA & Marder SR (1998). Tardive dyskinesia and serum iron indices. *Biol Psychiatry* **44**: 493–498.

Woodbury MM & Woodbury MA (1992). Neuroleptic-induced catatonia as a stage in the progression toward neuroleptic malignant syndrome. *J Am Acad Child Adolesc Psychiatry* **31**: 1161–1164.

World Health Organization (1992). *International Statistical Classification of Diseases and Related Health Problems*. 10th revision. Geneva: World Health Organization.

Yamaguchi S, Tsuchiya H & Kobayashi S (1998). Visuospatial attention shift and motor responses in cerebellar disorders. *J Cogn Neurosci* **1**: 95–107.

Yamawoki Y & Ogawa N (1992). Successful treatment of levodopa-induced neuroleptic malignant syndrome (NMS) and disseminated intravascular coagulation (DIC) in a patient with Parkinson's disease. *Inter Med* **31**: 1298–1302.

Yamawaki S, Yano E & Urchitomi Y (1990). Analysis of 497 cases of neuroleptic malignant syndrome in Japan. *Hiroshima J Anesthesia* **26**: 35–44.

Yoshino A, Yoshimasu H, Tatsuzawa Y, Asakura T & Hara T (1998). Nonconvulsive status epilepticus in two patients with neuroleptic malignant syndrome. (Letter.) *J Clin Psychopharmacol* **18**: 347–348.

Yudofsky SC, Silver, JM, Jackson W, Endicott J & Williams D (1986). The overt aggression scale for the objective rating of verbal and physical aggression. *Am J Psychiatry* **153**: 35–39.

Zalsman G, Hermesh H & Munitz H (1998). Alprazolam withdrawal delirium: A case report. *Clin Neuropharmacol* **21**: 201–202.

Zarr ML & Nowak T (1990). Catatonia and burns. *Burns* **16**: 133–134.

Zaw FK & Bates GD (1997). Replication of zolpidem test for catatonia in an adolescent. *Lancet* **349**: 1914.

Zaw FK, Bates GD, Murali V & Bentham P (1999). Catatonia, autism, and ECT. *Dev Med Child Neurol* **41**: 843–845.

Zawilska J & Nowak JZ (1986). Effect of electroconvulsive shock (ECS) treatment on the histaminergic system in rat brain: biochemical and behavioural studies. *Agents Actions* **18**: 222–225.

Zuddas A, Pintor M & Cianchetti C (1996). Risperidone for negative symptoms. (Letter.) *J Am Acad Child Adolesc Psychiatry* **35**: 838–839.

Index